REFLECTIONS TO
UNCONDITIONAL LOVE

I0458233

AIRE STILLMAN

ISBN: 978-1-960136-89-3

Table of Contents

Introduction

Embracing Unconditional Love to Transform Your Life:

Have you ever felt like you're searching for something more? Something deeper, something real that touches your soul? Something that connects you to your truest self and those around you? If you're reading this, you're probably on a journey to discover the power of love and how it can truly change your life.

As I reflect on my own experiences, one truth remains clear: **love—unconditional, unapologetic love—is the key to everything**. It's the force that drives us, heals us, and shapes our relationships with others and ourselves. But this isn't just a feel-good cliché. It's a transformative, life-altering energy that, when embraced fully, has the potential to reshape how we live, love, and connect.

I've spent years diving deep into what it means to love, not just in relationships, but in every aspect of life. Through personal struggles, triumphs, and the ups and downs of adult life, I've come to understand that love isn't always easy, but it's always worth it. My journey has taught me that to truly grow, heal, and succeed, we must start by loving ourselves, others, and the world around us in a way that is unconditional and pure.

In addition to my personal journey, I bring years of professional experience to this subject. As a coach, mentor, and advocate for personal development, I've worked with individuals from all walks of life, guiding them to understand their value, heal past wounds, and embrace love as a core principle for transformation. I've spent countless hours studying human relationships, emotional intelligence, and self-growth. My educational background in psychology and holistic wellness, coupled with years of hands-on experience, has given me a deep understanding of the inner workings of the heart and mind. This has allowed me to develop a comprehensive approach to love that not only heals but elevates those who embrace it.

This book is a reflection of my experiences, a guide to help others—whether women or men—tap into the incredible power of unconditional love. I want to show you how, by embracing love in all its forms, we can unlock deeper connections, personal growth, and lasting happiness. But more than that, I hope to remind you of something we often forget in the hustle of life: **love is the most powerful tool we have to create meaningful, fulfilling lives.**

But love isn't just about feeling good or being loved—it's about communication, connection, and community. These three elements are the heartbeat of healthy relationships and the foundation upon which unconditional love thrives.

- **Communication** is the bridge that connects our hearts and minds. It's through honest, open, and empathetic communication that we truly understand one another. This book will help you explore how to communicate with authenticity and vulnerability, creating stronger connections in every area of your life.
- **Connection** is at the core of human experience. We all yearn for meaningful relationships, and when we approach these connections with love, they deepen and flourish. By embracing the power of love, you'll learn how to connect with others on a profound level—whether in romantic relationships, friendships, or professional settings.
- **Community** is the space where we are seen, heard, and supported. We are all interwoven in the fabric of life, and the importance of a community that supports and uplifts one

another cannot be overstated. This book will encourage you to build your own community of love, where connection, communication, and unconditional support thrive.

Throughout this book, you'll explore the stories, lessons, and insights I've gathered from both my personal life and from others who have discovered the transformative power of love. This isn't just about romantic love—it's about love for yourself, for others, for the world, and ultimately for life itself. In the pages that follow, I'll show you how love can shift your perspective, empower you to make bold choices, and heal parts of you that may have been broken for far too long.

You will learn how to:

- Cultivate self-love and embrace your authentic self without apology
- Develop deeper connections with others by opening your heart
- Use love as a tool for personal growth and success
- Strengthen communication in your relationships to deepen understanding
- Build a supportive community where love and connection thrive
- Transform challenges into opportunities for learning and expansion
- Create a life rooted in unconditional love, compassion, and kindness

Each chapter is designed to help you embrace the fullness of love—how to give it, how to receive it, and how to let it guide you to your highest potential. Whether you're facing relationship struggles, personal setbacks, or simply seeking more meaning in your life, this book will provide practical tools and powerful insights to help you along the way.

I'm not here to tell you that love is easy or that it comes without its challenges, but I am here to show you how embracing love in all its forms can lead you to a life of peace, fulfillment, and joy.

So, as you turn these pages, I encourage you to open your heart and be ready to receive the love that is already around you—and that which is waiting to flow from you. This book is more than just words on a page; it's a call to action for anyone ready to transform their life through the most powerful force in existence: **unconditional love.**

Are you ready to embrace it?

Let's begin this journey together.

A MESSAGE TO THE READER

Dear friend,

I hope that wherever you are this message may be found. That no matter where in the world or what time zone you're in that this special message has found you for some specific purpose. Above all, you are special. You are *special* to me. My hopes and dreams of this book are to share my personal stories and other incredible human stories with you as a guide to which road map fits in your narrative. I wish to share my experiences with you as my most authentic version to be the most transparent, open and naked in hope that the pain and beauty I've felt can help you better navigate your own life. My goal for this book is to captivate you with raw emotions. I hope while reading, you smile. Not just that smile with your teeth, but the smile that lights up your eyes. The smile that gets your heart pumping out of your chest, while tears are streaming down your face as you reach to wipe away your eyes while your body is holding back its one emotional response.

I hope that this book makes at least a small impact in your life. That aspiration comes into action and follows your heart to its unconditional love, and dreams. **You deserve that too**. Through these trials and tribulations of my life, and those I've met along the way, I've learned that I can use my life lessons to help pave the way for others. I'll hold the flashlight for you as we travel down the dark tunnel. If I can make your steps a little bit easier, then I've done my job. I want you to know that I see you. I've dreamed of you holding this. I've dreamed of your beautiful face, and if I've made you cry, smile, sad, angry, or uplifted, know that you are seen. May my mirror resonate or trigger something inside of you that needs to be seen. May you walk alongside your shadows, in your own life. Please know that sometimes we are "the villain", the antagonist in our own stories, and sometimes in other people' stories too. The same can be said for the "hero", the protagonist. If you're lucky and you're truly living life, you'll be full of both. That's the delicate balance of duality on this planet we call home, Earth. I don't believe you're reading this by accident, in fact I don't believe in coincidences. Nothing is a coincidence, it's a synchronicity. In fact, I prayed you'd find this one day, when you were ready. It was created just for you. Please take the lessons I've learned and turn them into actionable steps. My goal is to help you transform into the best possible version of yourself and find your unconditional love along the way. May you always feel worthy. I love you.

Sincerely,

Aire Stillman

What is Unconditional Love?

Unconditional love is, at its core, love without any conditions or expectations. It is a pure form of love that is given freely, not contingent upon reciprocation or any specifications from the other person. This kind of love prioritizes the happiness of the loved one above all else. Loving them where they are at and needing nothing in return. Love with *no strings attached.*

How to Unconditionally Love Someone?

Unconditional love often manifests as a readiness to forgive minor transgressions and mistakes. It means not keeping tabs (score) of arguments and "one up's" or who has the upper hand in disputes. This type of love encourages humility, allowing individuals to acknowledge their own faults and seek forgiveness when necessary, without letting pride interfere. It gives individuals the opportunity to acknowledge disputes, rationalize and admit when "they" are wrong.

What are the Four types of Unconditional love?

"The four classic types of love- affection, friendship, passion, and selfless love- are represented by the Greek Terms; storage, philia, eros, and agape. These categories illustrate the diverse ways love can be expressed in our relationships."

The Four Essential Types of Love:

Physical Love: Involves touch, closeness, and presence.
Mental Love: Centered around understanding and thought-provoking conversations.
Emotional Love: Focuses on feeling seen, connected, and valued.

Spiritual Love: Encompasses chemistry, energy, and meaningful connections.

The Five Love Languages:

1. Physical Touch
2. Quality Time
3. Gift Giving
4. Words of Affirmation
5. Acts of Service

Eight Expressions of Love:

1. Nurturing Communication
2. Time Together- Quality Time
3. Actions
4. Thoughtful Gifts
5. Physical Affection
6. Emotional Connection
7. Intellectual Stimulation
8. Growth Support

The Importance of Definitions:

I hope that by providing definitions you're able to better understand my thought process. A deeper grasp of the words and their meaning allows you to engage more fully with the ideas presented, uncovering layers of meaning that go beyond surface interpretations. I strive for depth in my writing, while I may express one idea, there often exists a double entendre. Like an onion, I have many layers- each layer revealing new insights as you peel them back. I encourage you to read carefully, take a moment to reflect, and reconsider. Each word, sentence and story has been crafted thoughtfully, with paradoxical meanings that defy simple interpretation. There is always more than "meets the eye."

My Fascination with Psychology

My interest in psychology stems from a personal quest to comprehend the complexities of my own mind. I've dedicated my life to unraveling the thoughts and patterns that shape who we are, driven by a desire to understand phenomena that feels beyond the ordinary.

What Do We All Long For?

Ultimately, we yearn for connection, communication, and community. Some may even say that we seek creation, a life purpose or the act of being expansive. Through the essence of time we've seen that we are better as a human race together. Our villages, and communities have been major backbones in our history.

This journey to uncover the meaning of unconditional love has shown me there are countless directions, lanes, and moments of discovery waiting to unfold. It's not a straight path; it's a winding road full of surprises, challenges, and revelations.

As my journey began, I quickly realized I needed tools to help me along the way—a map to provide direction, a compass to guide me, and a vehicle to carry me forward. But even with these tools, the real challenge was learning to trust my intuition—God's compass—to steer me in the right direction. No matter what your faith is or isn't, something is helping steer the weather of the ship to refuge.

Join me as I continue this quest to explore the depths of unconditional love. There's so much more to discover, and I'd love for you to be part of this adventure.

THE COMPASS

CHAPTER ONE

UNCONDITIONAL?

I've been searching for the meaning of "unconditional" my entire life, both consciously and unknowingly. It's a word I've heard often, yet never fully understood. What does it really mean? Is it even real? For as long as I can remember, I've chased it like a mirage, hoping one day to get close enough to touch it, to experience it for myself.

Over the years, I've traveled across this vast country, from the crowded streets of the East Coast to the quiet expanses of the West, from the warmth of the South to the cool northern winds. Each place, each encounter has pulled me closer, piece by piece, to a deeper understanding of love, and what it means to love without limits. And yet, no matter where I go, I can't shake the feeling that I'm still missing something. The idea of "unconditional" feels just out of reach, like a puzzle with one missing piece.

So, where did this word even come from? Who decided it was a goal we should all strive for? Who decided that loving someone, or something, without conditions was even possible in this messy, complicated world we call "home"?

I'm about to take you on a journey through the highs and lows of my life and stories of people I've met along the way, across seasons, through cities, and beyond borders. Together, we'll unravel the meaning of unconditional love, and maybe even discover whether it's something we can really achieve, or just a dream we've all been sold. Hold tight – the answers might be more complicated than we imagined.

ROADMAP 1, LOCATOR STAMP/STOP:
43.04225°N 87.94063°W

Just a girl from Milwaukee, Wisconsin, making her debut at St. Luke's Hospital on a memorable August night. I was born at 10:05 PM on August 18, 1992. Yep, the cat's out of the bag—now you know my age. I hope you didn't expect to read this book without a dash of my humor. I've always had a bit of sarcasm up my sleeve, so if you were hoping to skip over that, well, bless your heart. 😊

And for those who aren't familiar, "bless your heart" can pack a punch down South. It's the sweeter way of saying "you dumba$$" when you want to be polite. Or it can just mean, "Oh sweet pea, you silly goose." Either way, I promise you're in for a ride!

I'm a small-town "Wisconsinite" with Southern roots. I grew up in Kansasville, a tiny town where you know just about everyone, from your neighbors to the folks at town hall. It's one of those places where everybody knows each other's business. Wisconsin is wide open, with land stretching for miles. At a four-way stop, you can spot a car coming from a long way off. The air is so fresh, blending the scents of freshly cut grass, blooming flowers, and the wind dancing through your nostrils.

Wisconsinites are social creatures. If you walk into a local tavern, grab a seat at the bar, and try to keep to yourself, Earl next to you will ask about your aunt Linda—and he'll actually care. Growing up in this kind of environment taught me that people love to share their unfiltered thoughts. Here's a key insight: people really LOVE to talk about themselves. Especially after a few drinks. 🍺 Ever had one of those nights where you spill your life's secrets to a stranger? Yeah, me too!

Real talk: people can be so open that they become incredibly vulnerable with strangers, spilling their entire lives only to wake up the next morning regretting it.

The human experience often leads us to confide in strangers about our "secrets" and personal realities. It's often easier to share our truths with them than with friends and family because strangers are less likely to judge us harshly. This can lead us to build mental walls—barriers that complicate our closest relationships, despite our best intentions.

For me, these childhood experiences were my first lessons in personal development because I learned the power of truly listening to someone's side of the story. The essence of active listening.

Active Listening: What Does It Mean?

"Active listening is about fully engaging with a speaker. It means listening attentively, understanding their message, responding thoughtfully, and reflecting on what's been said. This kind of interaction keeps both the listener and speaker engaged, making it a crucial component of compassionate leadership."

What Is Active Listening?

Google defines active listening as "when you not only hear what someone is saying, but also attune to their thoughts and feelings. It turns a conversation into an active, non-competitive, two-way interaction."

Robin Abrahams and Boris Groysberg from Harvard Business School describe "active listening as having three aspects: cognitive, emotional, and behavioral. Here's how they define each aspect in their article, "How to Become a Better Listener":

Cognitive: "Paying attention to all the information, both explicit and implicit, that you are receiving from the other person, comprehending, and integrating that information"

Emotional: "Staying calm and compassionate during the conversation, including managing any emotional reactions (annoyance, boredom) you might experience"

Behavioral: "Conveying interest and comprehension verbally and nonverbally"

From a young age, I realized that sharing my perspective and connecting with others came naturally to me. I loved telling stories to my parents and their friends—who, at that time, were practically my friends too since I hadn't really made my own yet. Many of my early memories are of hanging out with them at my dad's softball games and other sporting events.

These experiences taught me early on that humans have a deep need for connection. We all want to be heard and seen and it became clear to me that our voices, thoughts, and feelings genuinely matter. This insight highlights the importance of both active and passive listening.

According to the dictionary, **HEARING** is defined as "the process of perceiving a sound." On the other hand, the dictionary defines **LISTENING** as "to hear something with thoughtful attention." By their dictionary definitions, they have obvious differences.

Passive Listening:

"Listening without reacting. Using that time to do something else and not really paying attention to what's being said. Listening requires attention, meaning it's active. Hearing is passive-unless you close your ears, sounds will enter and be heard."

Active Listening:

"The listener is attempting to really internalize and understand what they are hearing. This requires motivation and purpose. The listener has an intention to connect and participate."

Comparison of Hearing vs. Listening

Comparison Point	Hearing	Listening
Meaning	Perception of sound	Active understanding of the sounds you hear
Process	Passive - Physical	Active - Mental
Senses	1	1<
Concentration	Not Necessary	Required

I've noticed that we often overshare or complain about our lives instead of taking real action. I can definitely relate—I've been guilty of spilling my secrets, indulging in gossip, and letting my emotions run wild. (Hey, I'm only human, and my healing journey has had its ups and downs, with plenty of room for growth.)

As a kid, I struggled with feelings of worthiness. I didn't always believe I deserved to be heard, listened to, or even have a love story of my own. I've always been a hopeless romantic, thanks to those feel-good romantic comedies from Hollywood. But as we continue this journey together, you'll see that the idea of "unconditional love" is a lot more complicated than it seems.

I've had a bumpy start, and sometimes I forget this truth. It feels a bit like living in "The Truman Show" with Jim Carrey—each day seems the same. I often feel like I'm going through life in a sort of daze, where my default patterns are stronger than my self-awareness. It's like navigating life with my eyes wide open while still half-asleep. This cycle has repeated itself many times over the years.

Here's something to keep in mind: when we get hurt or feel betrayed by someone we trusted, it's usually a sign that we're about to learn a pretty important life lesson. And as tempting as it is to immediately grab the metaphorical "fix-it" tool, sometimes it's better to just... pause. Take a breath.

Before you hit that "send" button on that angry text or start crafting your perfect "I'm right, you're wrong" speech, try to step back and look at the situation from a neutral angle. Think of it like a movie—except you're the main character, and the popcorn's for reflection, not drama. Connect with your higher self (yes, the one who knows how to chill), and ask yourself some tough questions:

What would it be like to see this whole situation from all sides?

How would I feel if I were in the other person's shoes—heels, sneakers, or flip-flops, whatever they're wearing?

Now, in all the self-help books I've read (and let's be honest, there's a lot), they all say the same thing: reflection is *key* during conflicts. So, instead of immediately jumping into defense mode, take a pause. Imagine you're in the middle of an out-of-body experience, watching yourself from above (without the creepy ghost vibe, I promise).

Here's the kicker: when you're looking down from this new vantage point, can you spot any of your own blind spots? Have you been completely honest with yourself about your role in all this? Are you the one stirring the pot, or is this just a classic case of two people with completely different communication styles, like trying to talk to your dog in French? What's going on in the other person's head? What are *they* feeling right now?

The truth is, more often than not, what feels like a big, personal attack is just a case of mismatched communication. It's not that they're out to get you. They're probably just trying to get their point across, and, well, it's not clicking.

Kinda like my friend.......

SHE'S A FIGHTER, NOT A LOVER:

34.1939° N, 77.8063° W

One Sunday afternoon, I ran into Michelle **(THE REMINDER)** in the hallway of a café. I casually asked how her day was going, and to my surprise, she started opening up about a major moment in her life. She began sharing her frustration over a recent argument with her husband, feeling deeply hurt. "He needs to apologize!" she said, clearly upset. When she confronted him later, he threw her for a loop by saying he wasn't sorry. It felt so one-sided—how could she possibly be at fault?

The next day, when Michelle asked him about their plans, he mentioned needing some alone time. Instead of taking this as a hint to give him space, she decided to stir the pot. She walked into the café where he was working, ordered her coffee, and made a beeline for his table. He looked up, surprised to see her, but all she got was a casual smile and silence. Deep down, she knew he wasn't going to enable her aortic behavior.

Frustrated, she stormed outside, expecting him to chase after her like in the movies. When he didn't act accordingly, she immediately called her friends to vent. "We had a fight! Can you believe what he said? I need to come over!" she said, and they quickly responded, "OMG! Where are you? we've got you, be there asap? See you soon!"

As she sat in her car, ready to drive to her friends' place, a deep question popped into her head: "What am I doing?" Sure, her friends would cheer her up temporarily, but this was her husband. How could she build a long, happy life together if she couldn't even confront her own feelings and figure out where they were coming from?

At that moment, Michelle realized she needed to sit with her emotions, stay present, and deal with the situation directly. She understood that this wasn't just her story—it was his too. There are three sides to every story, and she had been so focused on fighting him that she forgot they were supposed to be addressing the issue together, not battling each other.

She saw that the problem wasn't solely his fault; she was part of the conflict too. The only person not seeing this was her. Michelle learned that the power of words and how we use them can either create distance or foster connection in relationships. Once spoken, words can't be taken back.

While you might have the ability to apologize, remember that every action has consequences. Just saying "I'm sorry" doesn't guarantee things will get better. In fact, it can sometimes make it seem like your apology isn't sincere. If your words have caused deep hurt, how can others trust you not to repeat the same mistakes?

Trust is built on the consistency between what you say and what you do. If apologies become just empty phrases without real intent to change, they lose their meaning and make others question your integrity. Reflect on the impact of your words and make sure they align with your actions going forward.

She shared her story with me to explain how she saw her life from a fresh perspective, and it was genuinely transformative for her. I was pumped to see her break that cycle!

Her experience reminded me that communication goes beyond just the words we speak; it's also about what's conveyed without them. We express ourselves through body language, tone, attitude, and the overall vibe of our interactions.

As my Pastor Erwin McManus wisely said, "Language is not what you use to reveal yourself, but what you use to conceal yourself."

As women, we often say one thing while our feelings and body language might tell a completely different story. For example, when your partner asks if he can go somewhere, you might say, "Sure, honey," but your body language might be giving off a totally different vibe.

I once had a hilarious mix-up during a meal with a friend. He said, "I ordered food here yesterday," but I heard it as, "Oh, you don't eat every day?" We both cracked up when he clarified. That one word— "ordered"—made all the difference. The tones, attitudes, and how the words are projected determines how the message lands.

Another moment happened at the gym when my headphones fell and landed under the bathroom sink. Just then, a woman walked up to the sink and stepped in front of me. In my head, I thought I'd said, "Excuse me," as I bent down to reach under the sink to grab it. I looked up and realized I hadn't actually said anything out loud. She saw my headphones and gathered my experience. She asked, "Oh no, did you drop your headphones?" I laughed and realized she was worried she might have stepped on them. I replied, "Oh no, thank you! They're way under the sink."

This reminded me that real harmony in relationships comes from understanding each person's unique style of emotional communication. For me, I often use words to handle conflicts, but others might just need a simple wink and a beer to move on. Sometimes, tackling a conflict head-on can actually make things worse; often, resolutions can be found through non-verbal cues. The key word here is "sometimes."

In our interactions, everyone speaks their own language, and some of us are lucky enough to be multilingual. Here are the key lessons I've learned about communication throughout my life:

Effective Communication Tactics:

Learn the Other Person's Love Language:

We all give and receive love in different ways, like a game of emotional charades. Are they words of affirmation? Acts of service? Or maybe they just need you to *actually* listen when they talk. Once you figure it out, it's like finding the secret code to their heart.

Practice Active Listening:

Here's a pro tip: don't just nod and pretend you're listening. Engage! Be fully present in the conversation, and I mean truly *there*. That means no checking your phone or mentally drafting your response while they're still talking. If you can master this, you'll not only understand them better, but they'll appreciate you more too.

Recognize Passive Communication:

Not everything gets said out loud. Sometimes people communicate with their body language, facial expressions, or that uncomfortable silence. It's like trying to read between the lines of a text message—it's not always what's written, but what's *implied* that matters. Pay attention to those little signs—they're like hidden Spotify playlists. If you catch the vibe, you'll understand the full track, no drama required.

Meet Them Where They Are:

No, you don't have to actually meet them at their place (unless they're making dinner, in which case, yes, go). But when it comes to communication, adapt your style to fit theirs. Are they a detailed planner, or do they prefer big-picture ideas? Adjust accordingly, and you'll be speaking their language without even realizing it.

Know Your Audience:

Communication isn't one-size-fits-all. Whether you're talking to a friend, your significant other, or a client, the way you communicate should fit the situation. With friends, feel free to be a little sarcastic. With clients? Maybe tone it down on the sarcasm... just a little.

The Other Key Components of Love:

Empathy:

This is the golden ticket to building deeper connections. It's about understanding how others feel, even if you haven't walked in their shoes (and let's be real, those shoes might not even fit). Here's the breakdown:

Cognitive Empathy: This is knowing what someone else is feeling. It's like getting the CliffsNotes version of their emotions.

Emotional Empathy: Now, this is when you really connect. You feel their feelings—whether it's joy, sadness, or that weird sense of secondhand embarrassment.

Compassionate Empathy: This is where you take action. You don't just feel for them—you do something to help. It's the ultimate "I've got your back" move.

Sympathy:

This is when you feel bad for someone, like when your friend spills coffee on their new white shirt. You're like, "Ugh, that sucks, I feel for you." It's a caring gesture, but it's kind of like handing them a napkin and moving on. Sympathy shows you care, but **empathy** is where the magic happens. It's that deeper connection—especially when someone's going through something tough. You're not just nodding and saying "that's rough," you're really *feeling* it with them.

Examples:

"I totally get what you're going through." – Empathy

"Oh, I'm so sorry you're dealing with that." – Sympathy

Best Practice:

Mindfulness. It sounds all zen and like something you'd read on a yoga mat, but it's true. Being present and checking in with your own feelings is the first step in really tuning into someone else's. If you're aware of your own emotions, you'll be better at picking up on theirs—and creating a connection that goes beyond just "I feel bad for you."

CONNECTIONS:

According to "People Don't Meet Anyone By Accident – The 7 Types Of Cosmic Connections - Awareness Act"

Years ago, I stumbled upon a website that stated "**People Don't Meet Anyone By Accident**" really opened my eyes to something profound: we don't meet anyone by accident. Every person in our lives has a role to play, a purpose they're here to fulfill, whether they know it or not. This idea helped me see that we're all actors on the "world's stage." Our souls have already signed a kind of pre-life contract, agreeing on the lessons we need to learn and the people we need to encounter.

I believe we all come from the essence of unconditional love—whether you call it God, Source, the Universe, or something else. At our core, we are all connected, and we create our own realities based on our beliefs and habits. I've heard many stories where kids claim to have chosen their families in heaven, coming to Earth with a specific purpose in mind. The idea is that we've already agreed to help create a better world and raise the collective consciousness.

Every person we meet is here to teach us something. After reading this article, it all clicked for me in a way that felt both grounded and spiritual. It made sense of the complex web of connections we form throughout our lives. According to the article, there are seven types of people we encounter, each with their own unique role. Each one is an expression of unconditional love, even if we don't always see it in the moment.

"THE ETERNALS"

These are the people who walk into your life and just *stick*. They're the ones who become your ride-or-die friends or close family members, never backing down when you need them the most. They've got your back, and the universe seems to send them your way to offer comfort in all sorts of unexpected ways.

They're the ones who truly get you, who accept you for exactly who you are—flaws, quirks, and all. Through the highs and lows, they're by your side, unwavering. No storm can shake their loyalty. You always show up for each other, no matter the chaos. People like this? They're rare gems, and their love is a reflection of the unconditional love we all come from.

"THE HEARTBREAKERS"

These are the people who waltz into our lives, making us feel like we're on top of the world, only to send us plummeting off the edge. They manage to break us in ways we never thought possible, but in doing so, they teach us a tough lesson. And that lesson? Well, it's different for everyone. Each Heartbreaker brings something new to the table, leaving us to learn in our own way.

Now, while it's never okay for people to shatter our hearts, those wolves masquerading in sheep's clothing don't just appear out of nowhere. Sure, they're frustrating, and you might wish you'd never crossed paths with them, but in the end, they'll leave you with a lesson wrapped in pain. Don't let it consume you, but don't forget to take something valuable from the experience either. Move forward with whatever dignity you have left. Though it's never fun, they too play a part in your journey towards self-love and healing, which ultimately brings you closer to the essence of unconditional love.

"THE EMPOWERERS"

These are the people who really push you to become the person you've always wanted to be. They show up at just the right time and give you the boost you need to feel unstoppable. They make you believe you can tackle anything you set your mind to, and before you know it, you're soaring. There's something truly incredible about feeling like someone believes in you, and honestly, we all deserve that kind of experience. These empowerers are expressions of love that help you embrace your true potential.

"THE RUNNERS"

These are the people who waltz into your life and leave an impact sometimes for the better, sometimes not so much. The impact they leave is like a whirlwind, and before you know it, they're gone, leaving you with the feeling that they've taken a piece of you with them.

Learning to let go of these people is crucial. It can sting a little, but it's a different kind of sting than the one you feel from a Heartbreaker. This is more of a clean break—less messy, but still a little sharp. Their departure teaches you to accept that not every relationship is meant to last, but that doesn't diminish the love they brought into your life, even temporarily.

"THE REMINDERS"

These are the people who show up just to remind you of something important. They might only be in your life for a moment, but their impact is quietly profound. They offer nuggets of wisdom or prompt you to remember things you've forgotten. They help realign your perspective and nudge you back toward your purpose. They often go unnoticed, but they play a crucial role in helping you stay connected to the essence of unconditional love.

"THE TEACHERS"

These are the people who walk into your life with a lesson, whether they know it or not. They push you to accept yourself, to keep moving forward, and to evolve—even when it's tough. They may not always be easy to deal with, but their influence is undeniable. Through their actions, they help shape who you are becoming. These teachers are a vital part of your spiritual growth, bringing you closer to understanding unconditional love in its purest form.

"THE LEARNERS"

These are the people who come into your life to learn from you. Sometimes, we're not the only ones gaining wisdom—we're the ones teaching it. Our actions, words, and energy can pass on lessons that shape their lives, often in ways we don't fully understand. In teaching them, we, too, learn more about ourselves and our ability to love unconditionally. Their growth is a reflection of our own.

In the end, we're all here on Earth to help each other grow, to teach and to learn, to experience love in all its forms. Each person you encounter, whether they're an Eternal, a Heartbreaker, an Empowerer, or any of the others, is a piece of the puzzle in your journey toward understanding the true essence of unconditional love. It's a beautiful, messy, and transformative process that makes all of us who we are meant to be.

ROADBLOCKS- THE SET UPS

Sometimes, life takes us on detours we didn't plan for. But here's the thing—those unexpected turns, delays, and roadblocks? They're not setbacks, they're setups. They're teaching us something, preparing us for what's ahead. Even when we can't see where we're headed, trust that there are many roads leading to where we're meant to be.

This reminds me of those times I've been stuck at a random red light, feeling the clock ticking as I rush to work. It feels like eternity, right? You're already late, and you're watching the minutes slip by. But then, out of nowhere, I rolled up to a scene where a crash just happened—cars all tangled up. And I realize, if I'd been a few seconds earlier, I might have been caught right in the middle of that. Suddenly, being stuck at that light doesn't feel like a waste of time—it feels like a blessing. A quick pit stop to save me from something bigger.

It's kind of like that feeling when you walk into a room, ready to make something happen, only to forget why you're even there. It's like the universe—or God—wanted you to forget, because what you thought you were after wasn't meant for you. It's a little nudge to reflect, pause, and reconsider. Life knows what it's doing, even when we're too caught up in the moment to see it. So, trust those detours. They might just be keeping you safe, or pointing you in a better direction.

CHAPTER TWO

FAMILY ROOTS AND REFLECTIONS

Components of Love:

43.0389° N, 87.9065° W

My family tree is a bit of a mix-and-match—Norwegian, Swedish, Italian, and German—talk about a stubborn blend! As the youngest and only girl among four siblings, I've often felt the weight of family dynamics. My parents, married for 39 years and in the same house for 31, have provided a solid foundation amidst all the family chaos.

Recently, a friend told me, "You must come from a good family." I was genuinely touched and asked, "Wow, what makes you say that?" He simply replied, "You can just tell."

I have two half-brothers from my dad's previous marriage and one full-blooded brother, we often look like twins with our shared energy and vibe. We're six years apart. Then there's me—"the baby." Some might say I've enjoyed a bit of "princess treatment," but it's come with its own set of challenges in discovering my self-worth.

Growing up, I sought attention and validation, craving more from the men in my life. I wanted to bond with my brothers, but they were more interested in wrestling than hanging out. I remember coming home one day to find my life-size doll ripped to shreds. My brothers thought they were "teaching me a lesson," but all I wanted was to be as cool as they were.

As time went on, my brothers grew up, married wonderful women, and seeing them evolve into men of character has been one of my favorite experiences as the little sister. When my first niece, Esme Stillman, was born, I noticed her initials were the same as mine (ES). She radiated joy from the start, but as she grew, her parents noticed some developmental challenges.

To me, there are no "coincidences," and Esme seemed like a reflection of my own early struggles. While I faced developmental challenges that later became disabilities, Esme's experiences were more severe. She's had numerous hospital visits and battles with epilepsy, requiring constant monitoring and care.

Esme's developmental age doesn't match her cognitive abilities, so she communicates through sounds, noises, and body language instead of words. When I'd visit her, I could deeply feel her pain, relating to her struggles through my own experiences. What stands out the most is the incredible care her family provides. Their love is palpable, and they handle her challenges with patience and unconditional love.

However, Esme's frustration often stems from her inability to express herself, leading to temper tantrums. I once suggested learning sign language to better communicate with her. Life isn't just about us; it's about making things better for others. Esme shouldn't feel like an "exception" just for being herself. Society often expects conformity, but we should strive to meet her halfway.

Unfortunately, it wasn't that straightforward. A speech pathologist would need to teach us all, but Esme struggled to connect with those lessons. Watching her struggle to communicate is heartbreaking, but her resilience inspires me and has taught me valuable lessons about empathy and understanding.

Silent communication—through gestures, expressions, and emotional resonance—reminds me that while words matter, real connection often goes beyond them. It makes me ponder what life could be like without language barriers and how we might benefit from exploring ways to communicate beyond words.

Many situations reveal how communication barriers—whether cultural, personal, or physical—create misunderstandings and distance. Imagine a world where we truly grasp each other's emotions and experiences without language constraints. It could lead to deeper relationships, easier conflict resolution, and a more inclusive environment.

Reflecting on my experiences with Esme, I see the power of silent communication and the beauty of connecting on a deeper level. This idea inspires me to explore alternative communication methods and embrace the richness of connecting beyond words.

Sharing My Shadows:

Growing up, I was labeled "LD"—short for learning disabled. My biggest struggle? It was converting short-term facts into long- term memories. And if you've ever tried to remember someone's name just seconds after meeting them, you'll understand the kind of daily frustration I faced. Subjects like math and spelling felt like cruel jokes, but nothing hit harder than the social struggle. Remembering names? Forget it.

My lifes feels like living in the movie *50 First Dates*—except, instead of a romantic comedy, it was more like an endless loop of forgetting. Every morning, I woke up almost like a brand-new version of myself, with no recollection of what had happened the day before. My mind was like a leaky bucket, always losing pieces of yesterday, no matter how hard I tried to hold onto them.

And my classmates? Oh, they didn't miss a beat. They noticed the way I couldn't keep up, and they made sure to remind me—loudly and often. The teasing was relentless, and every cruel comment chipped away at my sense of self-worth. Instead of learning to love myself for who I was, I let their words define me. The result? Anxiety. Panic attacks. The feeling that something inside me was always on the verge of breaking.

Navigating the school hallways felt like a game of hide-and-seek. I'd dart through the crowds, head down, just to make it to the special education classroom. To me, it wasn't just a classroom—it was a place for the kids who were somehow "less than" the others. And the shame that came with it? It was like an anchor, dragging me deeper into the feeling that I wasn't enough. I carried that weight with me, day after day, through my entire elementary school life. Shame, frustration, sadness—it was the soundtrack of my early years.

Default Mode:

Looking back, I see how everything has come full circle. It's fascinating how the lessons we learn as kids shape us, and as adults, we need to actively work on shedding old patterns and replacing them with healthier ones. For me, this means unlearning the trauma that's been stored in my body and reprogramming my mind with new, positive pathways. **Rewire your brain and refresh your mental programming down to the cellular level.**

I think of this process as a "default mode" reset. Just like a software update, it's essential to refresh our internal systems. Without this reset, we risk sticking with outdated programming that might lead us to negative influences or environments—kind of like a virus messing with our mental software.

By recognizing these challenges and actively working to rewrite my story, I'm learning to embrace my journey and all its twists and turns.

"I'm in my healing era, or I'll do it for the plot." ;)

SPEAKING LIFE INTO THE YOUTH:

My mom never let me say "can't." If I even dared, she'd pounce on me like a lioness on a gazelle. She'd immediately remind me of Thomas the Train (yep, the little chugging engine from my childhood). He was the one who believed he "could." Mom was all about instilling that belief in me, and let me tell you, it stuck. Looking back, I can see how much that attitude shaped me, because I always knew deep down I was destined for something GREAT. I mean, how could I not, with Thomas in my corner?

It's funny—my childhood shadows revolved around this nagging belief that I wasn't "smart enough." I spent so many years thinking, "I'm just not good enough." But here's the thing—those shadows were lies. The truth is, I'm not stupid at all. In fact, I've often found that I'm in places where I'm not being challenged enough to grow. And no, I don't mean mathematically—I've *definitely* made peace with the fact that math and I are not BFFs. But in terms of career responsibilities, or challenging conversations, being around people who push me to think differently— that's where I'm craving growth.

Lately, I've been observing a pattern, watching people spin in their own little revolving loops. I see it week after week. I had been working in an environment mostly populated by men who are on a 24-hour cycle of the same conversations, the same arguments, the same old agreements— timed like clockwork. And for a while, I was stuck in my own disbelief, playing small and buying into my own excuses. I let the situation—and let's be honest, my body—hold me back. I was letting it be my crutch. *IRONICALLY I WAS ON CRUTCHES AT THE TIME OF THIS RELATION*, but here's the kicker: This is the *exact* moment where I needed to build real character.

Because the truth is, I'm *not* weak. So why was I acting like I was? I wasn't rising to the occasion. I wasn't putting all of the cards on the table and using my gifts. I wasn't stepping into the leader I'm meant to be. It's time to stop playing small. I'm not stuck in their little cycle. I'm not on the same life lesson level they're on. I was done letting myself be pulled into their traps based upon proximity. I needed to lead by example— show them what *greatness* looked like. Whether it's loud and proud or quiet and subtle, I needed to be my best self, because when I shine, they'll shine too. (Duh, it's a win-win!)

Here's the bottom line: The faster I take back my power, the faster I heal my mind and body, I'd move onto a better place. The right place. And the person I'll be in that next chapter will be stronger, wiser, and more *me*. It's not about who sees me or when—they don't have the keys to my kingdom. What matters is my integrity, the actions I take when no one's watching. That's the real power. True love for myself? That's the golden ticket. "I am enough, and I can do anything I put my mind to." Thanks mom for building that concept into my subconscious so young. I deserve to be challenged. I needed to challenge myself to the test first.

When you look inside your cranium, that's when you crack the code to the vault. You uncover both the treasure and the trauma within your mind.

Access granted. *I've unlocked a new version of myself.*

Shaky Moments:

44.4965° N, 73.2348° W

I vividly remember performing with my high school poms squad at a pep rally. We had choreographed a routine with some epic stunts that only a few of us could pull off. Being in the front row was a big deal— it's where you really shined and everyone could see you.

But on that day, I slipped out of my headstand and totally messed up the routine. Most of the audience and even some of my teammates didn't notice, but I did. My heart knew the truth. I was my own harshest critic, constantly beating myself up for what I perceived as failures. Dance was "my thing"; I was supposed to be **great** at it. No one could take that away from me—except me.

When I fell out of my headstand, trying to recover and finish the routine triggered a full-on panic attack. My body went into meltdown mode, shaking uncontrollably and gasping for air. I was whisked off to the sidelines, where Mr. Everson, my favorite teacher and a part-time paramedic, came to my rescue. His calm demeanor and quick thinking helped me regulate my breathing and get a grip.

To feel so out of control was a terrifying experience. Physically, I was fine, but my ego took a hit. I felt ashamed for messing up and went into overdrive. I realized later that the panic was fueled by anxiety, a craving for attention, and peer pressure. I had slipped into a victim mindset, believing that life was against me instead of working for me. When you're told you can't do something, you either fight to prove them wrong or end up feeling even more pressured when new expectations are thrust upon you.

I was struggling with a lack of control in my life, amplified by the labels of "disability" and "not good enough" that had been running like outdated software in my mind. This old narrative colored everything I experienced, creating an intense need to control every aspect of my life. This need spiraled into a cycle of anxiety that I began to crave, chasing the dopamine rush that came with it.

Victim Mentality:

A victim mentality is like always carrying around a "poor me" sign, even when the world is actually handing you opportunities. It's when you feel like life's always out to get you, even though the evidence is like, "Nah, you're good." You know the type—constantly blaming others for everything, from the bad coffee to the traffic jam, and somehow always dodging responsibility when things go south. No accountability

It's that feeling that you're completely powerless, like you're stuck on a ride you didn't sign up for. The thing is, this outlook can sneak into every part of your life—whether it's your relationships, your job, or even your health. It's like putting on blinders and refusing to see that you have the power to change the scenery.

"Victim mindsets can develop as a coping mechanism for previous traumatic experiences," says Dr. Julie Landry, PsyD - a clinical psychologist in San Antonio, Texas.

It may feel like you have little control or impact over external factors in your life. She explains that it commonly stems from:

1. Experiencing multiple situations where you lack control
2. Ongoing emotional pain that leads to learned helplessness

High School Highlight: My Friends

High school wasn't exactly the best time of my life. Honestly, I couldn't wait to move on and leave those miserable years behind- (yall, feel me?). Sure, being on the poms squad had its perks and social status within the high school hierarchy, but what really made high school bearable was my group of friends. We needed each other's support and a tight-knit community to get through those rough years. We made the best and worst decisions together. It didn't matter what trouble we were getting into, we were always laughing.

Now that I'm an adult, I look back and cherish those moments with my childhood besties. The connections we built back then are still strong and formed a foundation that continues to enrich my life today.

But let's rewind a bit—let's dive into the journey of becoming a dancer.

She's A Dancer:

33.5054° N, 84.1359° W

Around age seven, my family took me to a neighborhood parade. I remember watching the high school girls dancing down the streets, smiling, and me waving from the sidelines. They looked so beautiful and carefree that I was instantly captivated. It wasn't long before my mom picked up on my excitement and signed me up for dance classes at a downtown studio.

Sage Street became a major part of my life. I was thrilled by the opportunity to learn how to use my body to express myself through dance. Every class was a new adventure, and I fell in love with the rhythm and movement. I felt like I was born to be a star—dressing up, doing my makeup, and grabbing my cute little microphone to choreograph routines for my friends turned into one of my favorite pastimes.

My girl cousins from North Carolina were such a vital part of my childhood. They brought their "cool" Southern accents and high energy whenever they visited. We'd dress up in our wildest outfits, layer on goofy makeup, and grab our bright pink echo mic. The mic's echo effect was just the cherry on top of our fun. It wasn't just about the echo; it was about the laughter, the shared joy, and the carefree moments that made everything unforgettable.

We'd sing along to TLC, Britney Spears, Missy Elliott, and Christina Aguilera, making up dance routines and lip-syncing our hearts out. There are hilarious old photos of me in a feather boa–- always going all out with my outfits and performance style.

As high school rolled around, my friends and I kept the tradition alive. We'd take over the basement or my bedroom, come up with epic dance routines and create our own "music videos." I was often the main one curating the perfect playlist and playing DJ, with enthusiastic suggestions from my girlies. "Build Me Up Buttercup" became our staple anthem—just ask my dad! We'd belt out the lyrics in spirited acapella sessions, filling the house with our energetic performances. I didn't realize I was taking the lead; I just loved having fun and making the most of every moment.

One day, while we were in full performance mode in my bedroom, the peaceful house was abruptly interrupted by a loud, frustrated shout from the living room: "SHUT UP!" It was my dad, voice booming through the house. We all burst into laughter, trying to stifle our giggles as we attempted to quiet down.

SHE'S GOT THE CREATIVE BUG; Singing &, Creating Art.

Another wave of creativity began to wash over me as I dove headfirst into the arts. I was eager to explore everything—drawing, painting, singing, and playing instruments. As a kid, I tried my hand at four different instruments: the violin, clarinet, and drums, but my true passion was the saxophone. Playing it not only inspired me to sing, but also honed my breath control. However, the best instrument I had was my voice. I loved singing in church and at school, pouring my heart into every note. I'd sing in the shower, in the car, on the streets—I didn't care who was listening.

Choirs were incredibly special to me, thanks in large part to my choir teacher, Ms. Easter. She was a vibrant woman whose husband sold Dippin' Dots at fairs on the side. With her short, organized hair and quirky long dresses, she was hard to miss. She often encouraged me to take on solos, which I loved. Despite my enthusiasm, I was frustrated because I wanted to be a soprano, but she always saw me as an alto. Annoyed and stubborn, I fell in line, but still pushed the boundaries in the church choir.

Josh was another one of my choir teachers who made a big impact in my vocal range. He was a feminine male with a high-pitched range, sporting soft, fluffy brown hair and always dressed in white, resembling our pastors. I could never figure out how he hit those high notes so effortlessly! He crushed it. He would always encourage me to perhaps take up playing piano. When I saw his fingers tap the keys, I was seduced into another world. Their music notes took me far away.

Creating:

Whenever I went home, I found solace in creativity. My childhood mind was a whirlwind of imagination and I was always redesigning everything around me. I started by rearranging my room to shift the energy flow and my mom noticed my need for creative expression. She encouraged me to explore my talents and took me to the paint store to pick out new colors for my bedroom.

Every few years, as I went through growth spurts, my room evolved with me. It changed from light pink to lavender and red, eventually pushing the boundaries of design. I painted the ceiling dark blue and hand-painted glow-in-the-dark stars to mimic the night sky—a nod to my obsession with space. My curiosity led me to hunt down the coolest LED lights from Spencer's. With my brothers' growing interest in club vibes and black lights, my own fascination with lighting grew. My walls were light blue with hand-painted clouds, creating a dreamy atmosphere perfect for daydreaming and imagining that anything was possible. I even switched to hot pink and made a giant heart-shaped collage of photos featuring friends and family.

My love for music continued to grow. Every night before bed, I'd pop in my JLo cassette tape and dance myself to sleep, twirling in my sheets until I was dancing in my dreams. The next night, I'd flip the tape and fall asleep to the other songs, repeating the ritual. My days began with dancing, eagerly anticipating my classes and running the moves over in my head. The memories I cherish most are those of deep friendships, especially with Caroline.

Caroline came with another girl, Alexa, and the three of us instantly clicked. I loved dancing with them every week. One day, however, that class abruptly ended and we lost touch due to them going to different schools.

It wasn't until middle or high school, when our schools merged, that I saw them again. Recognizing them was a delightful surprise; it felt like they were destined to play a significant role in my life, even though I didn't know just how much. Their laughter and passion planted seeds that would flourish for years to come.

Another group of girls who meant a lot to me were a collective group: Jessi, Sammi, Krystal and Amanda.**(THE ETERNALS)** All women from different backgrounds, but we were just a hop- skip and a jump away. Our family homes were all near each other. We were always weaving in each other's lives.

Another group I idolized: my poms squad friends. I tried out for the squad in sixth grade and vividly remember bombing the dance tryout. I called my mom, crying because I didn't think I'd make the team and desperately wanted to be a part of it.

When I later received the callback that I'd made the team, I couldn't believe it. "THEY CHOSE ME!" It was a moment of pure joy and disbelief and these memories began to boost my self-esteem. I continued training at dance studios and with the poms squad over the next 5 1/2 years, nurturing my love for dance and the bonds I formed with my teammates.**

Conversations with G:

I owe so much of what I understand about unconditional love to a deeper connection with God, the Creator of this vast universe. I share this with love, not to impose on anyone's beliefs, but to honor my own journey—a journey that seeks to understand all that is. Through it all, I've learned that unconditional love is a force that points me back to myself, gently reminding me to remember what I've always known and to remember "*who we are.*"

Going in and out of religion has shaped my path, showing me what resonates and what doesn't. But no matter where my spiritual feet have wandered, I've always considered myself a seeker, a spiritual being longing to understand my place in this world. It was through reading **"*Complete Conversations with God*"** by Donald Walsh that my eyes opened to a perspective I never thought possible—one where I began to see life not just as a set of experiences, but as a profound, living conversation with the Divine.

The relationship I've built with God, with spirit, has become the most **invaluable** relationship I could ever imagine. Beautifully stated from the book: "My purpose in creating you, My spiritual offspring, was for me to know Myself as God." Life, at its core, is a journey of self-discovery, a journey where every relationship mirrors back to us the lessons we need to learn. And the most powerful lesson of all is this: "*We are here to create.*"

In the book, it's said that "In a moment you pledge your highest love, you reach your greatest fear." This hit me hard, like a soft whisper in my soul. The moment we say "I love you," we often brace ourselves for the echo of doubt—wondering if that love will be returned or if we'll lose it altogether. And so, we begin to defend ourselves with shields, protecting our hearts with armor from the pain of loss. But if we remembered who we truly are—if we truly knew our divine essence—we wouldn't **fear**.

Fear, after all, is the opposite of unconditional love. And so, I've decided to embark on this journey to untangle the knots of fear that have held me back, and in doing so, to break through to the greatest thing of all: *Unconditional Love*. It's a love that has no boundaries, no conditions, no expectations. It simply is.

So, with each step, I invite you to unshackle yourself too, to step into the freedom of unconditional love. May we all remember *who we are*— and allow that truth to guide us back to the love we've been searching for, all along.

CHAPTER THREE

THE BUILDING BLOCKS

Building an Entrepreneur:

43° 2' 20.0472" N and 87° 54' 23.2956" W.

Hau and Associates was like my second home as a child. My mom was the partner of the accounting firm there, so I grew up immersed in that environment. As a kid, I was always looking for ways to stay busy, which led me to start creating. I began drawing pictures, and soon enough, my mom's boss, Dan noticed my talent and started paying me for my work.

From a young age, he planted the seed that I could do anything and be anyone—even an entrepreneur. The thought of earning $5 for each picture I drew was thrilling. What started as a fun hobby quickly turned into an obsession. I would create drawings, eagerly hunt him down in the office, and wait to be paid for every new masterpiece.

Looking back, I didn't realize I wasn't entitled to payment for every drawing, but I believe he always saw the bigger picture. He created a little monster, craving revenue for my hard earned work. When I asked my mom if he knew what he was doing, she replied, "He knew exactly what he was doing—*he was creating an entrepreneur.*"

Blast from the Past: A Story of Blossoming

Let's call it second grade. Honestly, thinking back, I know exactly when it was—because that's when I ended up with two books. Not just any books, but the kind of books that would forever be tied to the heart of my story as an author.

The book came to life through a very special project my school system had, and looking back, I'm convinced it was a creative writing class for high schoolers that sparked it all. They came to visit us in second grade, with their clipboards and big smiles, interviewing us about our lives. They asked about our hobbies, our families, our friends—everything that made us who we were. They absorbed all the tiny details, and with that, they created personalized hardcover books just for each of us. It was like magic in the making.

A couple of months passed, and when they returned with our finished books, you could feel the excitement in the air. We were like kids on Christmas morning, waiting to unwrap our very own stories. My book was about a rainbow. But not just any rainbow—it was a hero's journey. The first story book followed me as I rode a golden rainbow, embarking on trials and tribulations along the way. As a second grader, I thought it was *incredible*—not only because it was about me, but because some stranger had taken the time to create something so special just for me.

In my story, I slid down the rainbow to find a leprechaun guarding the pot of gold. He gave me a riddle, and of course, I couldn't crack it, I'm not one for torture. But the lesson wasn't about the gold—it was about what I already had. The leprechaun told me that my life, *myself*, was the true pot of gold. That I should hold things close to my heart and appreciate the treasures within.

That book marked the beginning of my own story. It wasn't just a tale for second graders—it was a seed planted deep inside me, sparking something much bigger. My second book was all about friendship. It was based around my soccer team and the importance of scoring "the final goal." - The plot was to describe the importance of teamwork, companionship, and connections. I remember thinking, "I can't wait to write a book for a second grader one day."

And so, as time went on, I followed that thread. I took creative writing classes, dabbled in storytelling, and soon realized that I had a gift for it.

My imagination was a wellspring, always flowing with ideas. I had a way of weaving stories that made people feel something—whether it was wonder, joy, or even a little sadness.

That book, written by someone else for me, was a turning point in my life. It showed me the beauty of storytelling, but it also showed me something deeper: it revealed that sometimes, the greatest treasures are the lessons we learn and the love we have for ourselves. In the journey of life, we all have our own "pot of gold"—and it's not something we need to chase. It's already within us, just waiting to be discovered.

So, here I am, years later, telling stories—not just for others, but to remind myself of my own pot of gold. And just like that second-grade book, I hope to create something that will spark light in others' lives, reminding them of the magic within them, too.

The Sport Fanatic:

During my formative years, my parents focused on instilling good character traits in me. They assigned me chores around the house to earn my own money and enrolled me in various sports to teach goal-setting, discipline, and teamwork. I played soccer for about five or six years, starting on an all-girls team. There's something undeniably cute about little kids in jerseys, running around and kicking balls.

In middle school, I joined a co-ed team, playing alongside my friend Christina, whose dad was our coach. They owned a Spanish family grocery store we frequented after practice. They tried to teach me Spanish on our breaks. I wanted to be included in the gossip during practices. I loved learning from their fancy footwork, which connected with my passion for dance. The skills I picked up in soccer—moving the ball, dodging opponents—mirrored those in dance, and I enjoyed the power of kicking the ball from across the other side of the field.

My interests expanded to softball, track, tennis, and basketball. I joined summer camps for basketball and even made a traveling team. However, I quickly realized I didn't enjoy the competitive environment for a sport that wasn't the center of my heart beat and felt out of place. Plus, I'd always double dribbled and I've always been a traveler by heart. (not good for the game) The silver lining was forming a new best friend, Krystal, and spending time with Caroline (**THE ETERNALS**), who also played on the team. Eventually, I shifted my focus to softball, which, along with dance, became my main passion.

I played softball for seven years, and each moment was filled with adrenaline. It was a special time that allowed me to bond with my dad. He helped me pick out my first glove and spent hours practicing with me, focusing on batting and catching. I deeply cherish those moments now, especially as he had often been focused on my brothers during those years.

Softball became my way of seeking my dad's attention without relying on motorized toys. I had a need for speed; I loved our snowmobiles, jet skis, and boats. However, things changed when he became my coach. The pressure to excel increased and I had to learn multiple positions. While others might have seen it as just a game, for me, it was about winning and proving myself—if not better, then at least equal to my brothers. I dreamed of winning a championship, just like my brother who was on a traveling team.

Funny enough, Caroline reappeared in my life during this time; her dad was the coach of the only other team in our league that was just as good as ours. We assembled a strong team of new players and won our league division for the season. The championship game was intense. In the bottom of the seventh inning, their big hitter smacked the ball out of the park, bringing all the bases home. They won. My emotions were a mix of frustration and admiration. I was a sore loser, but respected their team.

After that game, I hung up my glove. I felt crushed and was dealing with the ups and downs of middle school. My dad wanted to bond, but it became tough for both of us to play together without affecting our spirits and harming our relationship in the process.

As middle school went on, I shifted my focus to track. With a lanky frame that seemed perfect for speed, I finally found my stride. The thrill of racing and feeling like a blur on the track was invigorating. Track didn't just boost my confidence—it taught me about teamwork and communication. I learned that there's no "I" in a team, and this lesson extended beyond sports.

Looking back, I see how crucial this training was for my future entrepreneurial journey. Initially, I thought success came from making solo decisions. But, I've since realized that a business thrives on the collective strengths and weaknesses of its team and effective communication. Building strong connections and understanding each team member's role are key to nurture growth, both in sports and in business.

Tattoo Tour:

One lazy college day, while chilling in the dorm rooms, my best friend, Caroline casually tossed out, "Let's get tattoos today." She said it so nonchalantly, like getting a permanent mark was just another spontaneous decision. Looking back, she had a talent for getting me into all sorts of mischief. We were always testing the limits and living life to the fullest, often making mistakes together. Most of those choices turned out to be some of the best decisions of my life. If you don't believe me, stay tuned.

After a brief moment of contemplation, I asked, "What do you mean, get tattoos?" She responded with excitement, "There's a tattoo parlor right across the street. Let's go!" I was intrigued, but nervous. "What should we even get tattooed on?" I asked. She grinned, "That's the fun part. Anything! And anywhere!"

When we walked into the shop, we were greeted by an explosion of art on the walls—designs ranging from stunningly intricate to ones I'd never consider putting on my body. The shop was like a gallery of vibrant lines and colors, each piece with its own flair. My friend emphasized the importance of connecting with the tattoo artist. In my opinion, that's crucial. Building rapport with the artist helps you understand their style, why you want their tattoo, and whether their art resonates with your vision.

After some thought, I decided on a cursive phrase in Italian. A nod to my heritage. The saying I wanted etched into my skin forever: "Veni, Vidi, Vici." In English, that translates to Julius Caesar's famous quote, "I came, I saw, I conquered." It's a mantra that reminds me of the times I've faced tough decisions and conquered obstacles. It's a reminder to keep pushing through, no matter how challenging the journey gets.

CHAPTER FOUR

ALWAYS MOVING ALONG.

COLLEGE & WILMINGTON CRAFT

34.0188° N, 77.8986° W:

I decided to go to college because society directs everyone to fall in line—finish high school, get that degree, and follow the expected path. But after a year and a half of struggling through art school classes and partying to mask my frustrations and negative feelings I harbored about myself, I realized it was time for a change.

With renewed determination, I packed up my car and headed straight for Wilmington, NC, ready for a fresh start. At first, I was all over the place, working a series of dead-end jobs: direct sales for Direct TV, creative design, t-shirt creation for an Amazon distributor, and eventually as a Verizon District Manager. During this period, I also experienced the profound loss of my eldest brother, Ben. He passed away from a pulmonary embolism on his way to work after a vacation—a trip I had declined to join with my family. At the time, I had just moved to North Carolina, and a trip to California felt both too distant and too costly. The regret and grief I felt were overwhelming, and it made me realize that I needed something more. None of the work I was doing felt fulfilling. In search of purpose, I dove into the healthcare field. I started by working in home healthcare for the elderly while earning my certifications. Thankfully, this led me to some meaningful friendships.

I met Issiah (**THE REMINDER**) while trying to get in shape at the gym with Caroline. Issiah was a big-hearted guy with a passion for reggae concerts and workout routines. We bonded when we found his wallet at a weight machine, and soon after, he became one of my closest friends and eventually a roommate. Issiah was also an amazing cook, which was a huge bonus for me!

At the same time, I met Kate (**THE REMINDER**) in my nursing assistant course. She was a tall, skinny, and quirky tomboy with a goofy personality. She had a hilarious personality that always carried me into seeing the bigger picture, while living joyfully through the crap of the present. Then there was Christy, who came into my life while covering for me at my elderly patients' home. She was a stunning blonde with an infectious smile and an even more infectious laugh. Originally from Boston, she playfully referred to herself as a "Masshole."

In a twist of fate, Christy (**THE ETERNAL**) went to the Verizon store to get a new phone and ended up meeting Issiah. They discovered they both knew me, and Issiah invited her to a concert we were supposedly attending. The funny part? I had never actually planned to go to that concert—I had a date with someone else- Issiah just hoped I'd come along! Despite the mix-up, it was clear that Christy and I were meant to be besties. Not long after, I landed a job at the hospital, and life started to fall into place.

For the next four years, I worked in the Cardiovascular Intensive Care Unit at the local hospital as a Tech and Unit Coordinator. There, I found my calling in helping patients recover and rebuild their strength after heart surgery.

Seeing patients bounce back and become stronger, both mentally and physically, sparked a deep passion in me. It became clear that my mission was to inspire others to be their best selves. This was a pivotal moment in my life, marking a shift toward a more fulfilling and purposeful path.

Happy Hospital:

34.2055. -77.9215

I once heard that a friend's voice can actually make your blood flow faster, which took me down memory lane to my time working in the Cardiovascular ICU. In that role, I helped patients recover from extensive heart surgery. It became clear to me that human connection is essential for feeling loved and supported. Patients who had family and friends visit or pray for them often experienced faster recoveries.

However, there was a paradox: after the intense emotional and physical strain of surgery, patients needed rest, which required a calm environment to support their healing. Fortunately, our unit had strict visitation hours, which helped create a more peaceful setting.

Initially, I didn't fully understand this necessity because, as an extrovert, I would want my family around me. I discovered that even well-meaning family members could inadvertently cause stress. For instance, I once had a patient whose heart rate would spike whenever his wife entered the room. Despite her intention to support him, her presence would trigger a stress response and made his recovery more challenging. This example highlighted the delicate balance needed between support and maintaining a stress-free environment for healing.

Sometimes, we think we're helping our loved ones, but our actions can inadvertently add stress. It's important to consider their perspective and understand that support doesn't mean overstepping boundaries. Instead of making assumptions or playing a guessing game, communicate openly and ask how you can best support them. Your intentions may be good and heartfelt, but the experience involves more than just your own perspective. Being mindful of this can prevent causing more harm than good and ensure that your support is genuinely beneficial.

"A Healthy Heartbeat—"

Finding Your Rhythm

Your heart is always sending signals, and understanding them can help you tune into your overall well-being.

Imagine this: You're cozied up, binge-watching your favorite series on Netflix. The show is flowing smoothly, no interruptions. But then, for some reason, the stream starts buffering, and suddenly it's like you're stuck in slow-motion, waiting for the video to catch up. That sluggish, choppy feeling is kind of like what happens when your heart rate slows down too much, a condition called bradycardia. When your heart beats slower than 60 beats per minute, it's like your heart's on a low-speed setting, trying to play catch-up. For athletes, though, this is usually no big deal—it's just their heart's way of saying, "I'm super chill because I'm fit." But for others, it might signal a need for attention.

Now, flip the script to the opposite problem—tachycardia. Imagine your phone is running too many apps at once. Everything starts off fine, but soon it overheats, slows down, and might even freeze. Tachycardia is like your heart being stuck in that overdrive mode, beating faster than 100 beats per minute, working harder than it should. It's your heart's version of having too many things running at once, struggling to keep up with the demands.

Then there's fibrillation. Picture trying to stream a live concert on your phone, but the connection is spotty. Instead of a clear, steady feed of your favorite band rocking out, you get glitches, pauses, and buffering every few seconds. Your heart should be like a steady, rhythmic playlist, each beat falling perfectly in line. But in fibrillation, it's more like a broken stream where the beats are disorganized, quivering, and out of sync. Your heart can't stay in rhythm, struggling to keep the flow going smoothly.

And finally, let's talk about premature contractions. Imagine you're at a party, vibing to a perfect playlist, and then—out of nowhere—the DJ plays the next track too early, totally throwing off the groove. Instead of a smooth transition, the beat drops too soon, disrupting the flow. That's what a premature contraction feels like for your heart—a beat that comes too early, throwing off your heart's regular rhythm, causing a brief hiccup in the steady flow of your pulse. It's like a brief, unexpected interruption that messes with the usual beat.

These different heart conditions are like the rhythm of a song—sometimes it's smooth, sometimes it's offbeat. But just like any good playlist, the goal is to find that perfect flow where everything is in sync.

"Life's rhythm is like waves on the shore—steady yet constantly shifting. Each day, we face the choice between growth and routine. Will we embrace new opportunities or cling to the comfort of what we already know?" —**Spiritual League**

NURSING PRO TIPS:

Let me share a few pro tips from my time in nursing that could come in handy if you're ever in a tough spot. These are tricks of the trade that I've picked up over the years and I hope you'll remember them when you need them most.

I'll start with something we all might face—anxiety or panic attacks. It's tough when your heart starts racing and your mind starts spinning, but there's a simple trick I use to help calm things down. Try drinking lukewarm water. It may seem small, but it helps calm your circulatory system, and it's amazing how staying hydrated with electrolytes can make a difference. Drink small amounts, and take slow deep breaths. I've used this tip countless times, whether I was working triage during an event or helping people stay grounded at music festivals.

Now, let's talk about cooling down if you're feeling overheated. We've all been there—too much sun or physical exertion, and your body starts to protest. Here's what I do: apply ice packs or cool water to major veins, like the ones on your wrists, and gently place a wet cloth on your neck's carotid artery. It's like giving your body a quick reset, and you'd be surprised how effective it is.

Lastly, I want to address a hydration warning that's often overlooked: don't overdo it with water. Yes, staying hydrated is crucial, but drinking too much water can actually be harmful if you're not balancing it out with the right amount of salt. Without sufficient salt in your system, your body can't manage hydration properly, and that can lead to dangerous conditions. So, next time you're reaching for that water bottle, just remember: balance is key.

These small but powerful tips have gotten me through some tough situations. Keep them in your back pocket—you never know when they might come in handy!

Warning: Graphic Content:

Full Circle Miracles

The patient's condition was dire. He was on ECMO, the most advanced life support machine we had. ECMO involves inserting a tube into the heart and other organs to transfuse old blood with new, keeping the body functioning while the patient remains immobile. At this stage, the body often appears severely swollen, with fluids accumulating like a balloon. A person who once weighed 140 pounds might balloon to over 200 pounds due to fluid retention and blood transfusions. The body becomes discolored and is filled with fluids, with blood seeping from the chest cavity and open wounds.

Lying in bed for such a long time requires constant monitoring of open wounds and pus. We followed strict protocols, rolling patients every hour to prevent bedsores and cleaning up feces and urine resulting from incontinence. This patient had undergone multiple surgeries and CPR several times, and he shouldn't have survived. Yet, through what seemed like miracles, he began to recover. After months of intensive care, physical therapy, and occupational therapy, he gradually moved to less critical care and eventually left the hospital.

The most moving moment came later when this patient walked into my then-partner's gym, seeking personal training to complement his ongoing rehabilitation. I was absolutely stunned to see him; I didn't even recognize him at first, but he recognized me from the days I took care of him in the unit. Witnessing him in those sessions and helping with his recovery was profoundly rewarding. It was incredible to see the tangible results of our hard work and care—saving a life not just in the immediate sense—but in a meaningful, long-term way. This is what I called "miracle territory."

Experiences like this reinforced my deep appreciation for the impact of compassionate care. It illuminated my commitment to loving and investing in others, reaffirming my passion for supporting and taking care of people. My years in serving in the ICU inspired a small tattoo behind my ear—a circle of life tree resembling an acorn –symbolizing "unexpected miracles." It's a permanent mark on my soul, a reminder of the profound moments that shape our lives.

Mannequin Hand

Due to HIPAA regulations, I'll share this story delicately, aiming to shed light on the feelings of shame, regret, and their ripple effects. Working in the hospital, particularly in the Cardiovascular ICU, was a space where I often found myself needing to disassociate. The job requirements were unique and the human aspect sometimes felt lost amid the clinical details.

I recall one patient was admitted under urgent circumstances due to an intimate incident involving him and his partner. Although this type of situation isn't uncommon—people experience a wide range of scenarios behind closed doors—this case became public in a way that the patient had never intended.

Throughout his treatment, this patient and his partner had to face not only the medical procedures, but also the scrutiny and questions from his family. It became evident that he had never come out to his family about his true identity or about his relationship with his partner. When his family was informed of his hospitalization, they naturally wanted to know all the details. But with the situation involving a sexual act, there was added guilt, shame, and discomfort.

During their visits to critical care, the family's questions were difficult, and again due to HIPAA agreements, we could only share what the patient was comfortable with. The patient's condition was dire—he was on the brink of death and his family was discovering for the first time that his partner was not just a friend, but his romantic partner, with whom he was living with.

As staff, we observed the unfolding drama, but remained neutral, staying focused on making the patient comfortable while respecting his privacy. Tragically, after just four days, the patient passed away. His body succumbed to multiple organ failures, and despite our best efforts, life support machines couldn't stabilize him.

Reflecting on this experience, I felt profound sadness. The patient's partner expressed visible grief while the family was left grappling with unanswered questions and the burden of hospital bills, potentially facing financial ruin. The situation was heart-wrenching.

Returning home that night, I clung to my significant other and our pets, contemplating the depth of human emotions and the harsh reality of unexpected events. Working in the hospital, I witnessed daily reminders of life's fragility. Even on the toughest days, I understood that life was a miracle.

This experience compelled me to reassess my own life and the areas where I might be hiding or avoiding truths, whether from others or myself. I began to explore wills, advance directives, and the importance of planning for unexpected situations. The patient's struggle with shame and secrecy left an indelible mark on me, highlighting the importance of addressing these difficult issues head-on.

In essence, the story reinforced that all actions have consequences, and the pain and struggle of hiding one's true self can be overwhelming. I hope it serves as a reminder to confront and plan for the uncomfortable realities of life, to avoid leaving behind unanswered questions and unresolved feelings.

We all have dirty laundry,
what matters is how you fold the clothes after.

CHAPTER FIVE

MEETING MY FUTURE.

Meeting Mr. J.

It was a Sunday afternoon, and I decided to meet up with a guy I'd been texting on and off for a month. Honestly, I wasn't that invested, but there was this cute bar called Satellite that locals loved for its folk music and great drink deals. I managed to convince my bestie, Christy (**THE ETERNAL**), to come along. We figured it would be a win-win: check out this guy and enjoy a few drinks—two birds, one stone.

Walking into the bar felt like a scene straight out of a movie. As I entered, the air conditioning was blowing my hair everywhere, making me feel like I was starring in my own dramatic movie-scenes entrance. The bar was dog-friendly, and it seemed like every dog in the place rushed over to greet me. I bent down to give them some love, basking in their affectionate energy. When I finally stood up, I noticed everyone in the bar was watching me.

I made my way to the bar and sat down next to a buff guy who was clearly my date. Mr. J. **(THE REMINDER)** he was smiling at me, obviously in awe of my entrance, and the vibe seemed promising. After some small chat and a drink, I could sense that something was off. I have this gift of being an empath, I can sense everything others are feeling. He was having these quiet moments, and I asked him, "What's wrong?"

He hesitated and said, "Well, let me put it this way. You probably have all your family with you, right?"

I replied, "Actually, no. My brother died. Why do you ask?"

He was visibly shocked and responded, "My dad passed away, and I'm actually supposed to be at the wake/funeral, but I'm here instead."

At that moment, I thought, "This guy is crazy." After some light banter, I told him, "We can reschedule for next week when you've got your life together and made the proper arrangements. Let's get you out of here." I walked him to the door, and as we said goodbye, I felt his pain and had a bit of pity. He asked if he could kiss me, and I said "Yes." His kiss was gentle, and I felt a small spark—one I knew I'd be chasing for a long time.

The following week, he took me out to dinner. Here's where it gets interesting: I had been chatting with my hairdresser about him and she suggested a double date. Her idea was to throw him into the deep end and see if he could keep his head above the water. I thought, "Why not?" and agreed.

Dinner was fun, and after a few drinks, we went to a place where we could dance. He had no idea that dancing was "my thing". We ended up having a blast. Eating my heart out on the dance floor, and watching his attempt to move his hips was entertaining enough. When it was time for him to take me home, we got into his gray truck, and he played a throwback CD. As we sang along, his music choice struck a chord I didn't know I needed. When Sheryl Crow's "My Favorite Mistake" came on, it was game over.

He didn't know it, but he passed the final test. The nostalgia of that song brought back old memories, with the present and the future merging into one moment. I made him pull over, come inside, and he never left.

I've come to realize that music has been the soundtrack of my life. It's like the universe communicates with me through these melodies, narrating my story in the background.

House of Hospital Aftermath

Looking back, I realize I seriously underestimated how much my job was wearing me down. After working 14-15 hour shifts—moving patients from exams to the cafeteria, stops to surgery, the blood bank, hospital laboratory, and even to the morgue—I was completely drained. I thought dealing with deceased patients and transporting them to the morgue was just part of the job, but as it turns out, it wasn't standard for my role and should have been handled by other specialized police staff.

Seeing the chaos and sometimes gruesome scenes in the hospital every day really took a toll on me. Our hospital served as the morgue for the entire city, so I'd encounter all sorts of body parts—everything from babies to adults—packed into body bags. It was as intense as it sounds. But you know what? What really got under my skin wasn't just the daily horrors of the job—it was the sheer waste of resources and the numbers game that healthcare institutions love to play.

When I first started in the unit, we were all looking forward to a humanitarian flight to Haiti with Doctors Without Borders. I'd been dreaming about this trip ever since I was a kid—mission trips with the church, peace corps aspirations, all of it. I thought, "This is it, this is my moment to actually make a difference." But, surprise, surprise, the trip got canceled. They said, "Maybe next year!" and left us hanging like the last season of a show that never gets renewed.

Now, I had a specialty role in my unit that gave me access to a whole lot of things most people didn't get to see. So one day, on a random errand from my manager, I ended up in the hospital warehouse and stumbled across all the supplies that were supposed to go on that Haiti mission trip. I couldn't believe my eyes. Here were these supplies, gathering dust, while people in Haiti—people who actually needed them—were waiting.

I was beyond furious. I started asking questions, like, "Why are these supplies just sitting here, rotting away?"

The answers were, of course, maddening. Apparently, after the trip got canceled, the supplies couldn't be redistributed. They were tied to the grant for the Haiti trip and couldn't be used for anything else. So, they just let everything expire. These were supplies we had been holding onto for years, promised to a community in desperate need of them. And instead of finding a way to deliver them, they just sat there, collecting dust and cobwebs. I was disgusted.

At that point, I decided I couldn't just sit back and accept this. I had to do more. I wanted to make it my mission to find out how I could help more, be more, and ultimately, make a bigger difference. It was around this time that I started responding to the inevitable question, "How's your day going?" with the deadpan answer, "Living the dream!" It was a bit of sarcasm, but also kind of true. I somehow managed to land my "dream jobs" more than once in my life. But you know what? The more I did, the bigger my dreams grew. And now, I'm just out here, chasing them down. Because why not? Unconditional love for what you do, the people you help, and the difference you make—that's what really drives me now.

Through the years at the hospital, I formed some deep friendships, all thanks to what I like to call our "trauma bonds" from the job. The chaos of the unit made us a tight-knit team—kind of like a dysfunctional but lovable family. My ride-or-die crew included Courtney, Nikki, and Brooke. (**THE EMPOWERERS**). We were basically the "dream team." And then there was Paul, our manager. Picture a tall, plump, older caucasian man with big round glasses. (**THE TEACHER**) He was like the dad of the group—kind, gentle, and always ready with a dad joke or a pat on the back when the days got tough. Together, we survived the worst days—being locked in during natural disasters, dealing with crazy patients, and navigating, patient family drama that would give any soap opera a run for its money. Honestly, I wouldn't have made it without them.

It kind of reminded me of the military. Seriously, it did. We were trained like soldiers, with the same 24-hour shifts and charting protocols that could've been straight out of a manual for battle. And you know, I've had my fair share of friends in different branches of the military, and they've all seen some serious stuff. When I think about it, it makes sense why they're bonded by life in a way that's hard to describe—like a brotherhood forged in fire. They have this "die-with-you" mentality, and sometimes, they really do go through hell, only to come out on the other side a little worse for wear, but somehow still standing.

I was reminiscing about these stories one day while editing these stories to my friend Daniel (**THE EMPOWER**), and he told me a story from his past that still blows my mind. The kind of deep-rooted trauma that stays with you forever. He described moments when death was literally knocking on the door, only to have the whole operation go sideways because someone didn't wake up in time. No, seriously. The whole team could be prepped, materials packed, everything ready to go, but if the captain or general didn't wake up at the crack of dawn to sign a piece of paper? The entire mission—saving women and children, bringing supplies, taking shelter—was called off. And this wasn't a one-time thing; it happened way more often than it should have.

Daniel told me, "Sometimes, you just have to laugh (and cry) at the absurdity of it all. But that's what bonded us. Through all the crazy, the frustrating, and the downright ridiculous moments, we stuck together. And in the end, that was the only thing that mattered."

At the time I was desperate for some meaning in my life. When I got home from work, I either talked non-stop to Mr. J about the day's intense experiences or stayed completely silent, not really processing my emotions. This took a heavy toll on my partner, who had to bear the brunt of it.

It wasn't until his mother brought it up in a casual conversation— they didn't fully grasp what I was going through—that it hit me. They didn't know how to comprehend the information that I was compartmentalizing. I had disconnected emotionally, focusing solely on getting the work done. I was functioning like a machine, handling the wear and tear of an intense workload. I juggled over 20 roles: patient care, assisting my manager, attending board meetings, organizing the unit, hiring, and staying on top of ongoing training and coursework.

When I got home, I was also responsible for walking, feeding, and taking care of our dogs—both of ours and any that belonged to his parents or friends. I managed household chores, tried to maintain my own mental and physical health. I felt overwhelmed.

Meanwhile, my partner was a personal trainer. His daily grind was vastly different from mine. Despite wanting to support him, I felt like I was carrying the weight of the world. I helped him secure an internship at my gym, which led to other opportunities and eventually to the launch of his own business. He saw my additional responsibilities as extra pressure.

Realizing that the stress and sacrifice weren't worth the modest paycheck I was earning, I decided to invest in a course to help him better manage his entrepreneurial efforts. I spent $5,000 on coaching from people I'd never met in California. It was a gamble, but one I hoped would pay off for the both of us.

While enrolled in the course, I started asking myself, "Why did I do all of this for him? What if I could be an entrepreneur?" I spent days— afternoons, evenings—immersed in personal development, determined to grow up and fast. And then, like a lightbulb turning on, it hit me: *I could do this!*

When I brought it up to my partner, he was totally on board. He was excited for me! (I couldn't help but wonder if that's what he had secretly been hoping for all along.) From that moment, I started taking the reins with a new level of confidence. I realized I was destined for more, and nothing was going to stop me now.

I showed up to every meeting, jumping on all the Zoom calls, marketing myself in any way I could, making content, and creating videos to *sell* myself and my services. I even enrolled in a personal training course to back up my experience with something a little more formal than just my nursing credentials. I wanted to help him market, but honestly, I had a bigger vision. I wasn't about to get stuck working in a hospital for the rest of my life.

There had to be more to life than working in the ICU forever. I needed to build an asset for myself—a business that could create long-term success, not just a paycheck. It was my "boss babe era." I hit the ground running, ready to make my mark.

"Infected during that era remained unheeled in the present'
—unknown

Compartmentalizing:

"Mental process of separating different aspects of one's life, emotions, or thoughts into distinct, isolated categories. This can be a coping mechanism where a person keeps conflicting feelings, responsibilities, or experiences separate in order to manage stress, avoid overwhelm, or maintain focus. While this can be helpful in certain situations, excessive compartmentalization can sometimes lead to emotional disconnection or difficulty processing feelings as a whole."

Working Around The Clock

I started working on my business both inside and outside of my hospital shifts, juggling two careers as best as I could. I didn't fully realize the balancing act I was signing up for—honestly, I kind of underestimated the hustle life. It wasn't just a 7-7 anymore; it was more like a 24/7 game of keeping all the plates spinning. But I was determined to make it work, even if I didn't always know how I was going to manage it all.

CHAPTER SIX

A DIFFERENT DIRECTION

The Time I Ran My Half Marathon:

34° 12.8' N, 77° 47.2' W

A long achievement, that one time I ran a half marathon. Yes, you read that right—a half marathon. It all started with this wild idea I had about moving to North Carolina. Now, I've always been a sprinter—like, short bursts of energy and *bam*—but for some reason, I wanted to push my body and mind in a completely different direction. When I was younger in gym class and track I was always the dasher, so pushing myself to a new limit was the goal. You know, the kind of direction that made me think, "Why not go longer? Why not test this whole 'mind over matter' thing?" And thus, the idea for a half marathon was born. I thought, *F-it*, I'm gonna see if I can actually do this!

While I was training, I swear this whole thing felt like it belonged to other people. The idea came from Caroline and Seia—they were my original inspiration. Their goals were kind of planted in my head, like little seeds of motivation. But, plot twist—I totally outran them. Yep, Caroline had other goals and achievements in life and didn't complete that goal of hers until much later in life. Seia made it all the way to a 10k, but never completed a half. (At least that I'm aware of.)

I started small, running around the neighborhood, doing little 5Ks here and there with a few girls. But those running groups? They were always changing. One day, someone would be in, the next day, they'd be out, depending on who was interested or who was part of the "friend group." Ah, the cosmic flow of running. It was all about that "runner's high at the end of the day." It's breathtaking!

Oh, and let's not forget Whitney,(**THE RUNNER**) who became the *ultimate* runner in our group. (Just wait for it) Seriously, cosmic connections all the way.

But anyway, Caroline—total (**THE ETERNAL**) vibes—and Seia—(**THE HEARTBREAKER**) well, I'm gonna call her the "heartbreaker" in this story, because that's what happened in the end. But they were both part of the inspiration of my long-distance running, but it became–"*my thing*". I was ready to take it to the next level.

I moved quickly from 5Ks to 10Ks, then finally to the big 13.1. And let me tell you, each step of the way had its pivotal moments. When I first started training, I did all the prep—studied the best techniques, got all the gear, new shoes, waxed all the "areas", got my headphones and water holder ready... you know, the essentials. But oh, the headphones—*they were key*. Running for hours is no joke, and I quickly realized that music was both a blessing and a curse. Sure, I love music—it's the beat of my soul—but running with music at a tempo, constantly matching rhythms for long distances? Not so fun.

So, I switched it up and started listening to podcasts. And, oh, what a game changer. Of course, everyone and their moms were obsessed with murder podcasts at the time, so I got hooked on "Crime Junkie." Nothing like running through the streets, dodging traffic, and listening to true crime, right? I found it oddly motivating—plus, it made me run faster. You know, just in case someone was lurking around being suspicious... Gotta stay alert! Let me tell you, when I thought someone was getting a little too close for comfort, my legs turned into *flash mode*—I was out of there like a superhero!

Now, around mile 9 of my half marathon, I had one of those *core memory* moments. (like the Emotions movie, a green one!) You know the kind—the ones that stick with you forever, the kind that shapes who you are. I remember thinking, *This is it. This is a new best moment.* I could feel my body pushing beyond limits, my mind locked into a new level of focus. It was like I was witnessing myself become something greater than I ever thought possible.

And that's when I realized that the journey wasn't just about finishing a race—it was about creating moments that would live on in my mind forever. I wanted to change the thought patterns that told me I couldn't do something, and turn them into "I can."

That's the magic of running a half marathon—it's not just a physical feat; it's a mind-over-matter, heart-and-soul kind of thing. And trust me, that core memory? It's *staying* with me. I thought I was just going to keep running like Forrest Gump all the way to the full marathon after that race. But I ended up hanging up on my running shoes, when I started to feel my knee bone chafing the skin. Time to take a rest on that hobby.

During that time, I felt so much joy seeing Whitney, cheering me on from the sidelines. Her presence filled my heart with warmth. Caroline couldn't be there in person, but I carried her spirit with me. Seia and I were caught in a series of disagreements, and I found myself leaning more on Whitney, almost pushing away the support from others. For some reason, I didn't even notice at the time—I was just so focused on Whitney being there. I remember feeling deeply grateful to see my friends and family waiting at the finish line, but Mr. J. and I weren't exactly in sync. There was tension between us, and I couldn't shake the feeling of annoyance when I stood next to him, though I didn't know why. Everything had been building up, years of unresolved issues simmering beneath the surface. Crossing that finish line felt like a huge achievement, and I tried to push aside the unspoken emotions, burying them in the rush of success.

Navigating the Discomfort of Sexuality

Have you ever felt ashamed for wanting a sexual experience with your partner? I totally get that feeling. It resonates with me on a profound level and it's why I've made it a part of my story.

I spent years in a relationship that suppressed my sexuality. Shame, trauma, and gut-wrenching emotions emerged from that experience. Now, I'm finally ready to confront those demons and share my journey, hoping it might help someone else.

When it came to intimacy, I felt like I wasn't good enough—hot, sexy, beautiful, or wanted. Being with my partner began to change me physically and the constant stream of negative thoughts and emotional abuse warped my psyche.

I felt damaged, trapped in the role of a victim. Honestly, some of the painful words and experiences from our sex life were repulsive. What should have been a euphoric part of intimacy turned into a huge trigger for me.

All I ever wanted was love and connection. I craved intimacy. Sexuality has always been a core part of who I am. I thrive on that energy; I create from it. I genuinely LOVE SEX. There's never been shame in my game—I've always been comfortable with my sexual experiences, no matter who my partners were. I embraced it all. Until I was so closed down my body wasn't able to endure it any longer.

Warning this part might be triggering:

However, the years of compounding trauma started to sink me deep into such a dark place. I was often left feeling manipulated or gaslighted. When you confuse love for *control*, harsh patterns begin to emerge. Painful words pushed me into a deep hole of insecurities. Phrases like "*I won't get hard if I touch you,"* or *"It takes you too long to cum, I don't want to waste my time."* Realizing later in my healing journey just how painful the power of words can be and the effect they can cause. Those phrases shouldn't be said to someone you "LOVE." Frankly, they shouldn't be told to anyone...

The amount of disrespect was unnerving.

I was always trying to overcome his constant excuses as to why we couldn't have sex. Morning, afternoon, and evenings, no matter what time of day it was, it wasn't ever a "good" enough time to pleasure each other. I'd often hide in our room masterbating on and off for hours. Feeling shameful, almost wishing he'd come in and I'd get caught, my body was screaming for sexual fantasies. At that point, the thoughts in my head started to be damning and pushed all the limits. Dreaming of hot sex fantasies, in the shower, in airplanes, in public spaces that could get you caught for indecent exposure

I once went to a women's event where there was a sex coach on stage, but you could find me in the back of the room hiding in my chair. When this topic came up I started to shut down. I didn't know how to handle myself; my heart and body pierced from shame. The therapist was telling a story all about how we shouldn't be afraid of a hot, sexy, orgasm. Hearing it, talking about it, felt like something taboo. She said "In fact her life got a hell of a lot better" when she discovered she had a ***generous lover***. She went on to state, "He gave me multiple orgasms. Three, four, sometimes even seven in one night's sitting - Talk about a full course meal). I literally thought I exploded and all the pieces of me melted into the floor. I couldn't wrap my brain around the fact I wasn't being emotionally or physically touched—at all—let alone having multiple orgasms. At the time, I'd never even heard of such a thing. I knew after that event, I had a new goal. I was destined to test these new waters and figure out how to crack that code.

Unfortunately, I racked my brain for every possible reason why he "didn't want me." "He must be cheating," "Maybe I smelled bad down there," or "Perhaps I just wasn't attractive anymore." I wondered if I was letting myself go or if he was secretly gay. My mind swirled with every negative thought imaginable. How did I, of all people, end up in this situation? "How did I get here?" "How did I become the man in the relationship with a grumpy wife who doesn't want to touch him."

Sexuality is a huge issue in our country, and honestly, it's kind of a mess. From a young age, we're told not to "play with our private parts," but then, when it comes to actually talking about our anatomy, it's like we're all supposed to act like we're in a game of *Twister*—avoid saying the "bad words" like "vagina" or "penis." We're taught to be embarrassed about our bodies, which creates this weird, uncomfortable relationship with our own selves.

Here's the thing—sex is supposed to be magical. Like, *really* magical. We're built to explore our desires, to let our bodies connect in passionate ways. Sex isn't just for the birds and the bees—it's about two people coming together in this beautiful alignment that feels like fireworks, and yes, it's also how our bloodlines keep going (yay biology!). Honestly, it's one of the most powerful human experiences we can have.

But here's the catch: when we suppress that natural desire, when we shame ourselves about our bodies or our sexuality, it can build up inside of us like emotional junk food. And that *stuff* tends to show up as misbehavior, anger, or worse, violence. Things like sex offenses, rape, and even gang violence—these are all twisted by the mind, often stemming from unaddressed emotional needs or frustrations.

So, here I was, in a partnership where sex had become practically nonexistent. No spark, no passion, no anything. I was frustrated and ready to find some *connection*—anywhere, really. After a lot of thinking,

I finally came to the decision that I wasn't going to put up with this *drought* any longer. But here's where things got tricky—what was supposed to be an intimate experience was now physically and emotionally painful. My body started to reject the idea of being with my partner altogether. It was like my soul was saying, "Nope, this is done."

And that was the moment I realized—this relationship had run its course. It was time for it to expire and for me to step fully into my healing era.

"Hard conversations, easy life. Easy conversations, hard life,"
—**Jerzy Gregorek**

CHAPTER SEVEN

PIVOTING

THE GREAT PAUSE:COVID CHRONICLES:

It was such a time to be alive! Everyone was locked in their houses, unable to work, shop, play, or just exist as a person in the 21st century. Honestly, it was the experience of a lifetime that affected everyone—no matter your age. It was like a natural disaster that we could all relate to, a shared milestone in the human experience. My emotions were all over the place, just like everyone else's.

At this point, I had just opened two new gym locations, and not long after, *bam*, COVID hit and put one location on pause. It was a total curveball. Suddenly, everything I was working toward had to be combined—business and personal life all tangled up. Conjoining business with my then-significant other was really the beginning of the end. We lived together, our best friends were dating, and we were confined to our house. There was no separation of individuality. Not to mention, the intense pressure of opening a new business as the world shuts down. It felt like we were living inside a pressure cooker.

Many businesses failed, and we went into a recession. People got sick, and some tragically passed away. Others placed all their hopes on a vaccine to save them. The world seemed to turn upside down, and the simple act of walking out the door without a mask on suddenly felt like a crime. The sight of someone wearing a mask became the new normal. If you weren't wearing one, it was like you had *something* wrong with you. The sheer delusion of it all was, in hindsight, kind of comical.

No matter what you did, you were doing it wrong. It became a game of who got COVID first and who was next in line. Everyone knew they'd eventually catch it—it was just a matter of time. But if you got it first, well, you could play the victim card. You had to call everyone you knew and tell them you had COVID, like it was some kind of badge of honor—or a sexually transmitted disease. If you didn't, well, you weren't taking accountability or responsibility for your actions. A general sense of shame and blame started to take root in a way that I had never seen before.

Other People's Life Stories:

Coming back to my passions during this time, I watched other people bloom in unexpected ways. It was like a collective rebirth, and even though things felt so out of control, I couldn't help but marvel at how people found their own paths forward. Even in the chaos, there was beauty in watching people evolve.

DODGED MY FRIST DIVORCE:

43°04'N. 98°34'W. 5552.

It's time for me to get brutally honest about my past. This is a flashback to moments I've tried to leave behind, but true healing means bringing out the raw, real emotions. When you really heal, you feel every part of it—every sense gets involved. After the chaos of COVID hit, things in our relationship went through too many unvictorious battles. We were fighting each other more than tackling the actual issues. COVID turned our world upside down. Our business merged, we got sick ourselves, and we tried to isolate—spending time only with each other and our two best friends.

Waves of depression hit us hard. Eventually, our best friends, "Seia & Lucia" broke up, and we found ourselves caught in the messy process of helping them heal while watching them trade partners like they were swapping outfits. It felt like a never-ending loop of new dynamics. My friendship with Seia had a hard break as she felt that was best for her sanctity and we were already on the rocks. His best friend Lucia (**THE REMINDER**)--started dating my new "best friend"--Mo (**THE STUDENT/ TEACHER**)—a coworker in our business (I became a matchmaker, dropping seeds). Before I knew it, trading the spaces of relationships was a better dynamic. Then seasons started to change and we were hosting all kinds of family and friends at our house, which only added more tension.

It was around this time that I really started to evolve into a new chapter of the woman I wanted to be. I was *sick and tired* of being sick and tired. I felt sexually deprived, emotionally drained, and physically and mentally exhausted. I couldn't take it anymore.

One night, lying awake with a gnawing pit in my stomach, I snapped. My heart felt shattered into a million pieces, like a punch to the gut. I had spent too many nights in bed, tears streaming, aching for something—a touch, a hug, anything to ease the pain. Instead, all I felt was anger, hurt, and complete exhaustion, just staring at the ceiling. I could sense him awake next to me, but neither of us made a move to reach out, to fix it. It was like we were miles apart, even though we were only centimeters away.

Finally, I made a decision: The next day, I was going to write a letter to my significant other about my feelings. Little did I know, that letter would change everything.

The next morning, I dragged myself out of bed and shuffled into the kitchen, dehydrated and searching for fluids like a wild animal. As I stood there, I heard my partner approaching. The conversation that followed is something I wish I could erase. I was met with hurtful words that left me feeling confused, sad, and frustrated. After a terse "See you later, girl," and a slammed door, I was left reeling. He had never called me "girl" ever in our entire time together. It was the moment I reached my breaking point.

Furious and broken, I grabbed a pen and some blank white computer pages. Before I knew it, years of unresolved trauma poured out of me like lava. Tears streamed down my face as I scribbled aggressively, my fingers blistering from the force. I ended up writing eight pages. I don't remember every detail, but I remember the essence: "We may not have been officially married, but consider this letter a subpoena for our divorce."

I knew I couldn't keep pretending to be happy in a life that felt like someone else's story. I didn't have a plan—no idea where I'd go, what I'd eat, or where I'd sleep. All I had was a mantra: "Big Breaths, Little Steps."

I called Mo for support, and she dropped everything to help me. I also canceled a lunch date with another friend who, though relatively new, showed incredible empathy and came to help me figure out the next steps.

Together, we packed what I'd need for a few days. I had to leave behind one of our two dogs, and I cried over the pup I couldn't take. It wouldn't have been fair to my partner to take both. We all piled into the car and headed to the beach, seeking solace in nature's healing powers and planning my next moves. We had crab dip and wine at one of my favorite waterfront spots, and decided that if I was going to cry and process, we'd do it with style, by the sunset.

The next 24 hours were a whirlwind of emotions—pain, tears, laughter, sadness, happiness, frustration, confusion, surprise, gladness, and joy. This life-altering experience was unforgettable. Writing that letter helped shed many toxic layers, but the real healing came from leaving the relationship behind. Something inside of me knew that he was never going to leave me, and if I wanted healing for both of us, it needed to be me. I needed to be the one who left. Our relationship became a long list of trauma bonds, from the passing of his father and COVID to running our business and natural disasters, so I knew it was time to step into the next chapter of my life. I was ready to evolve the relationship with myself.

Over the past year, processing this pain has propelled my spiritual growth from the early stages to a deeper level of –"awakening". Now, the phrase "Big Breaths, Little Steps" has evolved into "Big Steps, Little Breaths." The small breaths are more meaningful now that my feet are firmly on the ground. Breath work has become a vital part of my healing process, helping me inhale positivity and exhale the trauma and pain I no longer want to carry with me. I desperately wanted to learn what it meant to start "living" for the first time in my life.

UPCOUPLING:

After weeks of our "uncoupling," we'd been through a lot of therapy. I agreed to go, mostly because I wanted to end things with a little dignity and a lot of respect. We still had too many business entanglements and family matters that needed to be dealt with. In the months leading up to this, I had asked if we could go to therapy to battle out our differences. He wanted absolutely nothing to do with it. Until, of course, I was finally gone, and then—surprise!—he suggested we do therapy to put our lives back together. I knew I wasn't coming back, but at least I needed a healthy way to handle all our unresolved issues.

Then came the questionnaire. They asked me to fill one out beforehand, and let's just say it felt like the therapy had already started. I poured my heart into it, venting my frustrations, hopes, and wishes for a future—without him, but with closure. Honestly, that was therapy before therapy. The weeks we spent in sessions were... an awakening. It was like a newsflash to both of us: we weren't listening to each other, nor were we seeing eye to eye. Which, let's be real, I already knew. We were living on different planets. He was focused on our future, while I was stuck in the present, pointing out that, well, if you can't be present with me now, there might not be a future at all.

Our therapist, bless her heart, didn't pick sides but instead cleared the air on so many things. And that's when I realized—therapy is like a relationship cheat code. If you're dealing with heavy emotional baggage or have people in your life who know too much and have too many opinions, a third party can really help you see things clearly. Highly recommend it.

But still, the answer was clear to me: it was time to break up the business—literally. He was so sweet and offered to help me move my things out of the house, as if lifting my bed would somehow keep us tethered together. I was grateful, honestly, though I think he was just grasping at straws, hoping that somehow I'd stay—or at least stay in touch. He was holding on, but I was already moving forward.

I settled into my new home in the container district: a new development downtown built from shipping containers. During the environmentally friendly era of tiny houses--(which, by the way, I had already mentally dubbed "The New Me"), I spent months focusing on personal growth. I cleared out the old—literally and figuratively. It was emotional, to say the least. I was diving deep into self-development and bible study, trying to understand what forgiveness really meant, and how I could become the best version of myself.

Then, one day, I called him up and asked him to come over for a "talk." I sat him down and apologized for everything I had done wrong. I took responsibility for making him feel abandoned, and for all the other emotional landmines I might've triggered along the way. It was probably the most honest and loving conversation we had in a long time. He was shocked. I could tell he still had a glimmer of hope that I'd return, that the spark would reignite, and we'd get back together. But no. He eventually moved into a new apartment with his best friend, Lucia. Not exactly the romantic reunion I had in mind.

That wasn't my intention at all. I just wanted to make amends, send him love, and give him the healing I had worked so hard to find myself. It was time to let go, but in the most graceful, loving way possible.

Emergency Contact:

As I was trying to reconnect with myself, I came to face a very real situation. I had an experience that made me recognize that there's nothing quite as unsettling as realizing that, should something go wrong, no one knows who to call as my emergency contact.

On a sweltering 80-degree day, I was at a local brewery with about 20 friends—celebrating a friend's birthday and sipping prosecco. I had only planned on staying for one drink before heading out for a kayaking session. But suddenly, those plans were the last thing on my mind.

One moment, I was laughing and enjoying the party, and the next, my iwatch buzzed with a warning: "Heart rate elevated: 120 bpm." A chill ran through me as I felt my heart pounding against my chest. My initial thought was pure panic: "Why is my iwatch going off?" It was the emergency health setting, about crashing vitals of the body. Before I could process it, my body started to collapse.--I turned to my friend, the birthday girl, and begged for her water. The next thing I knew, I was slumped against her, unable to move. She thought I was just being cute by sleeping / cuddling on her shoulder– resting– but I was immobilized. When she shifted, I blacked out, and I slid off her arm onto the floor.

When I came to, I was disoriented, surrounded by a mix of friends and strangers. I could barely hear my name being shouted over the commotion.

Hands were everywhere, trying to stabilize me, and someone was patting my forehead with a cold rag. I overheard that 911 had been called, which only made my heart race even more. I was in disbelief and confusion, not able to fully understand that I had fainted. The realization that my friends were calling an ambulance sent me into a full-blown panic. I've worked at our city's hospital, I knew I didn't want to go there for help. The emergency room was its own form of tragedy. There's not enough staff and it's a world wind of chaos.

One of my friends, sensing my fear, stepped in to help. She guided my breathing and kept me focused, assuring me that the EMTs would just get fluids into me and ask a few questions. We attempted to move outside to wait for the ambulance, but my legs felt like jello and couldn't stand.

When the medical team finally arrived, they helped me to the ambulance truck. My friends asked, "Who is your emergency contact?"—a question they couldn't answer now that I was newly single. They said they thought of calling Mr. J., but weren't sure. After a moment of hesitation, I suggested they call one of my best friends, Caroline, who wasn't at the gathering. She was actually a paramedic at the time, I knew she'd have the answers I needed. The EMTs reassured me, hydrated me, and eventually sent me on my way.

A friend drove me home, and a few others came over to check on me that night. Everyone at the party kept in touch to make sure I was okay. We were all shaken by the day's events.

This experience made me realize the importance of knowing who to trust in emergencies. But it also highlighted something beautiful: the way strangers and friends can come together to support one another in times of need. We are all interconnected, and in those moments, it felt like a testament to the unity and compassion we share.

CHAPTER EIGHT

RELATIONSHIP WITH MYSELF.

I started diving into every aspect of myself that I could, determined to be as ready as possible for the next chapter of my life. I wanted to be the best version of myself, in every possible way. So, I went all in—healing exercises, therapies, you name it. I uncovered a lot—emotions I didn't know I had, old traumas I had buried deep, and a whole lot of personal growth. It wasn't always easy, but it was definitely worth it. I began to see the progress, even when it felt like I was wading through a sea of emotions. The more I explored, the more I realized just how much there was to heal and how many pieces of me were waiting to be put back together.

Ever Heard of Mirror Work?

Grab a favorite face mask and throw your hair into a messy bun, because you're about to confront a real mess. This can be an uncomfortable experience if you're genuinely looking at yourself in the mirror. As women, we often check the mirror to see how our outfits look, assess our makeup, or evaluate our hair. However, this exercise dives deeper, confronting those nagging thoughts that creep in. The thoughts that tell you, "No, Sally, you're not hot enough. Your lipstick isn't popping. You have bags under your eyes." You might even be worried about that gray hair sneaking into your beautiful summer locks.

How to Meet Yourself in the Mirror:

Okay, grab a mirror and sit in front of it—yep, the one you've been avoiding because your reflection sometimes feels like an honest friend you didn't ask for. Now, look yourself straight in the eyes. I mean, really look. Acknowledge both your soul and your body—yep, that beautiful package of skin, bones, and caffeine-fueled ambition.

Now, think about that thing you've been avoiding. You know, that little secret or thing you've been hiding from yourself. (It's okay, we all have one.) Now, say out loud: "I'm sorry for... [insert your secret here]." Yep, get it out, even if it feels awkward. Trust me, it's worth it.

Then, let's do this together: "I love you. I love you. I love you." (Say it like you mean it!)

And then, "I accept you. I accept you. I accept you." (Because you're a work in progress, and that's totally okay.)

But what if, instead of focusing on those whispers, you start to speak differently to yourself? What if you looked in the mirror and said, "I see you." "I forgive you for...." "You are worthy of love or that career choice". This is the essence of mirror work—noticing the narrative you've adopted and consciously choosing to rewrite it.

This practice can lead to a profound shift in your mindset. By facing yourself with compassion rather than criticism, you begin to rebuild the trust and connection you have with yourself. Over time, you will stop seeking validation solely from external sources and start recognizing your inherent worth. This is where true self-esteem begins—from the inside out.

This practice can lead to a profound shift—one that allows us to truly meet ourselves on a deeper level. Once we are aligned with our true selves, we are able to experience true fulfillment. When you lack a deep, meaningful relationship with yourself, you miss the basic magic of existence.

I'll admit, the first time I looked at myself in the mirror, I thought I looked like hot shit. I had on a cute outfit, my makeup was on point, and I was really feeling myself. But I was also trying to follow my coach's guidance to go deeper. When she insisted I take off the "mask" we wear, I realized I needed to find a version of myself that was more authentic. I began to ask myself a serious question I had no clear answer to, "Who am I without all these facades?" In fact what have I been hiding from myself?

What is self esteem: according to" Self-esteem - Definition, Meaning & Synonyms | Vocabulary.com"

Self-esteem:

"A feeling of pride in yourself."

Remember, self-esteem is not about perfection. It's about pride—pride in your resilience, your uniqueness, and your ability to face your reflection with love. When you embrace who you are, flaws and all, you unlock the deeper magic of existence. And that, dear reader, is where the journey to true fulfillment begins.

The Shadows

The shadows below represent the darkest, most hidden stories of my life. By bringing them to light, I'm not only freeing myself from their grip on my future but also hoping to inspire others to confront their own shadows.

For me, some of the shadows I've been fighting against for most of my life have been battles with my physical self. It's been a constant struggle—trying to erase, agree with, understand, shift my perspective, and adapt. It's like trying to wrestle with a ghost that keeps coming back in different forms.

Shadow RECAP #1: Labels

As a child, I was labeled "LD" (learning disabled). My specific challenge was converting short-term facts into long-term memory, making math and spelling particularly difficult. My parents faced a tough decision: hold me back a year or let me advance with my classmates. They eventually made a decision and chose to hold me back, repeating the same year twice. I had transferred in the middle of the year and missed too much primary schooling that it was too difficult for me to process and catch up. It was seemingly an "easier" decision based on long term effects. Kind of like giving me a "reset." I was devastated, and just had an emotional meltdown. I threw a heated tantrum, cried, stomped around, begged and pleaded for any mercy but that ruling.

The label of "LD" brought teasing from my peers, and I let their harsh comments define me. I perceived the special education classroom as a place for kids who were "less than" the others. I would sneak in, afraid of being seen, and eventually developed anxiety and panic attacks. Throughout my primary education, I felt ashamed, isolated, frustrated, and sad.

As an adult, I had to dig down deep and confront these repressed childhood emotions. Through a healing practice called "Inner Child Work," I revisited and felt those old wounds. By releasing these emotions, I realized they no longer weighed me down or defined my destiny. They had shaped who I was, but they didn't determine who I could become. I let go of the chains that had held me back for so long and embraced the freedom to evolve. Today, I am proud to say I love the version and person I've become. I've really accomplished a lot, and surpassed any label that once was held over my head. Fear isn't something I'll let stop me. I won't hide in a box any longer.

Shadow #2: Birthday Party

It was late summer, August, at my parents' ranch-style home in the countryside. I was about 10 years old and felt sad, confused, and lonely. My mom had invested time and money into organizing my birthday party, and I eagerly awaited my friends' arrival. As minutes ticked by with no sign of anyone, and after several fruitless phone calls, I realized that no one was coming. Everyone turned out to be busy, or they're plans changed.

The pain of rejection cut deep. I longed for connection but wondered if I had pushed people away with any lasting efforts. Maybe I was "too much" or just too mean, due to the bullying I'd experienced. I may have unintentionally projected my hurt onto others.

Shadow #3: Finding Myself

I spent most of my 20's in a relationship that was both beautiful and disastrous both physically and emotionally. It literally took stepping away to see it clearly. Removing myself to view it from a larger perspective. I had been blinded by love, unable to see the truth until I was outside of it.

Those years were challenging as I struggled to piece together who I wanted to be. Manipulation had suppressed my sexuality and stifled my happiness. Surrounded by negativity, my light had dimmed. I needed to rediscover my joy and let go of people, things, and emotions that no longer aligned with who I was becoming.

After months of crying, releasing, processing, and reflecting, I began to feel spontaneous again. My soul craved new experiences and the thrill of the unknown. I embraced euphoria, let go of regrets, guilts, and chased the excitement of the present. Craving joy from the inner child, and repairing all of the damage that had been masked.

Music started speaking to me on a deep level, reminding me of my passion for dancing. It was like my auditory sensors were blasting on the highest volume. I let myself get lost in the rhythm and movement, reconnecting with my creative side. I enjoyed painting–allowing the brush to flow freely on paper–watching the water be gentle, making waves, creating masterpieces with my fingertips.

Through various healing techniques, I realized that the only person who could truly lift me out of my funk was myself. While having a supportive network is invaluable, ultimately, healing comes from within. Today, I am able to help others on their own journey's and it has become my true passion.

CHAPTER NINE

A NEW COMPASS POINT.

VACATION STATION:

Vacations are supposed to be a break, right? The idea of escaping reality for a while sounds perfect, but soon you realize just how much work they really are. Ever heard the phrase "you need a vacation from your vacation"? It's true—especially when you factor in time changes, travel hiccups, layovers, lost luggage, and missed flights. The stress adds up quickly. But lucky for me, my vacations are often packed with extreme sports, so while they might sound glamorous, it's action from start to finish.

Take my dad, for example. He's such a sports enthusiast that he'd plan our family vacations based on which teams were playing in a particular state. If there was a sporting event in the country, we were there, no question. But even when there wasn't a game on the agenda, we'd find ourselves on some wild adventure. I remember when Ben and I were little, going white-water rafting in the Rockies. We were laughing, cruising down the river in our raft, when suddenly, we hit a bump. The raft swayed, and Ben lost his shoe—thankfully, not his head! The instructor's warnings echoed in my ears, but the thrill of the rapids kept our hearts racing.

And then there was the 4-wheeler ride in the chilly Rockies, racing over the rocky terrain with the mountain stretching out endlessly ahead. The thrill of freedom was intoxicating, but with every twist and turn, I thought I might be flying off the side of a cliff. It was the kind of adventure that left you feeling both terrified and exhilarated at the same time.

I'll never forget the time we went jet skiing in Mexico, the ocean waves splashing in our faces as we zipped through the water. Or the time my aunt burned her leg. on the exhaust of a 4-wheeler in Cabo, and we all wondered if she was going to make it through. But, of course, she powered through it like the tough woman she is. Family vacations are full of energy—everyone laughing, bonding, and, at times, worrying about each other.

One of my favorite memories was my adult trip to Arizona. I remember running, jumping, and climbing the mountains like I was in a parkour competition, hiding in the caves, getting lost in the woods, heading toward the top of a trail that led to a stunning view of Horseshoe Bend. Standing there on the edge, with the wind in my face and the world stretching out below me, I felt more alive than ever. It was the kind of experience you can only get when you push yourself past your limits.

Jamaica had its treasures—each one an adventure wrapped in paradise. My days there felt like a whirlwind of excitement and relaxation, a perfect blend of both. Mornings started with peaceful spa days on the cruise ship, where I'd unwind, surrounded by the soothing sounds of the ocean and the luxurious pampering of a massage. It was the kind of tranquility that made you feel like you were living in a dream.

But by mid-afternoon, the adventure kicked into high gear. I remember the thrill of riding bobsleds down the mountainsides, feeling the rush of wind in my hair as I zoomed through the winding tracks, taking in the island's beauty from a new perspective. Getting back onto the cruise ship to wake up in another location daily. And as if that wasn't enough, we explored Mayan caves—ancient and mysterious, offering a peek into history while surrounded by the cool, damp air of the caverns. It felt like stepping back in time, immersing myself in a world far removed from the one I knew.

Through all these trips, I've learned more than just the thrill of adventure. I've learned to appreciate different cultures, foods, and the lessons about safety, responsibility, and being present have stayed with me. So, the next time you book a vacation, just remember: It may be an adventure, but it's also a chance to grow. You might return with more stories and wisdom than you ever imagined.

In the end, no matter how wild the adventure or how chaotic the travel might seem, the moments that stick with you the most are the ones that teach you about yourself and the world around you. And sometimes, the biggest lesson is just learning to be present, in the moment, with the people you love. That's what makes every vacation unforgettable.

Girl Group:

After my whirlwind of crazy vacations and launching business ventures, while trying to figure out what on earth entrepreneurship actually was, I stumbled upon a group of girls in Wilmington who were all different business owners with one thing in common: we wanted to build community. Oh, and we also really wanted to do fun things together. If I remember correctly, one of the girls, Ivy, **(THE EMPOWER)** slid into my DMs on Instagram and invited me into the group. At the time, I had already been messaging another girl, Mer because I found her Insta and thought she *seemed cool*—plus, I was feeling a little lonely and just really wanted to connect.

Enter Mer. **(THE EMPOWER)** She was this fiery little ball of energy with blonde hair and muscles to spare. She was also building a business and, like me, trying to make waves in the coaching world. We spent countless coffee dates just tossing ideas around, pretending to actually get some work done (because that's what entrepreneurs *do*, right?). Then, out of nowhere, Ivy reached out to both of us. I was practically giddy at the thought of meeting new women and finally feeling like I wasn't the only one on this crazy journey.

So, one day, we all met at Casablanca—this gorgeous all-white building that looked like it belonged in Colombia but was actually tucked away on the outskirts of Wilmington. The coffee? Incredible. The avocado toast? Let's not even go there. They topped it with red onion, radishes, a sprinkle of salt and pepper, and a little dash of egg—pure perfection. As I waited in line to grab my food and find a seat, the girls began trickling in one by one.

First, Ivy walked in and introduced herself. She was the one who'd reached out to everyone, after all. Ivy had this smile that could light up a room, with cute dimples and blonde hair, and her bubbly personality was impossible to miss. Born in South Africa and having bounced around—most recently from California—she was basically the definition of a world traveler. She ran her own skincare business and was a master at making connections.

Ivy shared her story with us, explaining how she and Brittany (**THE STUDENT/ TEACHER**) had decided to start reaching out to other girls they thought they'd vibe with. "We wanted to be friends with these amazing women," she said. "So, why not start a group?" And just like that, our little crew began to form.

Brittany—this gorgeous redhead, ocean blue eyes with an eye for design and detail. She was absolutely gorgeous, but her self-doubt? Pretty loud. We spent a lot of time boosting her confidence, and I'm so glad we did because she became a total powerhouse in both her photography and real estate businesses. She was super helpful to help orchestrate any photoshoots we needed.

Next was Olivia (**THE EMPOWERER**)—sweetest heart ever, brunette with an athletic body. She came with a background in yoga, teaching at the Evolution Studio, run by another amazing entrepreneur Macy. But Olivia's career choice was photography, specifically weddings. Eventually, she had babies (and I got to watch it all happen!), and then she ventured into milestone photography. It was so beautiful to see her juggle both her business *and* her growing family. Her babyshower brought us all so close!

We tried to meet up every couple of weeks—sometimes more, depending on everyone's crazy schedules. Then, one day, we all decided to go work at this cute coffee shop by the beach. It was on top of a surf shop, with windows that looked straight out to the depths of the ocean. It almost immediately made you daydream, mesmerized by the vast beauty. We were all set up and ready to dive into group chats when Ivy, being Ivy, immediately made friends with a dog, Spaghetti. I mean, who could resist? She started chatting with the pup, and that's when we bumped into Mari (**THE TEACHER**)—a graphic designer who had just moved to Wilmington from Florida.

Mari had this totally unique vibe, with her adorable freckles and light blonde-brown hair. She was rocking a basic T-shirt and cute jeans, and of course, our genuine hospitality kicked in. We immediately invited her to join us and share her story so we could all bond.

That was the day we officially became friends. Sharing stories, being vulnerable—it's how you build real connections. It's how you learn about people and how to empathize with them. We wanted our group to be a safe, loving space where we could always be positive and supportive.

Mari and I ended up getting closer because of our living situations, social statuses, and, well, relationship statuses (we both had some interesting experiences in that area). Watching the lives we created together has been its own story. Finding each other was one of the healthiest things that's happened in my life—we learned a lot about each other and, more importantly, how to grow and love ourselves. This is where we really began to appreciate both ourselves and each other.

CHAPTER TEN

FORGIVENESS.

Mother-in-Law:

Ruth was a unique, loving firecracker of a woman. (**THE HEART BREAKER**) When I entered into my relationship with Mr. J, I quickly realized that it wasn't just about partnering with him; it also meant embracing his family. It's a package deal and I was committed to all of them.

At the time, Mr. J was navigating the difficult process of grieving his father's passing, which brought us into some heavy situations. Packing up his father's belongings and making decisions about his remains was tough, but I stepped in to offer my love and support. Having gone through similar experiences myself, I found it easier to be there for Mr. J and his family during such a challenging time. I wanted to make a good impression with his mother and hoped to truly get to get to know her.

Over the five years that followed, we had our share of ups and downs. In my own pain and discomfort, I sometimes felt that Ruth's love was conditional. Mr. J's parents had the financial means to support our goals, but it often came with strings attached. Much of this was self-imposed. I was naive at the time and I found joy in simple things like walking their dogs, painting fences, cleaning homes, and finding other creative ways to make a little extra cash.

Throughout our relationship, Ruth and I spent many days thrift shopping, getting our nails done, and enjoying fancy lunches and dinners together. She truly became like a second mother to me, especially since my own mom lived so far away. Those moments of quality time shaped how I viewed the world and helped us deepen our bond.

Ruth's generosity was endless, but I saw her heart shine after her ex-husband's death. Soon after, we found ourselves co-managing the power of attorney for Lewy, who was one of the most remarkable gifts that God brought into our lives. Lewy was a charming, mid-height elderly lady with soft white hair that compliments her warm personality. She was often seen wearing funny, colorful sweaters that reflect her playful spirit. Her sweet smile lit up her face, and her wide eyes seem to always be full of wonder and kindness. Patience radiates from her, and you can feel the warmth of her genuine, caring nature that shines from the inside out. The time I spent with her while she was a resident on this earth, I will always cherish. She was the definition of unconditional love. We did anything for her, treated her like she was our own granny, even with no blood relation at all. Spending holidays watching Hallmark, trips to the nail salon, bringing her restaurants, cooking for her, organizing the remains of her life. She holds a special place in my heart.

While Lewy and I grew closer, I'd care for Ruth's home while she was away traveling with Mr. J. However, when the family got the second mountain house in Virginia, it revealed both the best and worst of our family dynamics. At times, we even turned wealth and privilege into an ugly accessory. Don't get me wrong—the hot tub, family boat rides, mountain sunsets, game nights, facials, and the retreat from natural disasters were incredible blessings - but when it came to cleaning, or maintaining things, that was another story. I found out that things cost a lot of money, so when they became damaged, it was a huge deal. She'd get really upset and angry and show emotions to lash out at the family. The air grew thick with discomfort. We were constantly on edge, often worried about a drunken mistake or slip of the tongue uncovering our family's drama. I also really began to see which family members suddenly wanted to be included in our future plans. Every decision was mentored and shaped by her reasoning, which didn't seem to always have my best interest in mind, and most of the time, didn't have J's best interest in mind either. This trickled down into our relationship, like a wrecking ball in the process. I felt like I was in a throuple and whatever decisions we had between us, became decisions influenced by her.

When our relationship finally ended, she did something that felt deeply personal—she hid my plants under the kitchen sink. Those plants meant everything to me. During the COVID lockdowns, I had poured countless hours into studying and researching their care and species. They became a symbol of growth and hope for me, so seeing them shoved away like that felt like a deliberate wound. It was one of many stories of pain from our time together, but honestly, who wants to relive all of that?

As I was moving out, I noticed she had already made our once shared bed and rearranged the seats and even added a new comforter. It was such a gut punch—a total "ick" moment. I remember thinking "Wow, really? She just barged in here? Like he can't make his own bed, eww." That cemented how quickly she wanted to encourage him to move on. I felt like that could have been something that was adjusted after I'd fully moved out, but while I was still moving my things out of the house - yikes. (There is a time and a place) I could feel the resentment building inside me, and it began to consume me. I was still in my twenties, grappling with my identity and desperately clinging to the idea of being a good housewife—even though I knew I was so far from that ideal.

Looking back, I realized she really did try to keep me on the straight and narrow, but in ways that often felt stifling and at odds with who I was. The resentment I carried was as much about my own insecurities as it was about her actions. In those moments, I was lost—trying to navigate a version of myself I wasn't sure I could ever become. But maybe, just maybe, those painful experiences were planting seeds for the person I'd eventually grow into.

This relationship really challenged me in many ways and honestly I'm so thankful for all of the lessons. It's been extremely powerful to heal from this pain. I needed all of those tough lessons and I believe she did as well. I am blessed to mention that after we separated and I had the space to deal with my own sh*t, I was able to take accountability for my own actions. We've been able to reach out to each other over the years and catch up. Lewy's funeral was a monumental rekindle for us, it warms near and dear to my heart. We even wish each other many years of happiness. She'll always be a mother to my heart.

Even four years later, I'm still getting used to the healing it takes for my heart to be open. We often don't even realize that the pain, grief, and sorrow we feel only pains us. That person you're angry with might not even know you've been angry. Put down what you're carrying and realize that those subconscious patterns might still be playing a role in "upgrading your computer." Navigating these complexities taught me valuable lessons about love, family, and ultimately, forgiveness.

CHAPTER ELEVEN

MEMORY LANE.

CONSCIOUSNESS UNLOCKED: FIGHT OR FLIGHT.

33.6954° N, 78.8802° W

It was a summer afternoon, and a group of my friends had packed up the truck to head down to Myrtle Beach for some Topgolf fun. We thought it would be a nicc escape from our usual routine in Wilmington. I was in the backseat with the girls while the guys sat up front, not paying much attention to the road. Suddenly, I heard them shout, "Holy shit, did you just see that?"

"What?" I screamed back.

"There was this guy flying down the street in a Lambo, and he just hydroplaned!"

"What? Stop! Go back!" I urged. They pulled over, and without a second thought, my body jumped out of the car faster than I could process the situation. The next thing I knew, I was leaping over a stream of water flooding the ditch, getting as close to the overturned car as possible. My instincts and nursing experience kicked in, adrenaline rushing through my veins.

I started yelling to see if the driver was okay. "Are you okay?"

"Yeah, I can move; I'm not hurt!" he yelled back, luckily able to slide out of the car with no injuries.

Just then, a crowd gathered, and we struggled to get the butterfly doors open against gravity. Together, we helped guide him to safety. I quickly assessed the situation and realized we needed to get everyone away from the water. The car could explode, and with rain and lightning in the air, the risks were real. My critical thinking was on high alert.

As I helped people move to safety, the driver suddenly started screaming in agony. "FUCK! MY CAR!!!!!!" I thought it was insane he cared more about his car than his life, but who am I to judge. Thank god he was safe.

My friend who had rushed to the scene with me jumped over the danger zones and walked back to our vehicle like nothing had happened. I looked around at everyone's faces—they were in complete shock from what they'd just witnessed. It felt like I was a sleeper assassin who had just woken up and sprung into action. They all hugged me and offered me dry clothes since I was soaked from the pouring rain.

After we got our bearings and the ambulances arrived, we hopped back in the truck and continued our journey to Topgolf, as if nothing had happened.

Jumping to My Timely Death: Before the Jump
33.9285° N, 78.0736° W

I woke up bright and early on September 4th, around 5:45 AM. The night before had been riddled with restlessness and excitement about the day's skydiving adventure in Southport, NC. As soon as I got out of bed, I went through my morning routine, including a quick meditation session. I visualized the day ahead: a thrilling skydive with a hot, funny instructor to ease my nerves and an exhilarating freefall. By the time I finished meditating, I felt unstoppable. I got ready and awaited my ride.

When the car arrived, I joined a group of women—Taylor, a single girlfriend I'd often make arts and crafts with, and Jaya, my beautiful friend who was always there to help whether it was a business venture, volunteer act, or speaking engagement- (**THE EMPOWERERS**) and two others who were new acquaintances. We took turns sharing our reasons for skydiving. Taylor, whose 28th birthday was just around the corner, joked that if she didn't make it out safely at least she'd "join the 27 Club."

Why I Wanted to Jump:

When it was my turn, I explained that my birthday had been two weeks before hers, which was why I had agreed to go skydiving with Taylor for our birthdays. But after the COVID-19 lockdown, I realized how short and unpredictable life can be. I vowed to live every day fully, and the synchronicity of skydiving near the 7-year anniversary of my brother's death was a reminder to live boldly. "Here's to being fully alive!" Plus knocking another item off my bucket list! We all cheered.

Going Up:

We arrived so early that we beat the staff, excitement you could say. While waiting, we enjoyed the company of some friendly dogs and eventually went inside to check in. The paperwork was intimidating— one of the women, a lawyer, was uneasy about the waivers. We knew the risks, but after initialing and signing every line, I was ready for whatever came next.

In the locker room, I grabbed my photocard for the video shoot I'd paid for. When I emerged, my instructor, Tyler, (**THE TEACHER**) was waiting. Just as I had hoped, he was a hot guy with a great smile and a sense of humor. I was instantly at ease. As he hooked me into the harness, the chaos of the room made it hard to focus. I told him he'd need to explain things a few times—"repetition is key." With the plane in sight, Taylor decided to go first, and Tyler asked if we were ready to go second. I was thrilled!

The Jump

We climbed into the tiny plane, packed in tight. Tyler strapped my harness to his and pulled me onto his lap to tighten everything up. I laughed as he recorded me. As we ascended, Tyler gave a tour of the view, keeping me entertained. When the plane reached 4,000 feet, the door opened, and I was hit with a rush of adrenaline. I remembered Will Smith's skydiving video, and we all laughed about the open door.

At 14,000 feet, the door opened again. The first two teams of instructors jumped out, followed by Taylor. When it was our turn, Tyler and I moved to the edge. With a countdown of 3-2-1, we leaped into the sky. I was laughing, crying happy tears, and throwing peace signs. I had worn my Wonder Woman t-shirt for this very moment. The freefall was exhilarating.

Safe Landing

After 55 seconds of freefall, Tyler tapped my shoulder to signal the parachute launch. The sudden drop felt like a rollercoaster, but the view was magical. Gliding down with the ocean in sight, I felt like I was one with the atmosphere. Tyler checked in, and I told him I felt euphoric. I was ready to go again.

We spiraled through the sky for five minutes, making the most of every second. When it was time to land, the perfect weather allowed us to touch down safely on our feet. I looked around, watching the others land, feeling a mix of elation and disbelief. I thanked Tyler for keeping me safe—my life had literally been in his hands.

What This Experience Meant to Me

This experience taught me that fear can be paralyzing, but on the other side of that fear lies pure bliss. Fear can teach us to be cautious, but it can also hold us back from incredible experiences. Remember this the next time you're hesitant to start a new project, go on a date, or take a leap of faith. Stepping out of your comfort zone is where the magic happens. Life is too short not to be the best version of yourself and embrace all that the world has to offer. We're lucky to be alive and to experience what the physical world has to offer—so why not take the plunge?

My Pivotal Journey: Spreading Joy and Positivity:

34.22816,-77.92755

Let's be real—COVID was rough on all of us. But as I watched everyone struggle with the emotional aftermath, I decided to make it my personal mission to spread some joy around Wilmington. My relationship was ending, my business was shifting, and I found myself diving headfirst into something new: *mental health*. I wanted to take the *physical fitness business* and building it to create more overall success, not just for me, but for others. That's how *ES Lifestyle Consulting* was born.

There I was, witnessing people's dread about going back to the grind. The *"Sunday Scaries"* were real, and the Monday morning blues were hitting hard. As I drove down the street, I couldn't help but notice the homeless people on every corner, and I started thinking, *"How can I change this?"* How can I help shift people's mindsets to focus on something positive?

That's when I had an epiphany! Once a month, I'd hit the streets with a sign full of positive affirmations, dancing like nobody was watching (*because they probably weren't*), and handing out flowers to brighten someone's day. My good friend Erin **(THE EMPOWERER)** from *Petals to the People* was all in on my idea. She was my flower supplier and my partner in positivity. Erin is this amazing woman with short brown hair, a heart full of kindness, and a creative spark that could light up an entire city. She used to sell flowers out of a quirky bus, painted with murals that brought color and life to the streets, before moving back to her store. Every time I visited her, I left with a bundle of flowers and an inspiring quote to keep my spirits high.

When I got home, I couldn't wait to hit the streets and share that joy. I started creating affirmations like, "You are loved" and "Be the best you" on my sign, but I needed to take it up a notch. So, I started dancing in the street while handing out flowers. It was my way of giving instead of begging, shifting people's mindset from *wanting* to *giving*. Because, let's face it, if we can all shift our focus to positivity, maybe we'd have a better shot at breaking the cycle of negativity that was lingering everywhere.

And guess what? It caught quickly. People began tagging me on social media, sharing my joy in community pages, and even the news reached out for interviews. Here's what they captured:

"As long as I can make one person smile a day, I've done my job," "I've accomplished what fulfills me, and that's my purpose."

At that time, I had also started my own life coaching business, helping people shift their perspectives on life. My affirmations signs became a big part of my coaching approach. If you were stuck in the Monday driveline blues or felt like you were trapped in a daily grind, I wanted to sprinkle a little bit of sparkle into your day. My mission was simple: shift mindsets and tweak habits. Helping people see the world through a more positive lens was what drove me.

"We could all use a bit more light."

And just like that, what started as a little experiment to bring some joy turned into a movement. A movement of positivity, energy, and a whole lot of dance parties on street corners. And honestly, I couldn't be more grateful for how it all turned out. This was just the beginning of creating new energy and positive changes in the community—and I couldn't wait to see where it would lead next.

CHAPTER TWELVE

STABILIZING SHIFTS:

The Chemistry of Joy: Finding Balance in the Mind and Heart

Happiness. Joy. Love. These aren't just abstract concepts, but tangible emotions rooted in the very chemistry of our bodies. The natural chemicals in our brains—dopamine, serotonin, oxytocin, and endorphins—are the invisible forces that shape how we feel, act, and connect with others. These chemicals are the tools we have to navigate life's ups and downs, and when we understand how they work, we can better create a healthy, balanced life. We can lean into happiness, invite joy, and, most importantly, love ourselves and others in ways that foster connection and healing.

Dopamine: The Reward Chemical:

Dopamine is often called the "reward chemical" because it's what we feel when we accomplish something, big or small. It's the sensation we get after completing a task, treating ourselves with kindness, or celebrating a little victory. In a world that can sometimes feel chaotic or out of control, dopamine offers us a reminder that success is not just reserved for major life milestones but can be found in the simple moments of everyday life.

For me, happiness comes in many forms. The completion of a project, the act of self-care, and celebrating those little wins—like getting out of bed on a hard day or taking a moment to breathe—have become my daily practices. Every task, every step toward self-love is a reminder that I am worthy of joy. And as I celebrate those small victories, dopamine gently reminds me that I am moving forward, that progress is a beautiful journey, and that there is beauty in the little things.

Serotonin: The Mood Stabilizer:

Serotonin is often called the mood stabilizer, the chemical that helps us stay grounded, even in moments of chaos. It's the feeling of calm that washes over us when we soak up the sun's warmth, when we meditate, when we walk in nature, or when we journal our thoughts. It's the soothing balm for a troubled mind, the gentle force that reminds us to stay present, to stay grounded, and to find peace amidst the storm.

For me, serotonin has become my grounding tool in the midst of life's uncertainty. Walking in nature, basking in sunlight, and quieting my thoughts through journaling or meditation have become my essential rituals for emotional balance. These practices have allowed me to stabilize my emotions, find peace within myself, and regain control of my thoughts. They serve as constant reminders that joy doesn't have to come from external circumstances—it can emerge from the simple, steady rhythm of life.

Oxytocin: The Love Hormone

Oxytocin, the love hormone, is the chemical responsible for the bonds we share with others. It's the warmth we feel when we play with a pet, when we interact with a baby, or when we share a loving conversation with a friend. It's the deep connection that links us together, reminding us that we are not alone. Love—whether self-love, the love we give to others, or the love we receive—is the most powerful force that keeps us connected to ourselves and the world around us.

I've learned that in order to truly love others, I must first learn to love myself. This has meant taking time for nurturing relationships, practicing kindness, and opening my heart to both myself and others. Random acts of kindness, a smile from a stranger, or a simple moment of laughter with friends have been profound reminders that love is everywhere. And when we share it—whether through a hug, a conversation, or a thoughtful gesture—we invite others to do the same. Oxytocin has taught me that love is the glue that binds us, and it's through these connections that joy multiplies.

Endorphins: The Painkillers:

Endorphins are our body's natural painkillers, the chemicals that flood in after we exercise, eat nourishing foods, or indulge in a little pleasure. They are what we feel when we exercise, when we get a massage, or when we enjoy a rich, dark piece of chocolate. Endorphins are the feel-good chemicals that help us release the tension, stress, and pain that can weigh us down.

In my life, endorphins have become my relief in times of stress or sorrow. Physical activity—whether it's a brisk walk, a stretch, or a full workout—has been a way for me to release the built-up tension of grief or frustration. A nourishing meal, a moment of relaxation, or even indulging in a small treat has reminded me that pleasure, joy, and self-care are important tools in the healing process. Endorphins have shown me that joy can be found in the act of self-compassion—releasing the weight of pain and welcoming in the lightness of happiness.

Painful Experiences and Learning: The Tools in Our Toolbox:

Grief and pain are natural parts of the human experience. They shape us, challenge us, and ultimately teach us invaluable lessons. In many ways, the painful experiences we face—whether they are emotional, physical, or spiritual—act like tools in our toolbox. They sharpen us, they mold us, and they prepare us for the next chapter of our lives.

I've come to understand that avoidance only delays the healing process. Grief, trauma, and pain need to be felt, acknowledged, and released in order for us to heal. In this process, we learn to navigate the depths of our emotions, uncover the lessons hidden in our suffering, and begin to create a life of peace and resilience. It's not about suppressing pain—it's about using it as a tool to grow, to forgive, and to move forward with love.

Becoming Loving Through the Nature of Ourselves:

The balance of these chemicals—dopamine, serotonin, oxytocin, and endorphins—teaches us how to live fully, how to embrace joy, and how to love both ourselves and others. It is through understanding and nurturing these natural forces within us that we create a healthy, balanced mind. As we move through the highs and lows of life, we come to realize that joy is not a permanent state; it's a dynamic process, a blend of moments and emotions that flow through us.

Ultimately, it's about finding a healthy mix—allowing ourselves to experience pain, but also opening up to the beauty of love, joy, and connection. The natural chemicals in our brains aren't just about survival; they are about thriving. They guide us toward balance, toward healing, and toward a life filled with love and light.

Healing Leaves

34.2236° N, 77.9018° W

Starr—oh, Starr—was that kind of friend who exudes love from every pore. She was the kind of person who could light up a room with just a smile and a giggle. She was a creator, and her energy was pure magic. Starr (**THE EMPOWERER**) ran a holistic shop called *Healing Leaves*, and let me tell you, it was the kind of place where you could literally feel the positive vibes as soon as you walked in. The products, the energy, the peaceful ambiance—it was all so soothing.

I frequented *Healing Leaves* because I loved the products and, honestly, I just loved the energy Starr put into everything. She became a fast friend, and as fate would have it, her shop was just down the street from my gym. We originally met because she came to check out our personal training programs, and she casually mentioned that her store was just a stone's throw away.

After a year of running the business and watching her pour her heart into it, the universe decided it was time for a shift. My life was transitioning out of the gym and into my consulting business, and Starr, exhausted from the constant grind, ironically wanted to transition into working for another owner of a coffee shop: Grinders., offered me the opportunity to take over her store. The idea of managing *Healing Leaves* felt like the perfect distraction—and also a great way to market my other ventures. So, after a couple of rounds of negotiations (you know, the usual), I agreed.

The next nine months were a whirlwind. I became the proud new face of a space that was, well, *meant to last*—but let's be honest, wasn't. The main investor had only seen the business as a side project, and the store was kind of sinking into the abyss of COVID chaos. The pandemic did not make life easy for small businesses, let me tell you. But there I was, ready to breathe new life into it.

I jumped in headfirst, bringing on new employees, practitioners, and offering up space for massage therapists, acupuncturists, sound bath gurus, and other holistic wonders to rent out their spaces. It wasn't long before *Healing Leaves* became a thriving community. It was like a little wellness hub, and I was loving every minute of it.

So here I was, running a business that wasn't originally mine, turning it into something new, all while trying to balance my other ventures. Life was messy, but it was also kind of magic. Having this idea of turning it into a *"Hogwarts"* I wanted *Healing Leaves* to be healing and healthy in all avenues. However, when you level up in your life you're bound to have new obstacles.....My investor was a real nincompoop,- I'll just leave it at that.

I knew deep down that with this business, the foundation of who I was had been waiting to explode and capture the beauty of life and its journeys. When I finally started putting my actions into reality, I realized it was time to stop staring at the sticky notes that read "New York Times Best-Selling Author, Speaker, (secretly a Singer.)" It was time to let everything intertwine and flow together, showing that every step I've taken—no matter how small—has led me closer to where I'm meant to be. Every place I've been to has included a pivot, and each lesson seemed to hit me first, so I could turn around and help others navigate through it. It's like I've been walking around with a flashlight, lighting the way for others as I move forward, one baby step at a time..

I took the initiative and decided to start carrying a journal with me everywhere, so I could capture moments of joy and love—both big and small. I wanted to bask in the love around me, constantly searching for those moments of human connection, like the six degrees of Kevin Bacon, where every interaction holds a thread that ties us all together.

As we've explored throughout this chapter, understanding your health and wellness is a deeply personal journey. It requires patience, self-reflection, and a commitment to nourishing both your body and mind. Remember, true transformation begins with understanding where you are and taking actionable steps toward where you want to be.

For more information on analyzing your health and wellness, feel free to visit my website at Contact - Aire Stillman Lifestyle Consulting. There, you'll find valuable resources to help guide you on your journey to better health and a more balanced life.

CHAPTER THIRTEEN

YOU MAKE ME BRAVE.

It Pays to Be Brave:

32°43'37"N 117°12'1"W.

Oh, let me take you back to when I was living in California—yes, California! I like to call it my "3 C's trip"—California, Chicago, Cancun. Now, that sounds like an adventure, right? It all started in California. That's where I got to discover something incredible about myself, all thanks to one simple, yet life-changing phrase: It *"Pays To Be Brave."*

I was invited by this amazing woman named Hannah, (**THE REMINDER**) she was a part of a business mentorship program I was in. I spent all this money, I *didn't have* to become an entrepreneur by "accident." The program focused on personal development and growth and let me tell you, growth was exactly what I needed. It was like the universe handed me a golden ticket and said, '*You want change? Go for it, girl.*' So I made it happen! When she asked if I wanted to fly across the country and go to this event and meet her in real life, I said yes, without blinking an eyelash. I heard a whole body–gut reaction "YES! Sounds amazing, take my money." It was about to be a whole lot of travel and a whole lot of learning.

The event, *"It Pays to Be Brave,"* was hosted by the inspiring Angie Lee. (**THE ULTIMATE EMPOWERER**) The moment I walked in, something clicked. It was like a fog cleared in my mind, and I saw a vision I hadn't even known I was searching for—my purpose. I didn't even realize it until I saw it. I wanted to be *on stage*, in arenas, speaking to thousands of women, empowering them to love themselves and motivating them to push beyond their limits. *Bam*, there it was. That was my new dream. It wasn't just a thought; it was a full-on *vision*. And trust me, I never would've gotten there without being brave enough to step into that room.

Now, let's talk about the speakers. One after another, they ignited something inside me. There were talks about sex, self-love, and intimacy—things I didn't even know I was missing out on. Remember when I mentioned at the time, I couldn't even get one orgasm, let alone multiple (oops, TMI?). But hearing these women talk about what **was** possible, it hit me like a ton of bricks: "*Wow, what am I missing?*" I felt like I was a little deprived, but more than that, I felt a fire spark inside me. Their passion, their unapologetic energy to take up space—it was like a dopamine explosion in my brain. I needed ***that energy.*** I needed to feel that match start the fire within, and that's when I realized something important: "***IT PAYS TO BE BRAVE***". You have to step outside your comfort zone to ignite that kind of will power in your life. "It pays to play."

At the end of the event, Angie, a phenomenal hype-girl speaker and comedian spoke about "shitting her pants" with laughter. She handed out individual handwritten letters to us. Letters that we were to read six months later—letters for our future selves. The thought was, "How proud would we be of ourselves when we finally did the thing we've always dreamed of doing?" When I got that letter six months later, I won't lie, I cried. It was like the universe was giving me a hug, reminding me of how far I'd come. The whole room of 3,000+ women had that moment, and that was just... *wow.* I mean, some of them probably moved (granted, life happens), but knowing the impact of that experience and all the ripples it probably created? Incredible.

And then, I got the idea to have my clients write letters to their future selves. This became one of the most powerful exercises I could share with them. Watching the transformation in their lives—seeing them start to believe in themselves, act on their dreams, and grow into the women they were always meant to be—has been beyond rewarding.

That, my friends, is what I'm here for: helping people realize their potential and step into their power. It's a reminder that it truly pays to be brave. The bravery to love yourself, to step up on that stage, and to take action—because when you do, the universe has a way of unfolding everything you've always dreamed of.

Back in Chicago: A New Perspective

After my "California dreaming", stepping back into Chicago was like landing in a completely different world. The West Coast had stolen my heart with its breathtaking sunsets over the cliffs in San Diego, and those iconic, skinny palm trees standing like skyscrapers. Seriously, I could've stayed there forever. But when I flew into O'Hare, I had a little realization: I'd never actually explored Chicago *on my own*. Sure, I'd been there as a "little gremlin" and a young adult, but back then, I couldn't really appreciate it. The city's nickname, the "Windy City," was all I could think of—too many cold gusts of wind and not enough appreciation for what it really had to offer. But after everything that had shifted in my life, I knew I needed to change my perspective.

So, I decided to explore. While waiting for my next adventure—my mom and I were headed to Cancun to celebrate my future sister-in-law's bachelorette—I figured I might as well make the most of this Chicago stop.

I headed downtown, and this time, I was in awe of the city's vibe. The tall buildings, the bustling streets, the energy—it all felt so alive. I even stopped by Millennium Park like a total tourist, posing for photos at The Bean. Yes, I had a full-on photoshoot with myself using the self-timer, embracing the weirdness of it all. I was *that* tourist, and I didn't care.

Afterward, I ducked into a nearby coffee shop to catch up on my thoughts, do some admin work, and reflect on everything that had happened. Running my business was a whirlwind, and I had so many ideas and feelings to process. As I sipped my coffee, I really took the time to admire the city, appreciating it in a way I never had before. It wasn't just the Windy City anymore—it was a place of new beginnings, fresh starts, and endless possibilities.

Sometimes, it takes stepping away to truly see what's in front of you. Chicago? It had just become a lot more exciting than I remembered.

Cancun:

Flying into Cancun, I was ready for anything. I knew a bachelorette weekend could mean unpredictable chaos, but I wasn't quite prepared for the whirlwind of events about to unfold. My mom and I arrived, eager to experience a group of women from all walks of life. Once you're outside the country, you quickly learn about "island time"—where life moves at a pace that feels like molasses compared to the hustle of American life. Let's just say the communication gaps didn't help much either.

The night before our yacht outing, the group huddled together to finalize plans. We were buzzing with excitement for the adventure ahead. The next morning, my mom and I showed up ten minutes late— only to find the lobby completely deserted. Not one soul. Turns out, a quick stop at the food court had cost us dearly. Starting to panic, we knocked on doors, but no one answered. The thought of missing the yacht and being left behind was setting in. Running to the concierge, who spoke limited English, we desperately tried to explain the situation. After a few frustrating minutes, he managed to hail us a cab.

As we got into the cab, I couldn't help but think, "This is it. We're about to be kidnapped in Mexico." The driver didn't speak English, and the ride stretched on—10 minutes, then 20, then 30. Eventually, he pulled over at a random booth, where another attendant, also non-English-speaking, joined the confusion. Gestures, pointing, and frantic attempts at communication ensued. Finally, we piled back into the car, hoping we weren't headed to a scene straight out of a movie where things go horribly wrong.

When the cab finally pulled up to a dock, I could've kissed the ground. Relief washed over me as I spotted the yacht. But there was one problem—none of the girls were there. My heart sank. Had we missed them after all? The attendant, who spoke a smattering of English, reassured us: "Oh, you're here. The rest of your group isn't." Seriously? The group that I thought had left us behind was now late themselves.

Twenty minutes later, a shuttle bus arrived, and out poured my sister and her friends. The reunion was a mix of shock, relief, and a lot of "Where the heck were you?!" moments. Apparently, they had been searching for us while we were searching for them. None of our phones worked, and our attempts at communication had gone nowhere. But against all odds, we all made it—in one piece, no less.

Finally, we set off on the yacht into the open ocean. As the waves lapped against the hull, I couldn't help but feel a lingering paranoia. "What if we all get abducted?" I thought, but I kept that little gem to myself. The day unfolded beautifully. I even chatted with the captain about my boater's license, and he jokingly suggested I take the wheel—so without thinking, I leaped into the seat to take the reins. A moment that made me feel like I owned the seas. Jumping in the water to snorkel with the turtles was a breathtaking memory I won't ever forget. By the time we docked, I felt on top of the world.

When we got back to the hotel, our phones reconnected, and messages started flooding in. My brother was freaking out, blaming my mom and me for being late. But in reality, the group had been even later. It was a perfect example of how poor communication and lack of patience can spiral into chaos.

Unfortunately, my triumph was short-lived. Montezuma's revenge hit me hard. The last two days were a blur of misery—vomiting, diarrhea, and the kind of stomach pain that makes you rethink every sip of water you've ever taken. I couldn't eat, couldn't function, and was counting down the minutes until we could leave. On the morning of our departure, my mom looked at me with so much pity it was almost funny. The bumpy hour-long ride to the airport felt like torture. To top it off, an alkalizer I had brought to ease my stomach sprayed all over my belongings. At that point, all I could do was laugh. What else could go wrong?

As the plane took off, I felt a mix of relief and reflection. The trip was a rollercoaster of highs and lows—a cocktail of unforgettable memories and hard lessons. It taught me the importance of communication, patience, and, most importantly, being mindful of who you travel with. Because let's face it, bachelorette weekend or not, the unknown variables can make or break the experience.

"When was the last time you truly embraced yourself for who you are, without judgment?"

CHAPTER FOURTEEN

LETTING THE LOST GO.

My Bloody Valentine: Miller's Transition (My Pup)

Rest in peace, my sweet little soul, Miller.

From the moment I adopted him, he was one of the brightest lights in my life. I discovered the true meaning of "unconditional love" through him. We were inseparable companions for eight years, navigating the highs and lows together. I always knew I'd have to let him go someday, but I never imagined it would be so sudden and traumatic.

When I first brought him home at six months old, I learned he'd been previously adopted by someone who was abusive and then returned him. He came to me with separation anxiety and nervousness. He was a scared little pup, but I was determined to nurture and care for him.

He had such a wanderlust spirit, always finding opportunities to run free. He took advantage of those chances countless times in his eight years. Almost everyone who knew him had a story about his "great escapes." In hindsight, his wanderlust mirrored my own love for travel and new experiences. We were a perfect match.

The Final Moments: WARNING GRAPHIC:

On November 17, 2021, around 10:00 a.m. Miller (my pup) was with me at Healing Leaves (my holistic center). A client arrived for a foot bath, and he greeted her with kisses and cuddles. I went to prepare the service, and when I noticed he was missing, I saw the store door ajar. I immediately assumed he'd gone on one of his joy runs.

I ran outside to find him, knowing that if I couldn't spot him quickly, I'd wait for someone to call me with his whereabouts. But something felt different this time. My gut told me to search urgently, so I grabbed his extra leash and headed out.

In the distance, I saw commotion near a busy road. People were rushing in that direction, and I feared it might be him. A woman approached me as I held his leash, she uttered " You should hurry" and at that moment, I knew he was in an emergency. I rushed over to him lying in the grass, surrounded by people crying and trying to help. His left eye was bloody and swollen and popped out of socket, and he was in obvious pain. Blood was everywhere, lungs caving inside his body.

A group gathered around trying to console me, and usher his body to get him to the vet. We hurried to the truck of the woman who had hit him, and she drove us to the emergency vet. I knew in my heart he wouldn't make it. I kept whispering, "I'm so sorry," as I hoped he wouldn't suffer any longer. I called everyone I could think of, praying for his comfort.

When we arrived at the vet, I didn't want to move him. Holding him still, I just wanted him to rest peacefully in my arms. A man outside noticed our panic, the lady was screaming for support. He quickly attempted to help us get inside. A nurse took him from my arms, and I saw the blood covering my arm and white shirt. As the reality of the situation hit, I collapsed to the ground in tears. The woman who hit him lifted me up and comforted me, and we waited together for the results.

The doctor confirmed what I already knew: "He's passed on. The trauma to his brain was too severe." I took a deep breath and requested an immediate cremation for you.

Leaving the vet, I felt like my legs were made of jello, trembling. We walked back to the car and discovered that one of her child's car seats was lost during the ordeal. I shared stories about how happy he must be now, running wild and free. Despite the trauma, I felt a sense of inner peace. We chatted on the way back to Healing Leaves, and when we hugged goodbye, I noticed the time: exactly 11:11 a.m. It felt like a sign—a reminder of new beginnings and a connection to something greater.

One of my staff members had managed to check on the store and found it locked. The stranger who told me to "hurry", had indeed gone to the store. She left her business card and my keys under the driver's seat of my car. The footbath customer had even taken the initiative to lock up the store when she realized the dog and I had disappeared.

The outpouring of good karma and love from family, friends, acquaintances, and strangers was overwhelming, and I wanted to express my deep gratitude to everyone who helped and supported me during that time. I'm incredibly thankful for the bystanders who assisted at the scene, and for the lady who went to Healing Leaves to inform the waiting customer. I appreciate the customer who took the time to lock up the store, as well as the woman who drove us to the vet and offered her comfort. A heartfelt thanks goes to my family and friends who reached out to offer comfort over the phone, and to the vet staff who cared for both my pup and I with such compassion. I'm also grateful to the clientele in the waiting room who showed kindness and empathy during such a difficult moment. Lastly, I'm deeply touched by everyone who sent condolences or celebrated the life of my beloved pup. Your love and support mean more than words can express.

I am deeply grateful for all the love and support. Miller, you were a beautiful light in my life, and I'll love you forever. May you run free over the rainbow bridge. I look forward to the day we'll be reunited in the next life.

CELEBRATION OF LIFE: A Message in a Bottle

34.2085° N, 77.7962° W

It was time for me to honor Miller's life in a way that felt right, a moment to cherish our time together while he was with me on earth. I spent countless hours at the oceanfront, praying and reflecting, searching for some sign or symbol that would guide me. I started calling them "God winks"—those little moments where it felt like the universe was saying, "Hey, pay attention, this is the answer!"

One afternoon, driving down the street with the light blue sky above, not a cloud in sight, and the salty breeze hitting my sinuses (almost tasting it on my tongue), I felt a wave of clarity wash over me. The watercolor beach houses brought up all the joyful summer vibes, and suddenly, it hit me. Hearing the song come over the radiofrequency: "Message in a Bottle- The Police." I needed to create a *message in a bottle*. It would be filled with happy memories of Miller and my closest friends, and sent into the ocean—something timeless to mark the end of this chapter.

It reminded me of the mailboxes we used to see along the coast, where people would leave letters for anyone to find and read. This felt like my version of that, but with the ocean as the ultimate receiver. It was exactly the piece I needed to complete the puzzle.

Over the next couple of weeks, as I gathered the final touches for my plan, I ran into Erin, who happened to be checking out my shop. I told her all about my idea, and to my surprise, she revealed that she had found an old "Miller bottle" from back in the day. We both agreed it was the perfect fit.

I started crafting invites for the people who mattered most to me, those who had shared in Miller's life and love. I sent out a mass invite because Miller had touched so many hearts, and I wanted to share his energy with others. My closest girlfriends were all in, and I invited all my neighbors too, because Miller had left an impression wherever we went.

Living in the Container District meant we had plenty of business parties to celebrate our expansions—drinks, appetizers, games, and lots of marketing. Still, the women in the community suggested I get out of the house and bring some cheer into my life.

So, to my surprise, I walked into our business networking event, only to spot *him*—my ex Mr. J—standing across the room. I froze. I couldn't believe it. My first thoughts, "Why is he here?" Of course he's also a businessman.. but still. The moment he saw me, he practically sprinted over, smiling like it was the most normal thing in the world. He asked, "How are you? And then, out of nowhere, this woman appeared behind him, echoing his responses, introducing herself as his girlfriend.

I was *shocked*. I mean, seriously—My thoughts "Why hadn't he told me? Why hadn't he introduced her properly?" I was taken aback by the whole situation and the recent death of Miller. In the most awkward of ways, I said, "Oh, okay, cool. Well, welcome... Wait, why are you here?" In my mind I thought: "This is my territory. It was literally my backyard." He knew that, he helped me move here after all. "What was his ambush about?"

She explained she was renting some space in the co-working area, which left me floored. I was like, "Okay, sure, whatever." I couldn't understand why he'd act like this, and honestly, I was a bit annoyed. I walked away, found my friends, and carried on, but deep down, it just didn't sit right with me.

After some uncomfortable small talk, I decided to *"kill them with kindness."* I walked back over and, in my own way, extended an invite to the celebration I was planning for Miller. I mentioned it to both of them, hoping they might join in honoring his memory. The next day, he blocked me on every social media outlet, and I knew exactly what had happened. She definitely made him do that. But hey, I didn't blame her. Needless to say, in the end, they didn't show up to the celebration.

When the day arrived, I was shocked by who did show up: Eleven of my closest girlfriends, and—wait for it—a random guy I accidentally texted, thinking it was my friend Lucia (my ex's best friend). However, this guy and I had a brief fling during my "single-girl season" (don't judge), but he was a good guy and came to pay his respects. The funniest part? When I told my girls who he was and how the mix-up happened, we all laughed so hard. It was like the universe gave me a little masculine energy to balance out the day. (Shoutout to you, sir, for showing up!)

The celebration was beautiful. We all wrote heartfelt notes, placed them into the bottle, and sent it into the water. Afterward, we went to one of my favorite Mexican restaurants by the beach to wrap it all up. My accidental date didn't join us, and I never heard from him again (honestly, I didn't even remember his name until I saw the mistext— oops). But the whole experience turned out to be a healing moment, filled with love, laughter, and closure.

Kindness In Courtney:

After Miller had made his exit strategy, I found myself feeling very alone. The sting of leaving my old life had truly set in. Miller was the last piece connected to an old life I was desperately trying to move forward from. I didn't want to go home alone; I couldn't be. Thankfully, my nursing bestie from the heart unit, Courtney, lived just a few blocks away. During that season, we spent nearly every extra hour together— concerts, boat rides, lunches, beach walks. Those beach sunset walks became even more frequent after his passing.

Courtney's kindness knew no bounds. She opened her home to me, giving me my own room and even letting me watch the house when she was out of town. It became a home away from home. Courtney, **(THE ETERNAL)** a sweet, tall brunette with the essence of a country girl—dimples, Southern accent, and deep roots—was a constant source of comfort. She stood by me through thick and thin, as we had both weathered rough breakups over the years. We often shared silly stories to commiserate, but loneliness still crept in, wrapping itself around me like an unwelcome guest. Heartbreak seemed to be a recurring chapter in my story, and each day felt like a battle for my heart.

On the surface, I tried to appear strong as I ventured into new rounds of dating. But deep down, I felt unsure and unsafe. Without the protection of a strong, tough significant other or even two big dogs to guard the home, I decided to take control. I transferred that feeling with her home, and her two loving creatures. Those pups became such a light in the tunnel. I realized I needed to do something for my own safety. I began self-defense classes, determined to rebuild my sense of security. Through it all, Courtney's reassurance and support never wavered. I don't think I could have made it through that dark time without her.

Slowly, piece by piece, I worked to repair my heart. Courtney and I would sing our little hearts out to country songs, keeping our minds busy with house projects—painting, house repairs, puzzles, hanging decorations. Our shared story radiated a kind of magic, like the soundtrack of our lives. One song, in particular, will always remind me of her, even though she didn't like it: "You loved me when you didn't have to. But you did and you do, and he knew. Thank God for giving me you."

That's my ode to you, Courtney. Thank God for blessing me with you. You helped me stand when I couldn't find my feet. Our life together was sweet, filled with moments of joy and connection. Whether it was family time with the boys—Astro, Nickel, and Brain—or our little trips to the mountains, the Post Malone concert, or our cute girl's trip to Tennessee to support our dear friend Nikki in her hardship, every memory shines brightly. Seeing Lizzo together was unforgettable.

Thank you for always loving me unconditionally. You never judged me for who I was dating, what I was wearing, my actions, my words, where I was living, or what I was doing for a career. You loved me through all seasons of my life, and for that, I am eternally grateful.

"Who are the people, or what are the things, in your life that make you feel truly seen and loved?"

CHAPTER FIFTEEN

PARENTAL PROGRAMING.

Speaking Existence into Your Children:

A Collection of Stories from Parents and Observers

Let me start by saying—these stories are a collection of wisdom not coming from my own parenting experience (yet), but rather from the hearts of my friends and family. I don't have kids of my own—though I did have pets, and while many might whine they're "like children," I think we can all agree that when your pet has a bad day, it's a little easier to hand them a treat and call it even. But don't get me wrong, pets do teach you responsibility and love—just with fewer temper tantrums.

One of my best friends, Sammi, is one of those people who radiates beauty (and I'm not just talking about her golden-blonde hair, which was brunette until recently, but who's counting?). She's got these brown eyes that could melt any man's heart and freckles that make her look like she just stepped out of a fairytale. Recently, Sammi became a mother, and I'll tell you—watching her go through the transformation was nothing short of inspiring. She said to me one day, "I thought I knew why God placed me on this earth, but I had no idea what true purpose really felt like until I became a mother. Now I know, I was put here to be a mom." I almost teared up just hearing her say that. The love she had for her newborn son was pouring out of her like a fountain. It was so palpable I could feel it from across the room at our usual hangout spot on Highway 11.

Funny enough, my own mom once told me something similar. She wasn't what you'd call the "maternal type"—before she met my dad, that is—she was helping raise his two other sons when they got together, after my dad's first marriage ended in divorce. But then, when she had my brother Nick, she said she realized that she was destined to be a mother and love all of her kids endlessly. It was like she unlocked a new level of LOVE, herself—cue the heartwarming music.

Now, let's get into the real deal: My mom never let me say the words " I can't." If I even tried, she'd swoop in like a lioness on a gazelle. It was game over for me. She would immediately remind me of Thomas the Tank Engine—the little chugging engine from my childhood. You know, the one who thought "he could" he'd say "I think I can! I think I can!" and did (spoiler alert: it's a metaphor for life). Mom was all about instilling that mindset in me, and let me tell you, it worked. I grew up thinking, "If Thomas can pull that train up a mountain, I can do anything."

Looking back, it's clear how much that attitude shaped me. Somewhere deep down, I knew I was destined for something great. I mean, how could I not, with Thomas on my side? If that little engine can pull through against all odds, surely I could too.

One summer afternoon, I decided to take my journal downtown to a bar in Wilmington—anything to escape the loneliness of being cooped up in the tiny house. I thought, "I'll do some people-watching for character development!" But then an older man, probably in his late 60s, Allen **(THE REMINDER)** walked up to me. He looked like someone who might have a few interesting stories to tell, so naturally, I braced myself for what could be a great conversation. In his southern accent, he asked, "Whatcha writing in that journal of yours?"

I told him I was gathering ideas for a book on "Unconditional Love." He immediately leaned in like he was about to drop some life-changing knowledge. "Oh, I've got a story for you," he said.

Turns out, this man's love story was something straight out of a movie. He told me that the moment he laid eyes on his ex-wife, he knew she was "the one." They quickly started dating, got married, had a son, got divorced, got back together, and then, you guessed it—got divorced again. I empathize, "Tough break, man." But here's where it gets interesting. He said, "The greatest love I've ever known was when my son was born."

He went on to tell me about the moment he first held his baby boy in his arms. "From the second the nurse handed him to me, wrapped in a little baby blanket, crying his tiny heart out, I started crying, too. He smelled so indescribable—it's a scent I'll never forget." He paused for a second, and I could see the love in his eyes. "Watching him grow has been the greatest blessing. It made everything else—every relationship, every challenge—seem small. I'm grateful that, through all that pain, I got to experience the truest love of all."

The man wasn't just talking about love and passion between significant others; he was talking about that fierce, unconditional love you have for your child. That's the love that changes and challenges everything.

A few years later, I went to a networking event where a mentor of mine, PJ (**THE TEACHER**) was the keynote speaker. Watching him share his journey of struggle and success was amazing, but the part that really stuck with me was when he talked about fatherhood. He said there's nothing more joyful than seeing the joy in your child's eyes. He shared how he and his son were into wrestling (the WWF kind, of course) and at home they practiced all of the moves! He knows all the moves by name, he gets so excited to wrestle together. He went on to tell a story about how they had just gone on a family vacation, riding roller coasters. But the highlight of it all? Watching his son's face light up with pure joy on the rollercoaster.

What struck me even more was when he said, "The best part of being a father is raising him to be a little gentleman. Showing him how strong he is, how he can be like daddy and '***help the people***'—that's his way of understanding entrepreneurship. It's about helping others in business, and if he can do that with good posture, he'll ignite his little superpowers and grow into a hero."

Honestly, hearing these stories filled my heart with joy. One day, maybe I'll experience this kind of love myself. But for now, I get to be the "fun aunt" who gets to watch my brothers, friends, and family raise their "littles." It's like I'm getting a sneak peek at the magic of parenthood, and it's absolutely beautiful.

I've watched my dear friend Yaya, (**THE EMPOWERER**) who has the most beautiful patience with her son. His behavior in public is remarkable—it's like he has a built-in sense of respect.

I'm constantly in awe of my childhood best friend, Jessi, who has two almost middle schoolers. It's been a decade of watching them grow into young adults. What inspires them, who they hang out with, what they "love to do for fun"—who they're dating currently, it always leaves me speechless.

These moments make me feel incredibly lucky to be a part of their lives. The love I see from my friends and family is the most authentic kind of love, and it's a reminder of how important it is to raise kids with intentionality and positive influence. The way you speak life into your children, the way you guide them—it truly does shape their world. So, whether you're a parent or an aunt, a friend or a mentor, remember that love is the greatest gift you can give.

And one day, when I have my own little one (who will definitely know how to say "I can"), I'll remember all these lessons and pass them on.

Until then, I'll be over here, cheering on my friends and their beautiful families, soaking in all the love and wisdom.

You can imagine the joy I found in collecting moments of joy from children, but there was also a stark contrast when I lost my pup. The overwhelming devastation I felt in that moment was a reminder of life's duality. It shows us both sides—the good and the bad—to help us appreciate where we are and how alive we truly are. We can't have the good without the bad. And I believe it's those tough moments that make us love even harder. The loss of my pup left me in devastation, I couldn't even imagine the loss of a child.

Grief is such an interesting experience; it's like a veil that, when lifted, reveals the depth of unconditional love and the blessings we often take for granted. It reminds us of the connections we've had, the love we've given, and the strength we didn't know we had within us. Through grief, we learn to embrace life even more fully.

I encourage you to ponder this question:

"What have you learned about yourself in your quest for love, both from others and from within? Children are clones of us, what do we learn from them?"

CHAPTER SIXTEEN

FORK IN THE ROAD.

FRIENDSHIPS COLLIDE: A NEW WORLD:

Fawn—oh, Fawn (**THE REMINDER**)—what a quirky, vibrant soul she was. She was my neighbor, a recently divorced bisexual from Michigan, on the hunt for something new, something entertaining, something a little more exciting. She had that air of adventurous curiosity, and I couldn't help but get swept up in her energy.

One day, she invited me to a small music festival where she was helping a friend out with her hula hoops. We met her at a bar near our containers, where she was doing her thing—playing with fire. Yep, literal fire. Not metaphorical fire, like some people you know. No, she was twirling it around like it was a casual Tuesday. The bar was full of "freaks" of all shapes and sizes and I loved it! They had a lyra hanging from the roof, and I jumped inside and started spinning around upside down like a natural. She was shocked how easy it was for me, surprising both of us, but I had that dancer blood and yoga spirit. Twirling only seemed natural. Having such a blast, I knew the festival was going to be a blast too.

Weeks later, as soon as I got there, to the festival grounds, I was hit with an exhilarating wave of nostalgia. It had been years since I'd been to a music festival, and I had forgotten what it felt like to embrace that part of me—the part that had been quietly suppressed for too long. It was like a door had swung open, and a whole new world of possibilities and freedom was standing there, waiting to be explored. This festival wasn't just a fun weekend; it was the start of something much bigger, an introduction to a whole new circle of friends and adventures. The next couple of years? Well, let's just say Wilmington would never be the same.

Fawn and I wandered into a giant dome, and that's when we saw her—a blonde girl in the empty tent, lost in her bead making. I took one look at her and thought, "Yep, I'm sitting next to her." I plopped down beside her and said, "Hey, can I make a bracelet with you?" She laughed and introduced herself as Vanessa. I grinned and declared, "Hi, Vanessa, wanna be my 'bead bestie'?" From that moment on, we kept bumping into each other throughout the festival. It felt like the universe was nudging us to stay connected.

Between bracelet making and meeting new people, we had our fair share of fun. I ran into Megan, a yoga teacher, former military woman who had no clue I was doing promo work, so she introduced me to her husband. Turns out, I was the perfect person to help them out with some future promo gigs. So, just like that, more doors opened.

One night, while I was trying to catch some sleep in my tent, the sun was rising when I heard this incredible sound—music that tugged at my heartstrings and literally brought tears to my eyes. The pastels cascading in the sky and their melody's light up the stage for the sunrise set. It was *Krispy Biscuits*. If you've never heard them, trust me, they could bring down a crowd. I'll never forget that moment. Want to hear what they are made of? Head over to @Krispee_biscudits or soundcloud- DJ YK "Sound of Sunrise".

As if the universe wasn't already conspiring in the most delightful ways, I bumped into this fiery little woman named Lauren. (**THE RUNNER**) She was a ball of energy, always ready for an adventure. She had a brand new Bronco, and I remember thinking, "*this is a girl who knows how to live.*" She and I hit it off instantly, like old friends reunited. And then, just when I thought it couldn't get crazier, I got a text from her at the end of the festival. *Turns out, we had actually met the year before, when we were dating two completely different roommates.* We both laughed at the coincidence. Life sure knows how to bring people together in the most unexpected ways.

The whole experience was one wild ride, and coming back home was like pressing pause on the chaos. It just so happened to be close to Christy's birthday, so we rallied everyone together and went out to one of my favorite spots, Yosake. A local sushi spot downtown, Wilmington.

Now, let me paint the scene for you: Christy entered with her bright yellow sunshine aura. She has an eye for fashion, with her hippie, boho, mountain girl seek outfits. There I was, in all my energetic, colorful glory, across the table from none other than Chris—Christy's other best friend. Chris had been in Christy's life for just as long as I had, but somehow, our worlds had never really crossed. Over the years, we'd existed in the same orbit but never really collided. And that evening? Well, let's just say it was a colossal collision that neither of us had seen coming.

We didn't know much about each other at first. In fact, we weren't exactly intrigued by each other's existence. But as the night wore on, we started to see the similarities. Our energy, our philosophies—they were practically identical. Funny how life works out that way, right? The more time we spent together, the more we realized that we had this magnetic connection. We were like mirror images of each other, with a shared curiosity about the world and a love for finding the extraordinary in the everyday.

And as the night went on, I couldn't help but think: *"This is just the beginning."*

CHAPTER SEVENTEEN

THE GREAT EIGHT: INFINITY SYMBOL

THE GREAT 8:

34.2104° N, 77.8868° W

Why were there *eight* of them, you ask? Ah, the great "**eight**"—this was one of the more adventurous chapters of my adult dating life. At one point, I found myself juggling not one, not two, but **eight** different people. Now, some might call it a "roster," but it was so much more than that. These weren't just people I was casually cycling through. No, I was building real relationships with each of them, getting to know their personalities, quirks, and qualities. And, of course, managing all of this while running my business was its own unique challenge. Talk about multitasking!

But here's the thing: I genuinely wanted them all to be happy. I wanted to seek understanding of what each person brought into my life. Looking back, I see how each one mirrored something in me—whether it was a blind spot I needed to address or a strength I hadn't fully acknowledged. In a way, it became a crash course in self-discovery and personal growth. I mean, who needs therapy when you've got eight different perspectives on love and life, right?

The real triumph, though, came when all of them collided—*and* they became friends. Yes, you read that correctly. Instead of chaos, there was camaraderie. It was like a live-action networking event, except with a lot more emotional depth. I'm all about elevating the people around me, and seeing the connections bloom between them all was such a fulfilling moment. I thrive on connecting people, and to see that come full circle in such a surprising way made me proud. It wasn't just about me learning from them; it was about making sure everyone walked away from the experience better for having known each other.

I loved each of them in my own way. The truth is, I was learning to love *better*—not just them, but myself. By learning how to show up for each person, I was asking the most important question of all: *Am I deserving of love?* And more importantly, *how can I become the best version of myself to give love in return?* It was about growth, not perfection. Navigating the highs and lows of multiple relationships taught me resilience, patience, and the courage to face obstacles head-on.

Of course, for the sake of their privacy, I won't go into all the details here. But I will say this—none of these relationships were in any particular order. You can imagine them as pieces of a mystery puzzle, each with its own lesson, its own story. If you're into mysteries, maybe you'll enjoy figuring them out!

In the end, it was all about learning what binds us together. The beauty of love, in all its forms, is that it has the power to connect, heal, and teach us if we let it. And for that, I'm grateful.

According to <u>APA Dictionary of Psychology</u>

Ability grouping: "the assignment of pupils to school classes on the basis of their learning ability. Or another example: the practice of dividing a class into sections based on student ability in one area."

PRINCE CHARMING:

30.3322° N, 81.6557° W

I got a text from my neighbor, Fawn, that made me laugh out loud. She said, "I can't wait to hear about the sexy chocolate man in the red boxers you have on your balcony." Cue the words of the early 2000s hit by

Justin Timberlake and Timbaland: "I'm bringing sexy back." Our container district homes were small, with an open layout that left little to the imagination, but that was a detail too bold to miss.

Fawn and I spent a lot of time together. We'd giggle over life's quirks, binge-watch TV shows, indulge in delicious food (she'd cook, of course), or dance around with our hula hoops. Our friendship thrived on a mix of shared therapy sessions, endless gossip, and an undeniable love for music. We swapped playlists like love letters, always searching for the next perfect song to capture a moment. Sharing music playlists is my ultimate love language, and Fawn understood that perfectly.

As Prince (**THE REMINDER**) was gently taking the cigar out of his mouth and puffing his release of emotions, smoking into the city streets, a lot like last night's sweat and cologne.

Let's backtrack a bit. It all started out while I was sitting at the bar the night before at the "Reel Cafe" a third story bar. Each level had very different energy, underground little dump.

I feel a tap on my shoulder and turn to see this gorgeous dark chocolate man with striking green caramel eyes, a perfectly built muscular frame, and teeth so flawless they could rival a Spearmint gum ad. To my surprise, he asked me, "Can you do a backflip?"

Caught off guard but unwilling to back down, I respond, "Yes, of course I can." His eyes widen in shock as he says, "Oh, can you do it right now?"

I laugh and reply, "No way! Why the fu*k would I do that in a bar? That's not even safe or smart." He nods and says, "That's fair." But as he talks, I can't take my eyes off him. Something about him feels familiar, but I can't quite place it. Once he has my attention, I don't want the conversation to end—he's SEXY. Smooth-talking his way through the room, he's magnetic, but somehow, my casual charm keeps our conversation flowing all night.

Before I know it, he's kissing me, and things heat up fast. As we're walking out of the bar, his friends call out that it's time to head back to base. That's when I find out he's a military boy, and let's be real—up to no good. He asks me to come back with them, and I reply, "No chance. I live five minutes away, alone. There's no way I'm going all the way to your place."

He grins and says, "Fine, can I come with you?"

"Bold," I think, but hell yes. I'm not one for one-night stands, but this man is damn near a 10. If I had to envision my future husband, he'd look exactly like this guy. I couldn't pass up the chance to plant those seeds. He was, quite literally, the man of my dreams.

When the Uber pulled up, I said, *"Your chariot awaits"*. He smiled, leaned down to my face and kissed me hard and passionately. Whispering in my ear "You're gonna be soaking when I'm done with you." Sending sensual feelings down my spine, my skin crawled. When we got back to my container, he was shocked. "You're joking, you live here?" He had never seen anything like it obviously. Most people hadn't. It seemed to be a perk to everyone I dated. We headed upstairs to my bedroom. Stopping along to the fridge for some nightcaps. He pours the drink down his throat, then tries to pour it into mine, and throws me on the bed. Slowly kissing every area of my body, undressing me. His eyes widened "You're so hot." Little did he know, I was already intoxicated by him. The night got very hot and saltery. He pleased every button I had. In the morning I saw him smile and kiss me on the forehead. He leaned over to grab his red boxers, grabbing a cigar out of his pants. He asked if he could smoke, I replied, "Yeah, on the balcony. "

Later in the afternoon, after a few more pleasurable rounds, I finally asked him "Why did you ask me if I could do a backflip at the bar?" He laughed and replied, "Well, we were having a scavenger hunt, and the guys wanted to find someone to do it in person." Sadly enough we found one guy, and he said he could, but his friends said he couldn't. He gave it all his might and went for it, but fell and almost cracked his head open. He was bleeding, and we just ran away." My jaw hit the floor, I replied, "WTF, and then you decided to come ask me after?" He winced at me, "What, you were hot, I wanted to talk to you plus I still wanted to win the scangerhunt." I replied, "Clearly you won." I did a black flip in my bed and winked at him. Then we both started laughing.

We showered together and got ready. We built quite the appetite, we needed to grab food. His marine buddies were driving back up to get him from base. When they arrived, they joined us for some beers and games in the container district. Showing them all around while the sun was shining bright. I was so thrilled to parade around town with him on my side. Kissing me every chance he got. I was in awe, when it was finally time for them to leave. He leaned in, hugged me so tightly, and kissed me deep like no one has ever kissed me before. He left telling me he'd text me. I wasn't sure I'd actually ever even see him again.

A few days went by and a message popped up from him asking me what I was doing on a specific date in the future... I was like "Umm? Idk why?" He said "I want you to come to the marine ball with me, but first I want to see you again."

I couldn't help but smile.

Our dates were super cute, and fun every time. Then it was time to turn into a princess for the ball. Fawn came over to help me get ready. Really felt like she was my fairy god-mother trying to make sure I wouldn't turn into a pumpkin later. Getting all dolled up, dressed to the nines' with none other than my prince charming.

I drove down to his house early, to prepare. As I got out of the car he came out to grab hold of my car door, and help me out. He said "Wow, you cleaned up well." Smiling, and replying "Not sure I've ever seen anyone more handsome in blues." Peeping around the house I made myself at home.

We finally made our way to the ball, during the car ride, he explains "Hey, I've gotta tell you something.... I'm kinda doing this *thing* during the ceremony, so just chill." As he hands me a bottle of booze. I had no idea what that meant or how high his ranking really was. He just told me that he went to a military academy, so he bypassed a lot of the "grunt" work—meaning the lower-ranking soldiers doing the tough, thankless tasks.

Walking up to entertain his friends and captains, we casually chat as we find our tables. We sat down at our table. There was a red cloth material holding the carefully placed utensils in order. I was so thrilled for a six course meal, I knew they'd go all out with the buffet. It was a special ball for the Marines. It reminded me of a few past lovers that once were in the military. I had only been to one other ball. It was in a past life with a guy I dated for a short period, in the Navy. But this was a special night, and so was *THIS* man. Suddenly it was his time to shine, he got up with a group of other combat buddies to put on a whole show for everyone, he was the main hero, of course... and naturally the protagonist in me, wants what I want. I want the hero in my story too. My undercarriage went hot. I was so turned on, I have a knack for being attracted to the main characters in their environments, as I reflect the same qualities.

Heading to a country bar afterwards; he started singing to me, and line dancing along me, until he was spinning me around. A real little dosey-doe. He told me how much he loved spending all this time with me, he was sad he'd be deploying so soon.

Our evening came with a lot more playtime; however this felt a lot like love making, or at least wild animals. That night I asked him why he invited me to the ball like any "silly, lovesick girl," he was always so honest, that's what I loved the most. He replied "Well remember the night we met?" "Yeah," I said. He said, "One of my commanders told me not to show up to the ball without a date." He didn't originally want to because he didn't have a girl, but his commander told him, "Just go to the bar, find some random girl, make sure she's not crazy and bring her." Again, I'm slightly shocked. I replied, "Oh wow, well I guess I'm glad that worked out in your favor. And out of every girl you could have chosen, it was me." He replied, "I knew it was you the first moment I laid my eyes on you."

Moments with Prince set my heart on fire. He always made me feel like the most wanted person in the room, and didn't need to hide his excitement or love. It was loud, and proud. I was very happy to be loved so fast, deeply, passionately, and romantically. He checked off all the boxes. Although, I knew this love would not be my happily ever after, it was something more special than that. Because it was intentional, honest, and clear. No confusion, just sweet.

Meeting Him on My Boat:

34.225727, -77.944710

It was a gorgeous, blue-skied day with not a cloud in sight. The air was fresh, and as I walked down to the river dock, I felt a wave of excitement. I was about to go on a ride I wouldn't forget. Unlike all those other days I've been a mere passenger on a boat, *this* was special—it was my time to shine! Huge thanks to my friend, Megan for convincing her husband that I'd be the perfect fit as a promo girl. We were launching an EDM boat tour on the Wilmington River, and I was ready to make the most of it.

I walked onto the boat, grabbed my credentials (and perks: free drinks, of course), and made my way around, greeting people. Everyone started to settle in as we headed out on the water. I had a lot of "special guests" to look after—fun-loving girls with big social followings and bright energy that I could recruit for future rounds.

Then, I noticed a group of three on the top deck by the DJ booth. It felt like I had an angel and a devil on my shoulders. My gut was telling me, "Go talk to them," but I wasn't so sure. After a couple rounds of drinks, I finally found my way to them. Smiling, I did my job:

"Hey, y'all!" Then I turned my attention directly looking at the tall, brown– skinned man with dimples in the Coachella tie dye t-shirt. "Ahh Coachella, wish I could have gone that year, Beyonce made her debut. Bhive had a huge show with a drumline, incredible. I'm Erica, one of the promoters. Are we having a good time here? Any feedback?"

They all replied, "Yeah, it's great!" Introducing themselves, "I'm Mr. Killa, this is Quinn, and Fiona.

Then *Mr. Killa* locked eyes with me, grinning from ear to ear: "Yeah, Coachella was dope—I didn't go that year either.. Are you enjoying yourself?"

Laughing at his boldness, I replied, "Oh yeah, of course... what's y'all's plan for after this?"

He grinned and said, "I don't know, we didn't make any plans yet."

I shot back, "Ah, well, y'all should come to our afters! It's at a bar downtown."

He raised an eyebrow. "Are you going to be there?"

I smirked. "Most likely... I'm still gathering my options, but I might make a special appearance." We both laughed, I winked and said "Come find me." Then I bounced off to find more people to invite.

As the boat docked the herd of humans and the rest of the team headed toward the bar, Megan and I decided to make our own fun and leave the others behind. We hopped from bar to bar, having a blast. Then Megan's husband called.

She put him on speaker phone: "Where are you two? You're my wife, and she's the main promoter. We need you both here."

We reluctantly agreed, "Yeah, that's fair. We'll be right there."

We rushed back to the bar where the after-party was. And to my surprise, Mr. Killa was there, waiting for my arrival. His friends hung out in the background as he made a beeline straight for me. With a devilish smile, he said, "You're finally here!"

I replied, "You found me!" He offered to buy me a drink, and I was excited. At this point, it didn't matter where we were in the room—every time I turned around, I was colliding with him. The chemistry was undeniable. Everything else became a blur, except for when I told him a secret about his style and his mom, and some then random friend of his pretending to be a bodyguard kept bumping into us, as if I was up to no good.

I remember saying, "What's his deal? I don't even know who you are, and I *definitely* don't care. This is my party. I should be the one with a guard."

Cocky, I know. But that's just how the night felt.

I woke up the next day to find his number in my phone and a bunch of missed calls. His Instagram page was pulled up, and my notifications were blowing up—some of my photos had been liked, and I had no idea what had happened. I stared at my IG, thinking, "Who the heck is this guy, and what did I get myself into?"

After a few minutes of my own social media (private investor work), I realized he was an artist/musician... and kind of a big deal in England (which I thought was insanely hot).

Spiking my curiosity, I finally decided to message him. "Last night was fun, wish I remembered. :)"

Before I knew it, he was asking me on a date for the next day: "What are you doing tomorrow? Want to come by the music studio? I've got a session, and there's a photoshoot planned."

I almost dropped my panties. I ran over to my neighbor's place, Fawns, and told her all the juicy details, laughing about the whole thing. I was shocked that some stranger wanted to see me *immediately* the next day and do my two favorite things—music and photoshoots. Of course, I had to say yes. It was almost as if he knew the exact words to say to me.

The next day, he picked me up in an old beat up stick shift. To my surprise, he was the guy that didn't care about appearance as much as he did about investing in the business. I'd admired that. The music studio was just a block from my container house. We went inside, and I was introduced to everyone. Trying to play it cool, I observed the group like an undercover agent. Then, we headed to the back for the photoshoot.

He jumped on the keys, as I danced around, and posed with him, laughing the entire time. The chemistry between us was so obvious, it looked like we'd been dating forever—yet we were just two strangers.

LOVERS QUARREL:

Vanessa—Tessa, my "bead bestie" for short **(THE EMPOWERER)**—had come into town to visit me and see what life in Wilmington was like. Little did she know, she was about to get a front-row seat to the circus of chaos I'd been living in. Honestly, our lives were so parallel, it was like we'd been living in parallel universes. She hailed from Chattanooga and, let me tell you, Tessa had two sides—one bubbly, girly, loving-magical fairy dust sparkly side, and then there was the *other* side: a bad girl, dominant, wild, and ready for anything. I guess that's why she immediately got why my love life was a corral of eight different stories and counting.

And that's when the magic happened. After she came to visit, we discovered just how much we really had in common. Tessa stumbled upon an old page of hers that showed some *interesting* work she used to do, and in the weirdest twist of fate, she matched with someone who just so happened to be in Wilmington for the little festival. The kicker? We were both mutual friends with this guy. Enter Astro, **(THE REMINDER)** the guy who once made his way onto my roster and stayed there as a very close friend. He was aware of my new relationship status.

In a hilarious turn of events, Astro had messaged me once, sending a screenshot of Tessa's page and saying, "This girl is exactly like you!" Funny thing was, he had no idea that she and I had just met. Of course, I casually responded with, "Oh, yes. Tessa. She's a good friend of mine." Oh, how we love to entertain fate.

Naturally, we played along. Astro invited us to his boat, and, well... *Muscular physique, tattoos, no shirt?* We weren't saying no to that. But here's the thing—Tessa had no clue how many love stories were about to unfold in the space of 48 hours. She had no idea what she was getting into, but I was about to show her just how much fun Wilmington—and my life—could get.

Tessa arrived at my place, and it was like the world shifted. We immediately started giggling, blasting music, and doing all the dumb girl things we do best. We gossiped about everything in my life, making sure she was fully caught up on the ever-evolving saga of my love life. "Okay, so this is Mr. Killa, and this... well, this is just another one of my... situations." I had to keep her in the loop, so she wouldn't be completely lost when we met these characters.

One of the first stops was Mr. Killa's music studio. Naturally, being our contact-creating selves, we took full advantage of the green screen to work our "model" magic. I may have been a little shy with the microphone (I don't know why—I mean, the guy was used to it!), but when Mr. Killa and Quinn started talking about laser tag, my competitive side kicked in.

Laser tag, baby! We weren't missing that. Although, I did warn Mr. Killa that my eagerness to win exceeded all levels of sanity. Running, dodging, hiding—I didn't win the first round, but I sure as hell claimed victory in the second. Oh, and I may have turned it into a metaphor for my entire life.

We stayed up until 4 AM, and then the *big day* arrived: the boat trip. Lucky for me, I had already invited Prince to come along, and *wow*, nothing quite like going from one romance to another in the span of a few hours. The boat? Exhilarating. Prince and I were all over each other, making out, being ridiculous, and yes—tug-of-warring me into the water like we were two kids in love. It was a blast. But there was this feeling gnawing at me. This feeling that the clock was ticking—Prince's deployment was looming, and I couldn't shake the feeling that this could be the last time we'd see each other. So, we prayed together, and I sent him off with a prayer for protection.

Meanwhile, Tessa and I—well, let's just say we *owned* that boat. We were the center of attention, soaking up the sun in our swimsuits, both feeling like we could take over the world. I wore my bright yellow two-piece, looking like a sunshine beacon. Tessa, of course, turned heads in a royal blue suit, blonde hair gleaming as she glowed like the water itself.

As I looked at her, at Astro, and at Prince, I couldn't help but smile. This was a life. I turned to Tessa, beaming, and said, "I'm so happy right now." She laughed and said, "You know what? I watched the most beautiful love story I've ever seen." Naturally, I asked, "What do you mean?" And she replied, "It's you. The LOVE story is about you, silly. With all the people in between."

And that was it. I realized how tangled my life had become. These little love webs were everywhere. Could this really be my life? I looked into Tessa's eyes and whispered, "I just have this feeling, you know? Prince is my present... But Mr. Killa? I think he's my future." And just like that, I had a revelation.

The funny part is, after that night with Prince, I never physically saw him again. He'd said earlier that day, in a moment of drunken honesty, that he might tell me he loved me if he got too drunk. Guess what? He did. So, when I didn't hear from him afterward, I was left confused. But some time later, he came clean, apologizing and saying, "I was starting to really like you, but I couldn't let myself get attached." That was his way of self-preservation, but, let's face it—I wasn't ready to hear that. I was sad and hurt, but I was also distracted and entangled in others.

Still, I got over it. I had other priorities—other *stories* to focus on. But I can't help but think about what could've been with Prince. What would've happened if he came back from deployment?

And then, it hit me... I'm focused more on the future. Checkmate.

Psychological Perspective:

These ups and downs reflect how attachment styles (such as anxious, avoidant, or secure) can influence the way individuals navigate love and relationships. Unconditional love, especially self-love, requires recognizing these patterns without judgment. It's about acknowledging the ebb and flow of emotions and not letting temporary setbacks define one's worth or the potential for future relationships.

The eventual realization that being "focused more on the future" suggests an evolution of self-awareness. They are shifting from the pain of the past (with Prince) to a more secure, forward-looking perspective, which is akin to self-acceptance and self-love — a key element of unconditional love.

The Concept of "Love Webs" and Emotional Complexity

This describes life as a "web" of love stories—relationships that interweave and shift in meaning over time. This concept mirrors the idea that love, in its many forms, is not linear or one-dimensional. In psychology, relationships and attachments are often described as complex and multifaceted, with each connection serving different emotional needs and purposes.

Unconditional love is often thought to be expansive and accepting, allowing for multiple layers and forms of connection without judgment or the need for exclusivity. The way this embraces these relationships with friends, lovers, and companions shows a deep acceptance of the complexity of love. They are open to exploring these connections without forcing a singular narrative or outcome, which is similar to the acceptance inherent in unconditional love.

FULL FORCE :

Mr. Killa wanted to take me out on a proper date, all sweet and thoughtful, but we were low-maintenance, so we ended up at some bar on the outskirts of town. He promised it had the *best* wings. Funny thing, though—I couldn't even eat chicken, but I figured I'd humor him. Surely, I'd find something else to eat on the menu.

Our first date was all about figuring out who we were, chatting and laughing, the kind of easy conversation you expect when you're with someone brand new. But then, out of nowhere, he went quiet. And not the charming, mysterious kind of quiet either. He muttered something under his breath, and I squinted, trying to catch it. "What was that?" I asked.

He hesitated for a second, then mumbled again, "I'm gonna f*** this up."

In reference to me. To *us*.

I remember looking him dead in the eyes, giving him a little smirk, and without missing a beat, I said, "Red flag."

We both burst out laughing, but deep down, we both knew that wasn't exactly a glowing start. I mean, who admits that on a first date? But hey, we were intrigued. We were playing with fate, weren't we?

A week later, he showed up with a gift—my very own pair of shoes from his brand's store. He said it was for promotion, but I couldn't help but think: "*Why not have a hot girl wear his name around town?*" "You must've done this with all the girls, right?" At least, that's what my suspicious mind whispered. But I didn't mind. A girl's gotta have a little swag, right? Makes sense to me.

So there I was, wearing the shoes, trying to ignore the gnawing curiosity in the back of my mind. Oh, the tangled mess of attraction and intrigue. "Where would this go?"

The Complexity of Self-Sabotage and Vulnerability:

Mr. Killa's comment, "I'm gonna f*** this up," during the first date is an interesting psychological moment. It reflects a common tendency in people with an anxious or avoidant attachment style: **self-sabotage.** "This behavior often stems from deep-seated fears of rejection or inadequacy, leading individuals to preemptively distance themselves or create a reason for the relationship to fail before they feel vulnerable enough to be hurt."

The psychology of vulnerability plays a key role here. Unconditional love involves the ability to be vulnerable with others—allowing ourselves to be seen as we truly are, flaws and all. In this case, Mr. Killa's self-doubt and fear of failure may have been an unconscious attempt to prepare himself emotionally for the possibility of rejection or disappointment. The response of—calling it a **"red flag"** and laughing—may signal protective instincts and a recognition of vulnerability, but also the acknowledgment that love requires understanding and acceptance of those imperfections. Instead of dismissing him, choosing to engage with his vulnerability with humor, indicating an openness to both his flaws and potential.

THE PROMISE LANDS:

34' 12' 7.182 N and 77' 55' 16.8252 W

One morning, I woke up feeling incredibly grateful, just happy to be breathing. I started the day with my usual morning meditation, grounding myself in peace, but as the quiet settled, I felt the pull of the outdoors. A walk was in order—some fresh air, a little freedom to let my mind wander.

As I strolled aimlessly down the familiar streets, by Courtney's house I stumbled upon a hidden gem tucked away in Wilmington—a park that felt almost like a secret. It had that kind of energy, the kind of place that stays in the corners of your memory, like it's meant to show up at just the right time. Little did I know, this moment would be forever imprinted in both my memory and someone else's—a very special someone: Mr. Killa.

I shared the story of my accidental discovery with him, and that's when he told me about a cherished childhood memory of his. He grew up in our little town. He and his friends had spent time there in their youth, calling it the "promised land." It was a place where, on dark and moody days, the moment they stepped onto its grounds, the darkness began to melt away, replaced by pure light. It was a raw, real reminder of duality—the balance between dark and light, struggle and peace, bleeding through all of life's chapters.

And here's the serendipitous twist: He had shot his first music photo shoot there, in that sacred space. I couldn't help but smile, because—of all things—I just so happened to be wearing his t-shirt from his new song launch. So naturally, I figured I'd grab some content while I was there.

It's funny how the universe works, isn't it? When time and place align, and you find yourself caught up in a full circle of divine moments, everything just clicks. The past, the present, and the future all come together like a perfect snapshot. And I thought, yeah, this is the good part. After years of heartbreak, finally, something being created felt special. Almost as the story or soul connection was bigger than us.

According to <u>Catharsis - Definition, Meaning & Synonyms | Vocabulary.com</u>

Catharsis: "purging of emotional tensions."

I felt a sense of new relief flush over me, like a purifying dip in the ocean cleansing away any lingering virus in my body, heart, and mind. Blissful tears began to run down my cheeks as I carried my childlike heart to the swing set. I pumped my legs as high as they could go, trying to lift my body above the treeline. I was chasing that rush in my stomach, like the exhilarating drop on a rollercoaster. I wanted to feel everything exciting again—I wanted to feel alive.

Dream Girl:

One day, we found ourselves in the "red room"—MK's bedroom, which, let's be honest, always felt a little bit like a dungeon. With blackout curtains and red LED lights lining every corner, it wasn't exactly a place for the faint of heart. But there we were, perched on his royal throne—aka the bed—when he decided to show me his collection of video games.

"I've got something special to show you," he said, his voice full of mischief. Naturally, I was intrigued. MK pulled up a game and began telling me the story behind one of his creations. For reasons I still don't quite understand, MK liked to choose women as avatars in his games. So, one day, he'd crafted a bad-ass woman with an athletic build, brown hair, and a fierce fighting spirit. As he started describing her, I began to notice something... familiar.

I squinted at the screen, staring at her likeness. "MK, does she look like anyone you recognize?" I asked, already suspecting the answer.

He started giggling, that signature MK giggle, before he said, "Yeah, I think she does."

At that moment, without a word, we both knew. It was me. He had literally created a video game character that looked just like me—the "woman from his dreams." I couldn't believe it. He'd designed *his dream girl*, and it was... well, *me*.

I blinked, still in disbelief. "Wait, did you make her after we met?" I asked, hoping for some reassurance.

"No," he said, "I made her a long time ago."

But the excitement in his voice told me this wasn't just a coincidence— he was genuinely thrilled to show me.

And there I was, as his creation—fully equipped with the same abilities, the same bad-ass energy. I was a character in his world, in a way that felt... strangely intimate.

As we drove deeper into the game, he showed me how he could create anything he wanted in this digital universe. He was currently stuck in some enchanted desert, navigating ruins and chambers on a quest to find the Queen herself—Cleopatra. As he fumbled through the virtual world, I realized something: I had no idea you could go rogue in a game and just do whatever you felt like!

"Yeah, the metaverse is a fun place to be," MK exclaimed with a grin.

Honestly, I felt a little on edge. I couldn't help but think about all the kids glued to their screens, their brains rotting away, escaping into virtual worlds instead of living in reality. It was easy to get lost in these games, but what about the real world? What about *life* outside the screen?

Still, as MK rambled on about the tech behind it all, he had this way of making the digital realm seem a little less intimidating. In that moment, I realized something—he was teaching me a lot more than I ever thought possible about tech. But more importantly, he was showing me a side of himself I hadn't quite seen before. And, apparently, it was the side that wanted to create a *dream girl*... one who just so happened to be me.

Over the next couple of weeks a lot went on, but we grew more invested in each other- almost obsessive (def on my end) I couldn't have believed that many things could happen in a relationship with someone.

We returned to his bedroom where he excitedly exclaimed, where he excitedly exclaimed, "I FOUND HER!" I replied, "Who did you find"? He said "CLEOPATRA— we were both so excited, opening up the game to choose me as the avatar we jumped inside the metaverse. We entered a castle where she was. It was an outdoor room with people in robes dressed all around, men and women, and she got up to say a speech with a cup of wine in hand *"everyone here can have sex with me tonight, but tomorrow everyone will be EXECUTED!"* We both laughed so hard saying "*What a savage*" it seemed exactly like the badass move a queen of her caliber was in control of. In these moments she became a pinnacle for my curiosity for many years to come. I was almost inspired by being his dream girl, what that meant for our relationship, and why the name Cleo would echo and have so much significant importance in my life to come.

ELEPHANT SHOES:

It was a warm, sunny day in the Carolinas, the kind of day that lets you know summer's not just a season—it's a lifestyle. From April to October, the heat and humidity roll in like a never-ending embrace. It's like a sauna, but with more mosquitoes and less zen.

But this day? This day was special. It wasn't just the weather; it was *the moment*. It was Mr. Killa's best friend, an older, incredibly cool lesbian woman, who was throwing a birthday party for herself. And let me tell you, she was *the* coolest. If there were a gender-bender twin of him, it was her—she had that FUN gal energy. I adored her instantly, and she had always been the one to see through the artist persona he wore. She got him in a way that no one else really did. In the past, he'd brought a lot of women around her, all trying to play the role of 'the cool girl,' but none of them quite lasted—she admittedly didn't know who was who.

We were there, at her birthday bash, and as the night unfolded, he'd told me he'd been talking about me for months to her. I, on the other hand, was still wrapped up in my "cool girl" persona. You know the one—the detached, cold-hearted *bitch* who pretends she doesn't care, that she's just living her best life, doing whatever she wants, whenever she wants. It was a mask I wore well, like a bad habit that made me feel untouchable. But deep down, I think I knew what it was—just a front. In reality, I didn't care about looking cool. Drugs, drinking, reckless nights—none of that lifestyle mattered to me in the long run. I was surrounded by the music industry. The only opinion that really counted was *my own*. And that, my friends, was a realization I was yet to fully embrace.

Now, back to the party, where we both danced around the topic of "*I love you*" like it was the hottest potato in the room. We couldn't quite say it, yet it felt like perhaps it was too early to be that "emotional", so we got creative. I'd throw out lines like, "I love those bottles of booze you bought," or, "I love the way you do... whatever you do," as if those words could somehow hold the weight of all the things I couldn't quite say. And then, just to keep it playful, we both tried mouthing "elephant shoes," because, apparently, if you read lips the right way, it looks like "I love you."

Of course, it was ridiculous. But so *us*.

And then, in the midst of all this circling around the truth, he finally broke the silence. He looked at me, serious for a moment, and said, "I hate that we live in a world where we can't just be honest with our feelings. Why can't we just say what we mean?"

Cue the *game*—"Tell me you love me without telling me."

I could feel it—the weight of those words, the truth of it. I loved him. Or maybe it was more like *I love how easy he makes this feel*. So easy, so sincere. And yet, so unbelievably *difficult*.

After everything—after the "single girl era" with its chaos and uncertainty, after building walls to protect my heart from being too vulnerable—he made it feel like I could just be *me*. The past me was almost married, a housewife. I could jump into that role from time to time. Not just the cool girl. Not the tough girl. Just the girl who could *love* without all the complications.

And that, my dear friends, was the paradox of him. He made everything feel so simple, while simultaneously making everything so *complicated*. But what a beautiful complication it was.

THE LITTLE THINGS:

I remember the morning so clearly: walking up to him, a little plate of food in hand. He was sitting there, deep in his world, staring at his laptop like it was the most important thing in the universe. His "day job" was needy to say the least. I was just bringing breakfast, but it felt like a grand gesture, an offering in the middle of the mundane.

Later that same morning, I snuck downstairs, and from the top of the stairs, I heard him yell something. It was muffled, and I couldn't quite catch it. Curiosity got the best of me, so I hustled back up to his room, slipped back into bed, and, before I could even get comfortable, he looked me dead in the eyes and asked, "Did you really just walk all the way down there to throw that away... and check for more ketchup?" "Yeah", I replied. He replied, "You know you could have just looked in this little fridge, and this trash can."

I laughed so hard, almost choking on the hilarity of it. He had been working remotely, his eyes glued to his screen, and yet, somehow, he saw me. He noticed the little things—the way I'd sneak a glance at something, the tiny quirks I thought no one would care about. It was as if he studied me, like some kind of scientist observing a rare species in the wild.

At that moment, I realized: he wasn't just there beside me. He *saw* me. He knew my moves before I even made them, and it wasn't creepy or overwhelming—it was just... knowing. He paid attention to me like I mattered. And it was a beautiful kind of unsettling.

It made me think of the way I felt when I would fall asleep in his room, all tangled up in the sheets. I often couldn't quite get comfortable, restless in a way that's both physical and emotional, but when he was next to me, there was this feeling of safety I'd never known. With Mr. Killa, I didn't need to worry about anything. Or at least, that's what I told myself—when I wasn't worrying.

Most of the time, though, we didn't sleep. We pulled all-nighters, diving into everything life had to offer—parties, sex, promoting whatever dream we were chasing that week. The nights blurred into one, entangled with bad decisions and wild energy.

But in the quiet moments, when I did drift off, I could feel his eyes on me. He'd watch me sleep, his gaze soft, his face full of something I couldn't quite name. In the morning, he'd tell me how peaceful I looked, how sweet I seemed in my sleep. His words always held this layer of something deeper, like he wasn't sure whether it was love or fear or both. Was he falling for me, or was he just waiting for the moment it would all fall apart?

It's funny how someone can make you feel so safe and still leave you wondering if they're keeping one foot out the door.

THE HEARTBEAT MOMENT:

I'll never forget one of the most romantic days of my life—though, if you asked me to recount the week leading up to it, I'd probably be a bit fuzzy. There were promo events, video shoots, and a whirlwind of everything that falls under "too much to remember but somehow, it all mattered." But there's one moment that stands out, so vivid and real, like it was etched into my heart. I know I won't ever forget it, and, honestly, I don't think this type of love will come again—well, not until my future husband shows up, that is.

It was the kind of moment that stole my breath away. There I was, drifting into the deepest slumber, the kind where the world starts to melt away, and everything feels soft. And then, like some divine act of fate, MK gently laid his head on my chest, right above my heart. He was listening—no, really *listening*—to my heartbeat, as if it held the key to his peace. He closed his eyes, focused on the steady rhythm, hoping that it would help us both fall asleep together.

Now, here's the part that still makes my heart skip when I think of it: when I woke up, there was a sudden shout, a burst of energy that sliced through the stillness of the room. "I DID IT! OMG! I DID IT! THAT WAS SOOO DOPE!" He was so loud, I was half-dazed, still clinging to the remnants of sleep, trying to figure out what was happening.

He was grinning, wide-eyed, like he'd just solved the mystery of the universe. In his excitement, he told me that by listening to my heartbeat, he had somehow found me in our dreams. As soon as he shared that with me, something clicked—like a jolt of electricity, a flash of dream memories came rushing through me. And there it was: I saw him, holding me tightly, embracing me like nothing else in the world mattered.

For a brief moment, I could feel how deep that love was. How it was like a tether connecting us, even when we weren't awake. And in that instant, I was shaken, floored by the realization that someone—*someone*—could love me like that. It was the kind of love that didn't need words, only a heartbeat to say it all.

It's funny how love works, right? You never know when it's going to sneak up on you, or how it'll feel, but when it does... it's everything you never knew you needed.

Psychological Perspective:

This reflects the idea that love is not just a conscious experience but something that permeates our unconscious minds as well. This dream connection can be seen as a manifestation of emotional attunement—a concept central to unconditional love. Emotional attunement happens when one person is deeply in sync with another, not just in terms of our words, but in our feelings, emotions, and subconscious experiences. In this moment, MK feels so emotionally connected that it transcends the waking world, and he finds me, even in his dreams.

Unconditional love involves this kind of deep attunement—the sense that, no matter what happens in the waking world, the emotional connection is so strong and unwavering that it transcends space and time. MK's ability to feel connected to me in such an intimate way suggests a form of love that is stable, unshakeable, and capable of moving beyond ordinary limitations.

CHAPTER EIGHTEEN

REIGNITING THE PERFORMER WITHIN.

Tie Me Upside Down:

35.0458° N, 85.3094° W

One week during my summer travels, I decided to head to Tennessee to visit Tessa. We were off to perform and work as promo girls at a music festival. The festival was a whirlwind. We took it over like pros, handing out goodies, monitoring the bathroom showers (don't ask, it's a thing), and helping everyone have the best time while also enjoying the music ourselves. I quickly learned the pros and cons of the music scene, and oddly enough, how people can also use it for some pretty dark magic... but that's a whole other story.

Sharing a car, which, at that point, had turned into our "house," was hilarious. Between sunny days, rainy days, packing, and unpacking, we got used to surviving in whatever conditions we found ourselves in. We'd change outfits next to a car door and rush off to get in the middle of the sea of festival festivities. We'd weave through vendors, seeking out the best music lineups, the ones that made us forget we were drenched in sweat and long past needing a shower. It was the perfect job, right? A week of music, chaos, and no real cleanliness. By the end of the week, we were both so ready to head back to her place, where, unbeknownst to me, a surprise was waiting.

When we arrived back at Tessa's house, I had no idea what was coming. She looked at me with a glint in her eye and casually asked, "Ever heard of Shibari?"

I blinked. "Shibari? Is that like... a sushi dish?" I hadn't the faintest clue.

"Nope," she laughed. "Class is in session: you're about to get an education lesson."

Tessa proceeded to introduce me to something I'd never in a million years expected. *Shibari*, I learned, is an art form—a beautiful, intricate practice of rope art and engineering. It's a contemporary form of rope bondage that originated in Japan, and let me tell you, it's not what I thought it was at all. It's a whole world of aesthetics, knots, and intricate design that mixes craftsmanship with, well... a bit of magic.

It was a world I didn't know existed, but there I was, about to dive into it—of course, in Tessa's signature "we're doing this and it's going to be epic" style.

And, trust me, epic doesn't even begin to cover it.

Shibari is a Japanese word that broadly means "binding" or "tying" in most contexts, but is used in BDSM to refer to this style of decorative bondage.

In Japanese, "Shibari" simply means "to tie". I'd only seen her do it in photos a few times, and was immediately curious. I've been a dancer my entire life, and I had been actively practicing yoga over the last decade, and been practicing with various aerial objects, ie: lyra, pole, silks.

Shibari was the next step up in my practice of air apparatus. I had the pleasure of meeting @kinbaku_boyscout **(THE TEACHER)** who mentioned he's been practicing this art form for a little over a decade. He has been a photographer for most of his adult career. I really got to know his personality and hearing "why this niche has found him." He's exclaimed he's extremely passionate about the different styles of knots, and the mathematics it takes to correctly balance a body type from the sky or other environments. His left to right brain does a fantastic job processing, I might add. He described his love of the art form, how each piece is so delicate but easily fits together, like a puzzle. When we arrived, we enjoyed.

When we arrived, we enjoyed a charcuterie board, started to get dressed into the desired outfit of choice. Something I felt "sexy" in, plus I added a little face paint. (meaning my everyday makeup.) He immediately started asking me qualifying questions of positions and what my past experiences had been to get an idea of which styles we should start with for the basic mechanics.

Then before I knew it, I lifted off the floor. With a bit of breath work I was able to embrace all of the transitions effortlessly. The ropes didn't leave much markings or hurt me at all. I'd honestly say it was a 10/10 experience. I was really only in the whole experience for about 40 seconds. Once he started tying the knots and lifted me off the ground, captured the photos and was down. Anyone that is interested please reach out, or research where you might be able to do this experience.

The Journey Back to Wilmington

Tessa and I were on a mission—one that would take us from the lively hills of Tennessee all the way back to Wilmington, full of stories, laughter, and the kind of bond that only road trips can forge. We weren't just heading home; we were taking the car back by storm, like two free spirits with the whole world as our playground.

Our first stop? Asheville. Christy's house, to be exact. We pulled in for a pit stop and ended up staying overnight. Little did we know, the universe had a little surprise in store for us. As we got out of the car, we bumped into none other than *Chris*—our old friend, the wandering traveler, and someone whose life seemed to mirror our own in the most beautifully chaotic way.

We spent hours catching up, swapping stories like old friends do. It was as though every experience we'd been through—every lesson learned and mistake made—was an open book between us. We'd talk about our journeys, break down what had happened, and what we had *really* learned from it all. It wasn't just about the crazy stuff that went down. It was about the way we processed it, grew from it, and figured out what we'd carry forward into the next chapter.

It was the kind of friendship that's built on shared understanding, the kind where you don't have to explain your soul—because they just *get it*. And so, after hours of deep conversations and laughter, we did what any good road-trip buddies would do. We invited Chris to join us in Wilmington. After all, what's a journey without a few more stops along the way?

It felt like our own little tribe was coming together—one lesson, one pit stop at a time. And the adventure? Well, it was just beginning.

Secure Attachment:

"Individuals with secure attachments feel understood and valued without the need to constantly prove themselves. The unconditional aspect of the love here is evident in the way that Chris and I can just "be" with each other, without needing to perform or show any particular side of ourshelves. They are accepted as they are, flaws, mistakes, and all."

The Role of Acceptance in Unconditional Love:

This describes friendships where friends don't have to "explain their soul" and demonstrate a profound level of **acceptance**. Unconditional love is built on the idea of accepting someone fully without trying to change them or place conditions on their worth. The fact that Chris and I don't need to explain ourselves to one another shows that there's a deep level of comfort and trust in our relationship. This is a hallmark of unconditional love—the knowledge that you are seen and accepted for who you truly are.

Grizmas: The Ultimate Party Bus Adventure:

34.2000°, -77.9500°

It was just another day at CBT Studios—well, sort of. This time, Mr. Killa and I decided to take things to a whole new level. We were knee-deep in tour prep and event planning for what felt like an eternity, but there was one thing we *really* wanted to do: throw an epic celebration for our friends. Enter *GRIZMAS*.

Now, GRIZMAS isn't your typical Christmas. You see, Griz, the artist, comes to town in July, and that, my friends, is what we call "*half Christmas.*" So, naturally, as the ever-enthusiastic promoter I was, I hit up every single person I knew in the city who was planning to attend the concert—pretty much all my friends (because let's face it, who *isn't* going to a Griz show when you're in the same city?).

The idea we hatched? Well, gather up all the party people at the studio beforehand, pack them onto a party bus, and cart them to the event with style. Oh, and let's make it a *super fun* promo event for future artists, potential venue renters, and pretty much anyone who might want to throw a shindig there. Boom. Perfect. Easy.

Our music studio, however, was a bit of a hidden gem. It was *massive*—we're talking multiple rooms. There was the sound room, the podcast room, a huge space for a full-on band, and the pièce de résistance: the event space with a stage. Of course, it was the ultimate pre-game hangout for a Griz concert.

Tessa came along, to help me get the ball rolling, she came from out of town just to visit for the festivities. One by one, our party guests arrived.

With my world-renowned hosting skills (*cue dramatic music*), I made sure everyone had drinks, snacks, and a good vibe. Meanwhile, Willy was working his DJ magic, setting the tone for the night. It was the perfect party setup. The personalities were all over the place, but don't worry, *I* bridged the gaps. It was a social harmony symphony, if you will.

When it was finally time, we loaded half the crew onto the first party bus. I corralled all the little ravers, making sure they were comfortable and ready to go. And then—*BOOM*—I took the mic. "Let me tell you a tale," I said, *"Not a creature was stirring, not even a mouse..."*.

I wove an overly dramatic, delightfully expressive, and slightly over-the-top tale about the dreams and desires of every raver under the moonlight (because, let's face it, hype girl energy requires flair). Then, as if possessed by the spirit of a circus performer with a caffeine overdose, I cranked up the music, climbed onto the bus chairs, and transformed into a one-woman show. Spins, flips, and impromptu pole tricks— moves no one thought I had in me—had the crowd eating out of my hand. Most importantly, Mr. Killa was absolutely loving it.

He was upside down, recording every second of my antics, and later told me with the sweetest sincerity, "I was almost in tears watching you. I was so proud, like, that's my girl, damn!" Hearing those words from him was pure magic. Every moment with him felt like a celebration, like life itself was throwing us a party just for being us. And why not? Each weekend was a new triumph, both in love and business, and we reveled in it like it would never end.

After my grand finale, I'd leap off the bus, watching it disappear into the sea of lights and music at the fairgrounds, only to hear the call of the next bus and the next adventure. Rinse, repeat, and amplify. I was like the Energizer Bunny with no off switch—except this Bunny came with dance moves and zero chill.

After the show, the party didn't stop. I was still leading the charge through downtown, ushering people into bars, and if they were brave enough to keep the afterparty going, I welcomed them back to the studio. But, honestly, I had no idea how much of a good time they were having until much later.

Fast forward a few months, and people started sharing how they saw videos or heard stories about the wild, hype-filled event. Some even reached out to me personally. A few girls who I didn't even know, told me that my energy inspired them to step out of their comfort zones, just by watching me shine so brightly. *That* was the moment my heart did a little happy dance.

You see, I'm not just here to throw parties or put on a good show. What really matters to me is the ripple effect I can create—the way I can light up someone else's world. Hearing that I helped people push past their shyness and take on new opportunities? That's worth every flip, spin, and dance move.

In the end, that's why I keep doing this. I want to bring joy, excitement, and maybe a little bit of *GRIZMAS* energy into the world. Who knew that a party bus ride could change someone's life?

MY 30th BIRTHDAY, THE BUTTERFLY EFFECT:

I was in full-on *passion project* mode, working tirelessly on a vision that could make a difference, no matter how small. After creating my affirmations signs, I teamed up with a local video company **Bootstrap.** Justin, and I had one goal: helping humanity through positive art. Together, we came up with this wild, yet meaningful concept: "The 7 Deadly Sins," but with a twist. We turned them into "*The 7 Virtues.*" Each act of goodness would ripple out into the community, creating waves of kindness that expanded in ways we couldn't even imagine.

And, of course, I decided to center my birthday around this grand idea of **the butterfly effect**—the idea that small changes can have big consequences. You might have heard the saying: *"**A butterfly flaps its wings in Brazil and causes a tornado in Texas.**"* I wasn't sure if we were about to trigger a tornado or just some good vibes, but I loved the thought of being a part of something bigger than myself.

PRIDE INTO HUMILITY:

Humility: "The quality of having a modest or low view of one's own importance. It involves being humble, recognizing one's limitations, and being open to learning from others. Humility is characterized by a lack of arrogance or pride, and an awareness that everyone has value and contributes in their own unique way. It often includes being receptive to feedback, acknowledging mistakes, and showing respect for others, regardless of their status or differences."

To kick things off, Justin **(THE STUDENT/ TEACHER)**, my assistant Olive (**THE STUDENT/ TEACHER**), and I decided to tackle pride by *humbling* ourselves. It started simple. We posted on social media, asking, "Hey, anyone need help with anything?" Then we went out to actually help them! First stop: a lovely lady who needed some help watching her son while she got work done around the house. Her son had ADHD and required special attention, so we spent the afternoon playing with his trucks and having a blast. It was a glorious day to see his bright smile light up going around on his motorbike, and it was a rewarding one.

Then, we helped a military man turned artist clear out his home, removing old furniture and hauling things to the dump. Nothing feels quite as good as lending a hand in those small moments of service. Maybe *that's* the true meaning of pride—doing good without the need for recognition.

ENVY INTO KINDNESS:

Kindness: "The quality of being friendly, considerate, and compassionate toward others. It involves showing empathy, offering help, and acting with generosity and warmth, without expecting anything in return. Kindness can manifest in both small, everyday gestures—like offering a smile or helping someone in need—and larger acts of support or care. It is an attitude of goodwill and a genuine desire to make others feel valued and supported."

Next up: Envy. What better way to counter envy than by spreading kindness everywhere? I set out with my signature move—giving away flowers. But this time, I went the extra mile, attaching personal notes to each bouquet. I left them in public places—on tables, in libraries, on mailboxes, and doorsteps. I was a flower bomb of positivity. I even showed up at my friends Rachel and Erin's business and surprised them with congratulatory notes. The joy on their faces was priceless. You could almost feel our hearts *hugging* each other.

GLUTTONY INTO TEMPERANCE:

Temperance: "The practice of self-control, moderation, and restraint, particularly in relation to one's desires, emotions, or consumption of certain things (such as food, alcohol, or material goods). It involves avoiding excess and maintaining balance in one's actions and behaviors. Temperance is about making thoughtful, deliberate choices that promote long-term well-being, rather than acting impulsively or indulgently. It is often considered a virtue in moral and philosophical traditions, encouraging individuals to manage their impulses and live a balanced, harmonious life."

To balance out gluttony, Justin and I volunteered at *Nourish NC*, a local food charity. We spent the day inside the warehouse, packing over 1,000 family boxes to be shipped out to the less fortunate. We got dirty, we got sweaty, and we were *exhausted*. But when you're making a difference, none of that matters. Sharing food, collecting supplies, and donating to those in need was one of the most fulfilling experiences of my life.

LUST INTO EXUBERANCE:

Exuberance: "The state of being full of energy, excitement, and enthusiasm. It refers to a lively, cheerful, and overflowing expression of joy, often characterized by an energetic or exuberant attitude. Someone displaying exuberance tends to show a great deal of enthusiasm or vitality, often in a contagious way, that can uplift those around them."

Lust wasn't about indulgence—it was about exuberance and joy. Justin and I teamed up with ***Atlantic Boudoir's,*** Alisha (**THE EMPOWERER**), in Wilmington to create a day of celebration and self-love for women. We held a giveaway, inviting a group of ladies to experience a sustainable makeover, all while empowering them through meditation, a cleansing ceremony, and self-love rituals. The morning of my birthday, I took the time to lead them through an experience that was as much for me as it was for them. We wrote letters to our future selves, sharing dreams and hopes for what was to come. And yes, they got flowers—because I never left home without them.

ANGER INTO PATIENCE:

Patience: "The ability to wait calmly for something without getting frustrated or upset. It involves enduring difficult situations, delays, or challenges without reacting impulsively or becoming agitated. Patience is characterized by self-control, tolerance, and the capacity to remain calm in the face of adversity or discomfort, often with the understanding that good things may take time. It is an important quality for managing stress, handling uncertainty, and maintaining perspective in difficult circumstances."

When it came to anger, I knew the antidote was patience. One of the most rewarding things I've done was adopt a grandparent. When I worked in home healthcare, I had the honor of helping an elderly couple, Helen and Ed (**THE REMINDERS**). They lived in an upscale neighborhood by the beach and were simply the definition of the human spirit. I'd help them with tasks they couldn't do themselves, like cleaning their cat's litter box, and bringing them homemade goodies. The joy it brought them was contagious. Helen's tabby cat, who adored her rollator (that's a fancy walker with wheels), would take joy rides around the house. Every time I think of them, my heart bursts with love.

GREED INTO LIBERALITY:

Liberality: "The quality of being generous, open-handed, and willing to share resources, whether it's money, time, or support, without expecting anything in return. It also refers to the willingness to give freely and to be open-minded, tolerant, and fair toward others, particularly in terms of differing opinions or lifestyles. Liberality involves a spirit of kindness, generosity, and broad-mindedness, often associated with an open, giving attitude toward others and a desire to promote the well-being of those around you."

As my birthday approached, I decided to turn the typical "me, me, me" celebration into an opportunity to give back. I threw a talent show at the *Busher and Barrel Grill*, and let me tell you, it was a hit! They made a special cocktail for the event, and all the proceeds went to Edens Village and Nourish NC. The energy was electric—friends from all parts of my life came to show their support. I hosted the event, performed a *hula-hoop routine* (yes, I am HER), and shared the stage with Mr. Killa and the gang. We were *almost official* by then, and it felt so good to celebrate love in front of everyone. The theme was simple: black attire, as it symbolized the end of my 20s. My friend Jose (**THE REMINDER**), always the sweet soul, invited a date that wore a white shirt. Bless him—he didn't follow the dress code, but I actually appreciated the pop of contrast. Shoutout to my assistant Olive, who was a total rockstar in helping make this night a success.

SLOTH INTO DILIGENCE:

Diligence: "The quality of being persistent, careful, and hardworking in the pursuit of a task or goal. It involves showing consistent effort, attention to detail, and dedication to completing a task or achieving a result. Diligence is characterized by a strong work ethic, focus, and a willingness to put in the time and effort needed to succeed, even in the face of challenges or obstacles. It reflects a commitment to thoroughness and excellence in one's work or responsibilities."

Finally, we tackled sloth with a day of *diligence*. I teamed up with the *Plastic Ocean Project* to help clean up our local community. Armed with trash bags, gloves, and an unstoppable team, we scoured the container district and collected any litter we could find. The work was tough, but the cause was bigger than any of us. When people from different backgrounds come together for the common good, something magical happens. And let me tell you, this project brought out so much love. It felt like we were planting seeds—seeds of kindness, change, and action—for the future.

Love Beyond Borders: Unconditional Love in Action

This whole experience got me thinking about unconditional love—and how it's not limited by race, nationality, or social status. Love can extend beyond borders, bringing humanity together in the most unexpected and beautiful ways. Acts of kindness, no matter how small, create ripples that inspire others to pay it forward. Unconditional love isn't just for the people we know—it's for the planet, for the environment, and for every living thing that calls it home.

What's more, unconditional love can be a *radical* act in today's world—a revolutionary move in a society that often feels divided and cynical. But when you give love freely, without expectation, something incredible happens: You create a space where others feel safe enough to do the same.

And that, my friends, is how the butterfly effect works. It's the tiniest of changes—a simple act of love—that can create *huge* ripples in the world. And if I can be a part of that ripple? Well, I think I'm doing alright.

So, let's keep loving, shall we?

CHAPTER NINETEEN

ENDING THE ERA.

Addressing Your Heartbreak:

How can we help our souls through a lonely hour? This question lingers, especially when we can no longer run or hide from ourselves. It's one of those moments when the silence feels deafening, and the stillness of our surroundings only amplifies the restlessness within. We may find comfort in solitude, seek it out even, believing it offers us a sanctuary. Yet, there are times when solitude reveals its other face—the one that carries a weight of loneliness that settles deep inside our bones.

I remember a time when I thought I just wanted to curl up and retreat into myself. I imagined that being alone would give me the solace I craved. But as the hours stretched on, that very peace began to unravel, leaving behind an emptiness I didn't know how to fill. The darkness crept in, subtle at first, but then it began to swell—thoughts that I had long avoided now swirling in my mind, tugging at me from every direction. I had overcompensated for so long, filling my days with noise, people, and distractions to stave off the reality of the loneliness I couldn't escape. It was easy to pretend everything was fine, to convince myself that I didn't need anything, that I didn't need anyone. But the truth was there all along, sitting quietly just beneath the surface.

And in that quiet, as uncomfortable as it was, I had no choice but to face myself. No more running. No more hiding. It was in those moments of raw stillness that I realized how much I had been avoiding—not just the loneliness, but the parts of me that were crying out for attention. The emptiness wasn't something to be feared. It wasn't something I had to numb or push away. Instead, it was an invitation to explore what I truly needed, to sit with myself and ask, *"What is this really about?"*

In the dark stirrings of that loneliness, I found something unexpected—an opportunity for growth. I realized that loneliness wasn't an enemy to be fought, but a teacher in disguise. It revealed the parts of myself that I had neglected, the feelings I had pushed aside. It wasn't comfortable, and it certainly wasn't easy, but it was necessary. And in those quiet, lonely hours, I learned how to meet myself where I was.

It wasn't about escaping the loneliness—it was about letting it wash over me, feeling it, acknowledging it, and then gently shifting my focus to what I needed to heal. Slowly, I began to reach for the small acts of self-compassion that would help me move through it. The simple comforts, like a cup of tea, a long walk, or a journal entry that poured my heart onto the page. These were the ways I began to care for my soul in the midst of the lonely hour.

When we face the silence, when we stop running, we are given the chance to reconnect with who we really are. It's in those dark moments that we can finally start to see the light—not as something we need to escape to, but as something we hold within. It's there, in the heart of loneliness, that we learn how to love ourselves in ways we've never known before.

The loneliness may not disappear overnight, but we can learn to live with it, to find meaning in it. In time, we come to understand that sometimes, being alone isn't a curse—it's a moment of clarity. A moment to remember that we are whole, even in our solitude, and that our souls can be nurtured even in the loneliest of hours.

CUTTING THE CORD:

So, remember when I mentioned dating a coil of people all at once? Well, the funny thing is, I think the reason my and Mr. Killa's relationship thrived so much was because we were utterly, painfully, and beautifully honest with each other about everything. It was like a secret we both kept without saying a word—we were mirrors, reflecting the same deviant, yet honest energy. He knew that, deep down, I must have been doing the same devilish things he was, living in the same chaotic space, making the same mistakes, and somehow, it worked. Early in our experience we were able to lay it all bare.

It was early in the relationship when I learned about his past/present. There was another girl—Fiona, **(THE RUNNER)** one he had deeply cared for, someone who had been through the same struggles he had. They had bonded over the lack of family, the absence of support. Their connection was forged through shared trauma long before me. But when she found out about me, it wasn't the right way. It should've been a conversation, a confrontation, but no, it was messy. It wasn't the way things were supposed to unfold, and, as usual, we had let things spiral.

In the end, we were all aware of each other and the roles we were playing. We tried to intertwine our lives—he and I, me and her, all of us together.

I even introduced him to Astro for a boat day, they became friends. Everyone else in my entangled conclave met him, everyone became friends, but somewhere in all of that, the tangled web of love and jealousy couldn't be untangled. We were all too invested, too intertwined, and it was never going to work. I had too many other energies in the mix, and he and her were connected in a very strong bond.

And no matter how badly I wanted to be the MAIN woman in his eyes, our lifestyles required an open relationship. No matter how deeply I felt that we belonged together, she wanted to be his one and only. And I *knew* that. Deep down, I knew she wasn't going to let him go, and honestly, neither was I. After all, I was his "dream girl." The moment he asked me to be his actual girlfriend, just after my birthday bash, it felt like a promise we both believed in. We were ***madly in love***, or at least, we thought we were. We thought nothing could break us. But then one night we all went out to the club together, everything changed. The dynamic was off. We had too many extra energies around us, most of them rooting for me. In her experience I was shifting too much attention, which might have been the truth. However, the only person's attention I wanted was his, and all of it was on her.

There was drinking, a storm of jealousy, and an unraveling of all the ties we had built. She thought I had a "superiority complex" –which at the time was laughable to me, but I did believe that I was, in many ways, fit to be the better match. Perhaps, maybe she was right. I did have a sense of ownership. Then, in the chaos of it all, Mr. Killa looked me dead in the eyes and said, "I choose her."

(THE HEARTBREAKER)

It was like a dagger through my heart. All the time, the energy, the love I poured into him, into us—trying to make our lives better, trying to make our work better, trying to make our dreams better—suddenly felt insignificant. I thought we had something real, something worth fighting for. But that moment proved it wasn't enough. It never was.

I had spent so much time imagining a future for us. We were literally going to roadtrip to Wisconsin for my childhood friend's wedding. I had all of the arrangements made for the event, and planned everything out. He was supposed to be my date, and I was the maid of honor. But now, everything was falling apart. I couldn't believe what was happening, couldn't grasp the way things were spiraling.

I made him drive me home. At first, he said he'd get me an Uber, and I snapped. "*Absolutely not. You owe me a ride at the very least.*" Stubborn on my own part, yes, but I deserved more than that shame. He had been so absent in so many ways that night, but I still needed him to do this one thing for me. We barely spoke on the way home, and I was so devastated, I couldn't even find the words. It felt like someone had suffocated me, leaving me breathless and lost. He apologized, but that wasn't enough. *"Sorry" wasn't* going to fix this. I was shook to my core, that in the end, the decision wasn't me. I wasn't successful in winning the fight to the death for the one I loved. He didn't choose me.

I spent the whole evening in tears, alone in the silence of my room, broken, confused, lost. I had known deep down this moment was coming, but I wasn't ready for it. I had convinced myself that this love, this deep love I had found with him, would last. I never thought I could find something like it again—not after I almost married someone else. A love like that was special. But here we were, and all of it was slipping away.

Days passed, and reality settled in like an uninvited houseguest. I had to cancel the plans I'd so meticulously crafted, swapping our grand road trip for a solo flight back to Wisconsin for the wedding. As fate would have it, just as I was about to board my plane, he called. Of course, he would. Timing was his specialty.

He was kind—annoyingly so—open and honest in a way that made my heart ache all over again. We danced around the inevitable, trying to untangle the mess of our shared future. There was still that festival looming in a few weeks. "We'll figure it out when you're back," he said. His words were steady, but my heart felt like it had been thrown into a blender.

Somehow, through all the chaos, my friends became my lifeline. They pulled me out of my heartbreak haze, shook me by the shoulders (metaphorically and maybe once literally), and reminded me that this weekend wasn't about me. It was about love—the kind I wasn't feeling, but had to celebrate anyway.

And so, I showed up. Not for myself, but for them. I watched them exchange vows, promising forever in a way that felt raw and real, even if my own love story was unraveling at the seams. I clapped, I cheered, I even smiled, though my heart felt like it was wearing a bandage made of duct tape.

It wasn't the love I had dreamed of, not the fairy tale ending I had clung to in my head. But maybe that's the lesson I needed. Letting go of what wasn't meant to be. Or, perhaps, letting go of my stubborn need to win. Because deep down, I couldn't tell if I was mourning him or the fact that I'd lost the fight.

I had played every card I had, stacked the deck in my favor, and still, somehow, I lost. She had won—victorious in a battle I didn't even realize I was fully fighting. And there I was, left with the bittersweet truth that I'd lost my best friend and the most romantically dramatic chapter of my adult life.

But hey, at least the wedding had an open bar.

Psychological Take Away:

The Importance of Self-Worth:

Pain highlights a reliance on external validation for self-worth. Psychologically, unconditional love starts with self-love—recognizing one's inherent value regardless of external circumstances.

The lesson of "letting go" becomes a critical turning point, underscoring the need to find wholeness within oneself before seeking it in another.

Growth Through Heartbreak:

The heartbreak, though painful, becomes a catalyst for growth. Reflecting on the need to reassess motivations and approach to love, transforming a painful experience into an opportunity for self-discovery and future resilience.

Selflessness in Moments: Despite the heartbreak, trying to show up for a friend's wedding, shifting focus from personal pain to celebrating others. This reflects a selfless aspect of love, a hallmark of unconditional love.

Acceptance of Loss: Over time, accepting that the relationship wasn't the right fit. This acceptance, though painful, mirrors the way unconditional love lets go when holding on causes harm.

Possession vs. Freedom: The sense of ownership and competition contrasts with unconditional love, which emphasizes freedom and non-attachment. The desire to be "the main woman" and "win" suggests love intertwined with ego and pride.

This encapsulates the messy, beautiful complexity of love, highlighting both the yearning for unconditional connection and the human challenges that often make it elusive. The experience taught me profound lessons about self-worth, acceptance, and the necessity of letting go when love is no longer mutual or healthy.

Trust the Signs, Follow the Beats:

So, here's a funny thing about how life works—and how it sometimes communicates with you through the most random ways. Let me take you back a bit, to my childhood. Picture this: me, in my brother's basement bedroom, jamming out to some Dr. Dre. The beats were bumping, the computer monitor was flickering with some strobe light settings (I swear, my brother was into all kinds of light shows and music), and the colorful desktop swirls were just as mesmerizing as the music itself. We were living our best life, no care in the world, just vibing to Cholo, Eminem, and the best tunes from his college years.

Little did I know that the song "Still DRE" would go on to foreshadow my future.

Fast forward to 2022. I had a goal. A very specific goal. "I'm going to learn to play the piano," I said. Don't ask me why it took me so long, but here we are. And guess what happens next? The piano version of *Still DRE* drops, and I'm hooked. I mean, I've never had a song speak to me like that before (besides all the 90s rap I grew up with, of course). Mr. Killa had let me borrow all of this music equipment and a keyboard was one of them. I was so excited, I couldn't wait to learn the keys.

Now, here's where the magic truly begins. I had just posted this beautiful piano version of a song on my Instagram, claiming it as my "theme song for California" because, well, it perfectly captured my vibe. A few days later, I'm in the sauna at the gym, about to warm up (because yes, I'm basically a fitness goddess in training), when something incredible happens.

My friend Kathryn—my gym buddy and low-key life coach, (***THE EMPOWERER)***—sits down and starts playing *that very same piano version*. In the sauna. I froze. "WHAT?! I just posted that song! Are you kidding me?" I blurted out. We both stared at each other, wide-eyed, like we'd just uncovered some cosmic conspiracy. She just laughed and said, "It randomly got stuck in my head, so I played it."

Kathryn was my saving grace, the kind of friend who enters your life right when you need them most. We'd been orbiting around each other for years, but during this particular season of transition, we finally collided. She was about to launch into her political career, a trajectory as bold and determined as she was, while I was gearing up to leap across the country.

Our gym dates were more than workouts—they were therapy sessions, filled with laughter, dreams, and the occasional venting session about life's chaos. And those cozy meals around the fire at her house? Absolute heart-savers. In those moments, surrounded by warmth and her steady encouragement, it felt like we were both gearing up for something bigger, something that would finally make all the waiting and longing worth it.

Now, fast forward again, to a week later. Kathryn and I are cruising to the woods for some much-needed R&R, just chatting away about my California dreams, and how we were obsessed with the dancers at "Playground LA" on Instagram. They were showing off moves at this dance studio, and we were imagining what it might be like for me to be part of that world. Suddenly, *the song* starts blaring through the radio. Mind you, we were listening to some old-school classical music station, so it *definitely* wasn't supposed to happen. We both froze. We looked at each other, and BAM—goosebumps everywhere. It was like the universe was yelling, "Hey, you're on the right path, keep going!"

And there it was, clear as day: a sign. A very funky, piano-filled, Dr. Dre-themed sign telling me that California was waiting for me, and I just had to follow that inner compass. The universe had spoken in the only way it knew how—through music, synchronicity, and a seriously random but somehow *perfect* moment.

Lesson learned: Trust those little moments. Follow the signs. If it feels right, go for it. And most importantly, never underestimate how much of life's clues are wrapped up in a song you *didn't* expect to hear on the radio at that exact moment. Trust your intuition. Keep moving forward. And trust the journey.

Take Inspired Action

When things start lining up, whether it's through music, signs, or random encounters, don't just brush them off. Start paying attention to what feels aligned. If you get a gut feeling, a nudge, or if you keep hearing the same song over and over again in random places (like I did!), take it as a sign to act. If you're unsure, ask yourself, "What does my heart say?" Then make the next move. Whether it's taking a leap of faith or a tiny step forward, let it move you. Let the universe show you the way.

How Does This Connect to Unconditional Love?

Well, let's talk about it. Just like that song kept popping up, unconditional love works in much the same way. It's there for you, consistently, without judgment or expectations. Unconditional love doesn't need to make sense; it just is. It's about trusting the journey, even when you can't see the full picture yet. It's about believing in yourself, even when things feel uncertain, and knowing that the universe (or love, or fate) has got your back. Much like my piano version of *Still DRE*, life has a funny way of sending you exactly what you need at the exact right time. You just have to be open to receiving it and follow the flow.

So, keep your ears open for your version of *Still DRE*—whether it's a song, a moment, or a feeling—and trust that it's leading you exactly where you need to go. Because just like California, your dreams are waiting for you.

NEW LIGHT.

It felt like a miracle wrapped in chaos, the way we kept orbiting each other, like two stars caught in a gravitational pull the universe couldn't resist. After everything, we always found our way back—sometimes as friends, sometimes as something messier, fueled by late-night "I miss you" texts that hit like whispers from fate.

When we were together, I'd hear this quiet voice in my head, stern but tired, like a wise old friend saying, *"This isn't right. You need to let go."* But my heart? Oh, it loved the drama, the misery, the bittersweet tension that seemed to spark a flood of creativity. Breakups became symphonies, heartbreaks birthed art.

I joked with him once, "I break up with you, in my head, every time we're together." He laughed, that easy, maddening laugh of his, and said, "That's great content."

We'd both laugh, and like a bad romantic comedy, the cycle started all over again. The real turning point came when I told him I was finally leaving—packing up my life and heading for California. He was thrilled for me, beaming with pride as he launched into one of his signature pep talks, the kind only he could deliver.

But just as I was preparing to slip away to Atlanta for a detour—to help a friend through a divorce—he stopped me dead in my tracks. With that piercing, no-nonsense look in his eyes, he asked, "What are you talking about? You belong in California. Why are you going to put that off? When are you going to live for yourself, or are you just going to let fear win?"

His words hit like a gut punch, but they were exactly what I needed to hear. I had been so focused on escaping that I hadn't stopped to think about embracing something just for me. I was always helping others first. For the first time, I realized he was right—I deserved to live for myself. Ironically, the guy who once told me, "You don't need me," was the one who pushed me to see that I needed *me.*

It was a lightbulb moment. I started shedding my old life, quite literally, selling him a bunch of my stuff—including my car, which he desperately needed. "Can I paint it matte black?" he asked with a grin. "Of course, it's your car now. Do whatever you want," I replied. Without missing a beat, he smirked and said, "Our baby—since we never had one" with a wink.

In those final hours of packing, when I was knee-deep in my suitcases and stress, he showed up again. This time, not as the person I used to lean on for love, but as someone empowering me to fly. He even offered to ship some of my things to Cali when I was completely stuck. His role in my life had shifted: he was no longer my partner, or (**THE HEARTBREAKER**) but (*THE EMPOWERER.*) And in some twisted, poetic way, that made all the difference.

"The end is never the end, A new challenge awaits, a test no man could be prepared for a new hell he must conquer and destroy, a new level of growth he must confront himself, the machine, and the ghost within, this is the journey —Kid Cudi

CHAPTER TWENTY

CALIFORNIA

"Feeling like I'm constantly being challenged into insanity."

Energy is communication, right? I try to tune into my soul and listen to the signs from the universe. When I started considering a move from North Carolina to LA, everything seemed to point in that direction. I saw signs everywhere—movies, conversations, spiritual nudges, even in emails. My eyes and ears were wide open, soaking it all in.

But, it felt like I was constantly navigating a maze. I'd hear "go right," then hit a roadblock, and suddenly it was "go left." So, I'd pivot and get stuck again. "Go up." Stuck again! I was like, "Seriously? I'm listening and following, why am I getting all these mixed signals?" Finally, I hit pause. I became still, listened, and prayed. I told myself, ***"This is meant for me; the way will be paved."*** And then, just like that, it started to happen.

After Wilmington, I found myself nestled in my parent's home, a brief pause in December's embrace. It seemed a perfect middle ground—coming back after ten years, a time to reconnect, reflect, and share the holiday warmth. I'd missed so much—especially my nephew's and niece's childhoods, watching from a distance as life spun its own story, miles and miles away. And as December unfolded, it became the canvas for my own *reset*.

I wandered through familiar streets, revisiting old haunts, letting memories whisper through the spaces that shaped me. My secret hiding place down by the lake behind and opening in the woods brought a lot of solace. This gem specifically hit "home" for me during bad decisions, emotional turmoils, happy existences. Each step back was a chance to appreciate the journey I'd taken—past decisions, triumphs, and lessons learned. Still, there was something inside, a pull to keep moving. My soul, restless, longed for the sun and salt of California.

The search was on. Applications sent, interviews stacked high like promises on a shelf. But finding a home? That was like chasing shadows. Until one call finally came through, a flicker of hope. A job in LA at a music store—a start. The pay wasn't lavish, but it didn't need to be. It was a doorway opening. The next challenge was a roof over my head.

At first, I'd brushed off a listing. But the phone rang again, and this time, a perfect room waited—well, *almost* perfect. The first one slipped away, but luck was on my side. A second room was available—this one even better. A room with a view, a patio, and a new chapter unfolding in front of me.

Like a whirlwind, everything clicked into place. A new path laid out before me, stretching westward, where the sun kissed the coast. My dad, always the master of planning, packed up my two suitcases with precision—along with my new recently purchased piano, a little piece of my heart and soul that I promised would follow me wherever I went. I'd bought that piano unaware that it would connect the dots to the job. Music would be my constant companion, guiding me on every road.

With a final hug and kiss, I said goodbye, *"See ya later,"* not knowing when or how the next chapter would unfold, but certain it was time to go. The journey stretched ahead, taking about a week, the road winding through winter's fury—snowstorms, freezing temperatures, and closed highways. The route I'd planned had to change, like life itself, constantly rerouting.

But the pit stops? Oh, they were magical. Each destination felt grander than the last. Photos were taken—my tears fell not from sadness, but from sheer awe. The world, vast and sprawling, seemed to take my worries and lift them into the air, reminding me how small we are in the grand scheme. Driving through the states, I realized that every road can be rerouted, every detour is a chance to grow. Forks in the road—decisions made on instinct, based only on what felt right. Was the road paved, or was it rocky? Smooth, or bumpy? Every road had a lesson to teach.

I checked in with family at every stop, keeping the thread of connection alive. The mountains, valleys, sunsets, and sunrises whispered their stories to me. I cried—not just from the weight of everything that had been, but from the quiet joy of knowing I was exactly where I was meant to be. There's no better place to hear God's voice than when you're on the path he's paving for you, moving mountains and making miracles along the way.

And then—California. A burst of sunshine, the promise of the West. I arrived at the hotel, a humble but welcoming Quality Inn. The bed was warm, the room a sanctuary after the long journey. I couldn't help but smile, knowing I was about to sleep in one state, and wake up in another—*California*. It was as if I had *finally* arrived. "California dreaming" they say..

I jumped on that bed like a child, laughing with joy. I wanted to shout, to scream, dancing to share the moment with the world. But for now, I just let myself be. The journey was only just beginning, but for the first time in a long time, I felt like I'd *made it*.

My apartment was incredible. From my window, I could see the Hollywood sign just 50 feet away! The building was a *smart building*—nothing like I'd ever experienced before. Everything was tech-driven; I needed my phone to access the locks, garage, gates, you name it. It was a bit surreal—there were hardly any humans around because it was all about the gadgets.

The best part? The rooftop. It offered breathtaking 360-degree views of the city. I could see the Hollywood Hills, Downtown, and the surrounding suburbs. It was exactly what I needed to shake things up. My word for the year was "breathtaking," and this place delivered. And let me tell you, the next chapter of my living experience was even more insane!

STARS ABOVE AND STARS BELOW:

The month prior passed, while I found myself at my parents' house, just days away from my big move to California. Mr. Killa had reached out to me, telling me he had a show in California—*LA*. I was shaking, literally trembling. To make it even more insane, his show was just a few blocks away from my new apartment. And, of course, it was happening *the very day* I arrived. The universe was just out here showing off at this point.

The first day I was moving into my new place, he asked for a ride from the airport, I couldn't believe it. I never imagined we'd be reunited so soon, but here we were, spending a week together in California, laughing, catching up, and having a blast. It was like time rewound itself, but this time, we were just...better. More honest. More ourselves. Even more loving, getting to explore the town together. Korean BBQ on the rooftop, burgers around the corner, trips to Target. Then his big show felt natural. Like nothing was different, except everything was— we were literally across the country together.

One evening, as we were winding down our adventure, he suggested, "Let's go for a hike." And we found ourselves asking, "Why didn't we do this while we were dating?" Funny how the world works.

So, naturally, we found ourselves climbing to the top of the observatory, AirPods in, jamming to music as we made our way up the mountain, stopping to snap goofy photos along the way. We laughed until we couldn't breathe. Then, just as we hit the top during golden hour, something magical happened.

As the sun dipped below the horizon, the sky erupted into a masterpiece of orange, pink, and purple—a breathtaking display that felt like it had been painted just for us. The glow stretched across the city below, casting everything in a warm, golden light. It was one of those rare moments that begged you to pause, to let time stand still, and simply *be*.

As night fell, the city lights began to twinkle like tiny stars scattered across the earth, mirroring the universe above us. There we were, caught between the sparkling lights of Hollywood superstars below and the shimmering constellations above, suspended in a magical in-between.

In that moment, it hit us: *we* were the stars in the middle, ready to shine, ready to glisten with our own light. It was poetic, cosmic, and just the right kind of dramatic—the perfect Hollywood moment, but somehow even better because it was real.

In that moment, with the world beneath us and the sky above, we made a prayer—a wish for our futures, for our paths to reveal themselves. MK always had a way of making life feel like a movie. I knew, even then, that there was no other person who could make an experience feel this special. It was more than just a night out, more than just a hike—it was a moment of pure magic.

Between the champagne showers, the red-room sushi nights, days spent in music studios with famous DJs, and excelling in my promo jobs, life felt like it was unfolding exactly as it should. We had been through so much together—pain, love, heartbreak, but somehow, in the chaos, we found peace. That peace was this: a new chapter, a new friendship, and a whole lot of blissful relief, coming together at the perfect time.

This story illustrates a **complex and layered relationship** that embodies aspects of unconditional love but remains grounded in human realities, such as personal growth, timing, and mutual benefit.

Unconditional Elements:

Forgiveness, joy, and shared elevation are at the core of their connection.

The ability to find peace and connection despite past heartbreak demonstrates a love that transcends specific conditions.

Blending of Unconditional Love and Personal Growth:

This relationship serves as a **catalyst for healing and transformation**, blending unconditional affection with the realistic boundaries needed to maintain emotional health.

NEW LOVE ON THE HORIZON:

Chi was the definition of tall, dark, and handsome—a 6'5" Nigerian man with an eight-pack in all the right places. He was a retired football athlete, effortlessly radiating strength and confidence. Fortunately for me, our paths crossed early on, when I pulled into my parking space in the underground apartment garage. God blessed me with a spot right next to the elevators, and on the other side of those elevators stood *him*.

I remember the first time I laid eyes on him. I saw him from behind, wearing a tan trench coat, with a woman lingering in the shadows nearby. At first, we didn't really pay attention to each other. Our interactions were brief and fleeting, but that was about to change.

One day, I parked a little too far back. I had just gotten a new car and wasn't completely aware of the surrounding space. The compact parking spot was a bit too tight, but I thought nothing of it. The next morning, I found a note on my windshield. "Learn how to park!," it read, and immediately, I felt guilty. "Welcome to LA, already pissing people off..." I thought.

I tried to push the thought away, but the next day, I stepped off the elevator, only to see him standing there—*Chi*. He was looking at me, then glancing at my car. With his thick Nigerian accent, he said, "This is your car, for you?"

I felt terrible, but I smiled brightly and responded, "Ah, yes, I apologize."

That's when it happened. I saw him fully for the first time. His gaze locked with mine, and in that moment, I realized just how gorgeous he was. There was an undeniable chemistry, something electric in the air. We both hurried into the elevator—he was on the third floor, I was on the second.

From that day on, I made a promise to myself and told my friends, "That man will be mine."

TRYOUTS TO THE FUTURE:

As I settled into California, just seven days after arriving, the excitement of my goals and dreams started to take shape. One of the first big steps was the tryout for Insomniac. I could feel the buzz in the air, but my stomach was in knots. I made sure to print out my headshots and set off on my journey downtown.

I arrived around noon, and the line was already wrapped around the building twice. I joined the crowd, quickly striking up conversations with the people around me. In front of me, there was a couple—the girl was sweet but visibly nervous, while her boyfriend was just there for moral support. He was even kind enough to grab us Starbucks, they paid for me. It was such a kind gesture, I knew it was going to be a fantastic day. Behind me, I recognized a familiar face: it was the girl I'd bumped into at the parking meter earlier. There was also a mother nearby, though she was dressed in fancy heels that seemed a little out of place.

Despite the long wait, the group around us became fast friends, sharing stories and laughter. Hours passed, but finally, it was time to step up to my box. By then, I was feeling prepared. A redheaded girl, who had previously worked for the company, had shared plenty of helpful tips, and I felt ready to take on the challenge.

As I walked toward the three boxes, I danced down the stairs into position, feeling the rhythm take over. Freestyling, glowing, and radiant, I forgot what it felt like to be in the spotlight. For a moment, I felt like I was "home," as if everything I had worked for had led to this very moment. I blacked out briefly, overwhelmed by the excitement of what my future was about to bring. My life was about to change again.

A few days after the tryouts, I was thrilled to get an interview with the company to join "Ground Control." With my ICU background, it felt like the perfect fit. I was excited that this company could offer an umbrella under which I could work all of my talents in one place. The idea of being able to choose which shows I wanted to perform at while also being a first responder was a dream come true, hitting every angle of what I wanted to do.

My first show was Wonderland, which was based around an Alice in Wonderland theme. I remember stumbling into the food line where I bumped into a gentleman wearing a bucket hat who offered me his little duckies. Funny enough, he had seen my partner and me at the parking lot earlier. It turned out that we were both working at Oasis, a safe place for festival-goers to take a break if the crowd got too overwhelming.

Daniel **(THE EMPOWERER)** and I spent the whole weekend together, laughing, touring the festival, and chasing the lineups. His military background and my nursing background gave us an unspoken understanding of each other. We connected instantly, going from strangers to the best of friends.

Weeks went by, and we realized we were both going to be performing at the biggest show together. By then, we knew we had to ride together.

Fawn decided to swoop into my life in LA just a week before my big debut, as if the universe thought I needed a little extra chaos to spice things up. I knew this was about to be an exciting and fast-paced season! We had a jam-packed week planned: giggling like schoolgirls, exploring the city, and indulging in far too much junk food—our usual brand of friendship.

We'd bought tickets to the RuPaul Drag Show, but in true *us* fashion, we rolled in so late that first day, we missed half the razzle-dazzle. Still, we made the best of it in our comic book girl outfits, strutting around like we owned the place. I have to admit, pink hair *really* works for me—there's something magical about stepping into a whole new character.

Somewhere in the middle of all the fun, Vanessa decided she wanted to come visit too. Her timing? Impeccably chaotic, overlapping with Fawn. So, the three of us juggled sushi girlie dates, belly laughs, and whirlwind catch-ups. After brushing Fawn off to the airport, Vanessa and I dove headfirst into life updates and transitions. Showing her my new LA world was an absolute blast.

A couple of nights before my big performance, the producer sent me a ridiculous video of the 80's dance routine we were supposed to learn. Cue rooftop rehearsals, hula hoops in hand, under a canopy of glittering stars and the dazzling LA skyline. Practicing up there felt like a scene from a movie—dreamy, chaotic, and absolutely unforgettable.

Finally, it was showtime. We packed up and hit the road, heading to Daniel's place for what promised to be an unforgettable weekend of camping adventures. On the way out, we bumped into Chi. Flashing my signature charm and a beaming smile, I fielded his curious glance at my ridiculous pile of luggage. "I'm off to perform in Las Vegas," I said breezily, "but Vanessa's holding down the fort here. Catch you later!"

He smiled back, and just like that, we were off—speeding toward what felt like Neverland, ready for magic, mayhem, and memories.

Similarity to Unconditional Love:

These relationships showcase acceptance, joy, and support, essential elements of unconditional love.

The friends offer presence and encouragement, creating a foundation of trust and safety.

Unconditional love, as understood in psychology, may look different when applied to friendships versus romantic or familial contexts. Here, it is less about sacrifice and more about *shared empowerment and mutual celebration*—a modern take on love that honors individuality alongside connection.

CHAPTER TWENTY ONE

PERFORMING FEELS.

Las Vegas: the city that never sleeps, where dreams are made, and anything can happen. I had been granted the right of passage, and let me tell you, when I got the call to be part of one of the biggest EDM music tours of my career, as a professional dancer, I could barely believe it. Vegas had a special place in my heart because, every time I've stepped foot in that city, something big happens in my life. (My 21'st, Friends bachelorette, Performing EDC, Author Book PR, Business Conventions)

It was the night of my first showcase, and I had prepared for this moment long before I even landed in Vegas. (Thanks to Venessa she came to visit me in LA ahead of time). We'd been rehearsing non-stop for a day. We literally thought we'd have the whole routine, but when it was time to rehearse we realized, we got to choreograph our own parts, and all shows would be different based on which girl was hosting the round, so I knew I was ready. But still, as I stood backstage, getting mic'd up, the butterflies hit me like a tidal wave. And you know what? I've come to love that feeling. If your dreams don't make you nervous, they're just not big enough, right?

When the DJ and producer cued me to enter the stage, I bolted into the spotlight. That's when it hit me: this is where I was meant to be. It felt like *home.* There's something magical about being on stage, knowing you're about to do what you love in front of a crowd, and that sense of calm that washes over you as you realize you're built for this.

I live to entertain, whether it's telling a joke, sharing a wild story, or getting the crowd to dance. The most important thing to me? Making people smile. That's the real magic. The energy from the crowd is like a drug, and the more I interact with them, the more alive the show becomes. It's a beautiful cycle: the audience feeds me their energy, and I return it tenfold. I was in my zone, and nothing was going to stop me now.

As the night went on, I wasn't just dancing—I was hosting, too. And let me tell you, hosting an event is where I truly shine! I helped run a dating game called "*Up to Date*," where I pulled audience members on stage to try and find their "true love." We were the matchmakers. It was a huge hit! We laughed, joked, and the energy was electric. I could feel the magic in the air as the crowd cheered and got into it.

But just when I thought the night couldn't get any better, *bam*—the finale arrived. The desert rain started pouring down, drenching everything in sight, but I wasn't about to let that ruin my vibe. I was on stage, laughing and twirling in the rain, feeling like the luckiest person in the world. And then, as if the universe was in on the fun, the fireworks went off—*and wow*, they were absolutely breathtaking. I've worked at a firework store before, I've seen dozens of shows, but nothing compared to the beauty of those fireworks lighting up the desert sky. It felt like a 15 minute finale, but the whole experience, which made the finale even more insane.

That moment, standing in the rain with fireworks above me, filled my heart and soul in a way I'll never forget. It was a full-circle moment that made me feel like I was exactly where I was supposed to be and every hurdle I handled to get to that moment was worth it. I'll always cherish that memory and the reminder that when you follow your dreams, life gives you moments that take your breath away.

Married Under the Electric Sky:

36.2725° N, 115.0104° W

Sara, my metaphorical "wife". (**THE EMPOWERER**) This bombshell of a woman entered my life like a surprise plot twist—unexpected yet undeniably perfect. Beneath her incredible exterior, I sensed a quiet plea for help, a longing that spoke to my soul. It was as if fate had handed us a script and said, "You two are meant to coexist together." And let me tell you, I needed that. I was struggling, drowning in the chaos of my own life when we met on the set of what was supposed to be my career-defining performance.

Returning to the professional dance world had felt like stepping into a battlefield, and the experience? Well, let's just say it was more abusive than a toddler with a crayon in a white room. From the company's growing pains to the complete neglect of the staff, it felt like the wheels were coming off every moment. They say managing a massive event is like wrestling a monster—many moving parts and far too many people to disappoint. But somehow, we all kept holding on, even when the basics were forgotten. I went two days without a meal ticket, sweating in the desert heat, while the transport broke down, leaving us to walk miles just to reach the location. Dehydrated, frustrated, and struggling to remember my dance moves, I could barely keep it together.

Then, amidst this circus of chaos, I caught a glimpse of her—my first round partner. There were two other girls I'd be with in the next rounds. She shot me a look, probably wondering who this overly dramatic mess of a dancer was. I gasped, desperate for anything to pull me out of my downward spiral. "What do you need?" she asked, her voice like a lifeline thrown into a storm. I looked at her, barely holding on, and whispered, "I need hydration, electronics, and light. It's too dark back here... I swear the energy vampires are coming for me."

Without skipping a beat, she handed me water, plugged in my electronics, and grabbed my hand. "Let's go get you some light, girl," she said with a grin.

We ran, half-laughing, half-breathing heavily, and stumbled next door to the nearby chapel. It was an all white chapel with bright lights, walking down a red carpet. In our delirious state, we joked, "We're gonna get married." A voice from behind us answered, "Ah. No, you're not!"

As luck would have it, we were standing in the way of a real wedding— one that wasn't ours but belonged to a friend of the festival's founder. "Time to go!" we laughed, scrambling out before anyone could think we were serious. But the light we had found in that chapel stayed with us, and with it, laughter became our armor. We took our newly energized selves to the rides, where we bonded with patients and joked, "Is this seriously our job right now?" Riding on the rides with them, attempting to recruit people to be on our show.

That weekend, we became more than friends. We became partners in crime.

Sara was going through her own journey of learning to trust. As we got split from the group, she handed me all her things, a silent plea for reassurance. She wondered to herself, *"What would I do if we got separated?"* She had assumed I'd be just another flaky friend, lost in the crowd. But I looked her dead in the eyes, my voice steady, "Bitch, there's no way that's going to happen. I'm sticking to the buddy system—this festival's a beast, and I'm not letting us get lost." We set up a prayer circle, protecting ourselves from bad energy and making sure no negativity could mess with us.

We were just two souls, having fun, doing good work, and celebrating life.

After our vows, life with Sara only got wilder. We dove headfirst into future business plans, which turned into a ridiculous, hilarious adventure all on its own. We called it "our plans for world domination, how we were going to take over the world. (Cue evil laugh) But that's a whole other story—one that could only be called: BOSS BABE Chronicles.

Death to Erica: To the Woman I've Become:

In 2023, I stood at a crossroads in Las Vegas—an unexpected place for a deep transformation to unfold. That was when I realized that the version of me I had been holding onto, the person I once knew, was no longer who I wanted to be. Vegas, for all its lights and chaos, became a place where the old me had to say goodbye. It wasn't just the glitz and glamour of the city, but the magnitude of what I had just achieved—performing at the biggest show of my life underneath the electric sky. Five million people. I had just stood on a stage, performing for a sea of faces, and it was there, in that moment, that I felt something shift deep inside me.

The old Erica died that night. I felt it in my bones, in my heart. She had tried to live here, to function in this new world, but the version of me that left Vegas wasn't the same. I wasn't Erica anymore. I had become something else. I left as *Aire*, a name that reflected the new energy I was embracing. A nickname I had been called my whole life by many-especially Caroline and my dad. I just changed the spelling later. The fiery, youthful vision that had once defined me was no longer the driving force. I had come to understand that I wasn't just meant to burn with passion—I was meant to harness the wind, to use the air to light the fire and change the very color of the flame.

The grief I felt as I left behind the old Erica was real. I mourned the version of myself that had lived in fear, in confusion, in a constant state of "trying." But I also felt relief. *Aire* was born from the ashes of who I was, and with that rebirth, came a sense of clarity. A sense of purpose. A sense of freedom.

I know it may sound strange to some, but in California it's more accepted for people to change their names. When I say I don't go by Erica anymore, I mean it. It's not just a preference; it's an acknowledgment of who I am now and the person I am no longer. If someone calls out that name, I don't even hear it. I almost forgot it for a brief moment. If I've asked you as a friend to stop calling me by that old name, I'm not doing it for dramatic effect or to make a point. I'm doing it because that version of me—*Erica*—died in Vegas. And in her place, someone new was born.

And it's okay to grieve that loss. We all have our moments where we need to shed old skins. It's in that grief, in the letting go, that we make space for something better, something truer.

This brings me to my mentor, Ty. His journey, like mine, was filled with ego deaths—those pivotal moments when the old versions of ourselves have to die for us to evolve. Ty had to confront his own ego, his own limitations, and ultimately, he was re-humbled by the need to heal and grow. He couldn't continue living the life he had been living. The man he had been had to be laid to rest so that a new version of him could rise—one led not by pride, but by character, by humility, and by a deeper understanding of what it meant to truly be a man of integrity.

In some ways, I see my own journey reflected in his. It's not just about shedding the past; it's about becoming the best version of ourselves. It's about understanding that sometimes, the hardest moments in life—the ones that feel like they're breaking us—are actually the moments that make us whole.

So, to the woman I've become: Thank you for choosing to rise. Thank you for embracing the grief and the healing, the shedding of old layers, and the courage to be reborn. It wasn't easy, and it wasn't comfortable. But it was necessary.

As I continue to move forward, I know that *Aire* is just getting started. The flame that was lit in Vegas is burning brighter than ever, and it's powered by the wind beneath it. With each step I take, I'm not just walking away from the past—I'm flying toward a future that's waiting to be fully embraced.

This speaks to a profound psychological and emotional transformation, capturing the essence of unconditional love toward oneself, particularly through the lens of self-acceptance and rebirth. Let's break it down in psychological terms.

Ego Death and Identity Reformation: "The concept of "**ego death**" is central here, where the old version of Erica—previous self-concept— was shed in favor of a completely new identity. This is akin to the idea of *"psychological death and rebirth,"* a common theme in both psychoanalytic theory and spiritual development. When a protagonist refers to leaving behind the old name and adopting the new name it is symbolic of a *self-reclamation* process. In many ways, this is an expression of what Carl Jung called the *"individuation process,"* where an individual confronts and integrates various aspects of the unconscious to become a more authentic self."

The passage highlights how shedding an old identity—no matter how painful—creates space for growth, much like the phoenix rising from the ashes. The grief experienced during this shedding is not a sign of weakness but a necessary step in transformation. This parallels the *mourning* process that comes with the acceptance of deep personal change, which in itself can be viewed as an act of *"unconditional love."*

Grief as a Necessary Part of Healing: The grief felt during this transition is significant. In psychology, grief is seen as a vital process that accompanies any significant loss, whether it's a person, a life situation, or, in this case, a former self. Acknowledge this grief and allow it to exist. There is no avoidance here—only acceptance and understanding that letting *go* is a part of personal evolution. This acceptance of grief ties back to the notion of unconditional love, where we allow ourselves to feel pain in order to move forward, knowing that this discomfort ultimately leads to *healing*.

AFTERGLOW:

Returning to my civilian life between gigs, I found myself entangled in an unexpected encounter with Chi. Our paths crossed again in the elevator, and I could tell that my energy and bright smile caught his attention. There was something about him that intrigued me, and I couldn't shake the feeling that the universe was pushing us together.

Then, one day, I bumped into him again at LA Fitness, just down the street from our apartments. It felt like fate had given us another nudge, so I took matters into my own hands and texted him, asking if he wanted to carpool to the gym next time. From that moment on, our connection blossomed quickly.

One evening, after we'd gotten home from the gym, I invited him into my room. As he looked around, admiring the family photos and how I'd designed the space, he suddenly lifted me off my feet and onto the bed. The passion was immediate, a hot, electric energy between us that felt completely natural. It was the start of a whirlwind romance. Before I knew it, we were spending all our time together. We began doing everything together. After work, he'd come home in his sexy suit, grab my hand, and lead me to his room upstairs. The chemistry between us was undeniable.

As our leases came to an end, something strange and wonderful happened: we realized we were both moving to the same street, just a few blocks over from one another. It felt like the next chapter of our story was unfolding perfectly. Around this time, I became completely obsessed with my hula hoop (thanks to Mr. Killa, who had bought me the top-of-the-line hoop for my birthday). I wanted to take my passion for dance, yoga, and hula hooping to the next level, so I reached out to some friends from the festival and started training in aerial apparatus and fire play. I was in my element, spending the next six months pushing myself to grow and expand in ways I'd never imagined.

When it came time to help Chi move into his new place, we were both thrilled. We celebrated by properly christening his new apartment, indulging in each other's company and enjoying every moment together. But then, things took a turn.

Right before I was supposed to move out of my place, the building started drilling and making noise, which delayed my move. I ended up spending almost every night at Chi's, but then his behavior started to change. He told me he was getting a roommate and that I couldn't come over anymore. It was such strange, confusing behavior, and I couldn't understand what was happening. It left me feeling unsure about where we stood and what was going on between us.

Second-Handed Season:

I was all set to move into this gorgeous condo—high ceilings, a pool, bright and airy vibes, mirrored doors, bathtubs, master closets, and vanities. A friend of mine and I had the perfect plan. We were going to transform the master bedroom into a music studio/green room, combining all our experiences and content creation gear to turn our home into a full-sized creative hub. We envisioned dancing, making music, and filming videos for our YouTube channel.

But then, on move-in day—after paying the deposit and everything—the landlord pulls the apartment because of my roommate's credit. It felt like a total betrayal. "That's the excuse they gave," I thought, but let's be real—it was Hollywood, and I suspected the owner just wanted to give it to a friend or someone with a sob story. Either way, I suddenly found myself homeless.

Looking back, I had made myself homeless the summer before by living in a container, selling my stuff, and renting a unit to travel for music promos. This time it felt different; it was like the universe kicked me into gear to explore. I thought I had all the green lights for that condo, but clearly, I was meant to be on a different path.

During this time, I called another friend who was going through a breakup. I shared my apartment saga, and she excitedly offered her big mansion since she was hardly ever there. I started moving my stuff in, making all the perfect arrangements, but then her much older boyfriend came back into the picture. He wasn't thrilled about us moving in to help her through her next chapter.

Looking back, it felt like a way for her to reclaim control over her relationship. She was the rich type who treated her mansion like a museum: "You can look but don't touch." It reminded me again of my ex's-mother, who owned that million-dollar mansion in the mountains and freaked out if anything got damaged. It was fair, but to the point where you felt like you couldn't even breathe in the house. Felt like you were walking on eggshells. It wasn't a home. Moral of the story? I had to move out abruptly again after some family wedding sob story. I wasn't welcome to stay, I knew there had to be a bigger blessing for this terrible repeating house cycle. That was the third or fourth place I wasn't "supposed" to live in. Perhaps, in hindsight, I was just reliving experiences and seeing how I would respond and react. Had I learned the lessons of the past, and let things go? Listen more to my intuition and with flow? Crazy enough, but she called to tell me a couple of weeks later that her house had got broken into. It was a nice and safe neighborhood. It had gunshots and bullet impressions on the garage door. I couldn't help but laugh when I processed the situation, "Wow, I literally dodged a bullet." God didn't really want me there, it was just a temporary pit stop.

So, I packed my things into a storage container and decided to embrace the freedom of being a free spirit once again. Living out of my car, I made spontaneous trips to San Diego, soaked up the sun on the beaches, watched meteor showers in Joshua Tree, and played volleyball by the ocean. I loved the freedom, the ability to go wherever the wind took me. But, as life often goes, my relationship with Chi continued to fade away. Life's chaos kept us from seeing each other as much, and the distance between us only grew.

We had planned a special vacation for our birthdays in August, a trip to Catalina, a place I had connections with through my travels. But when I brought it up to confirm the details, Chi dropped a bombshell—he didn't want to go anymore. It was one of many disappointments that seemed to pile up during my birthday month. I still didn't have a place to call my own, and my two best friends, Christy and Nikki, were flying out to visit me in California. But the trip turned into a disaster. Nikki and I checked into an Airbnb, only to have the hosts report a crime the night before we arrived. Christy's arrival was met with the shocking news that Los Angeles was expecting a hurricane. It felt like everything was falling apart.

On my birthday, as if things weren't already messy enough, Chi called me to wish me a "happy birthday." Then, with no hesitation, he casually dropped that he had bought a ticket to Catalina for the weekend— without me. I couldn't believe it. The discomfort in my stomach was overwhelming. How could he do this, especially on my birthday? I didn't call him after that. Our relationship, it seemed, had simply ceased to exist.

Then there was Ka'ila, an old apartment neighbor of mine. She was a stunning beauty with dark hair, olive skin, and a floral sleeve tattoo. Over the years, we became long-time friends, sharing many experiences together—getting tattoos, having coffee dates, exchanging houseplants, cooking homemade meals, and offering each other a place to crash during tough times. She made a deep impact on my life: always showing me grace, support, and love. Never any judgment. **(THE EMPOWERER)** One day, she suggested I stay with a guy she had met while working at the coffee shop. He seemed cool, chill, and we all thought it was going to be a good fit.

BOY, was that a nightmare! He turned out to be one of the most disrespectful roommates ever. And I once lived with five other girls in a house with **one bathroom,** in college! (Imagine that disaster.) It was originally his house, so he'd just walk into my room unannounced, eat all my food, and then send me passive-aggressive texts about nonsense, acting like everything was fine when he got home. **THE WORST!**

I'll admit I'm definitely not blameless in our situation either, but it was clear we clashed because he thought he had to be right about everything. I tried to be mindful of everything I did, the dishes, cleaning up after myself, not taking too much "space". I really set him off one day, after I texted to ask if he'd mind if I rearranged our kitchen a bit differently. It made more room for the bikes and fridge. He agreed, told me he liked it, and a few days later when I was gone, everything went back to his original way. (Yikes) The biggest lesson I learned from all this was about respect—The lack of it, disrespect.

Amid all these experiences, I began to reflect: Was I being respectful of his things? Was he respecting mine? Was I feeling frustrated anywhere else? Other friendships? Work? And then it hit me—I needed to ask myself, *"Was I respecting myself?"*

Elysium Park, Life's Mirroring:

34.086288, -118.237869

How many minutes do I need to spend wishing for the things I want in life? I realized today that I need to stop waiting for things to fall into place and take the bull by the horns. It's time to create my own path, to make things happen, not just dream about them.

I've found myself at a crossroads today, sitting at a familiar park—a place I've been to many times before, yet each visit feels new, like it's meant to teach me something. Elysium Park. The air here feels different, charged with possibilities. Over the past year of living in LA, I've joined a group called the "Gratitude Group." They host free sound baths and journaling sessions in the park, offering a peaceful retreat for anyone who wants to embrace mindfulness. They meet on Sundays, sometimes Saturdays, in a sober, joyful space to nurture the soul rather than harm the body. This group became my anchor in LA—my "church" without being a church, where I could just be, without pretense or expectation.

But today, as I drove down the street toward the park for a solo retreat, I felt a pull, a desire to connect with nature and detox my mind. Even though I arrived late, the energy in the park was palpable. The chimes from the sound healer filled the air, and I felt the sun on my skin, bringing a sense of calm and bliss. Laying my things down on the grass, I looked up at the sky and felt at peace, surrounded by towering trees and the soothing sounds of the world around me.

After the sound healing, something unexpected happened: a neighbor lent me a pen. I had forgotten mine, which is rare, but I've learned to trust these little "coincidences." To me, it's a sign from the universe to engage, to connect. And so, I did. As I walked over to a table with a giant coloring sheet for the community project, I was introduced to someone. A man, I was told, was a famous DJ who had toured the world. My first instinct was to feel curious—what could this person offer me? But, as I've been practicing, I reminded myself that everyone is simply human, just like me. "We're all special," I thought. Some of us just have a little more star power. He's not here to offer me anything, I should be offering something to him in service.

We started chatting, and I listened as he shared his journey. He spoke of the places he's toured, the people he's met, and the music he's created. Then, he said something that echoed in my spine: "I've played with the greats, taught for 15 years, but the doubts still creep in. Am I big enough? Should I be here? What's next?" It struck me deeply. He had everything—success, recognition, a career to envy. And yet, the doubts still lingered. When do we ever feel like we've "arrived"? When is it ever *enough*?" This insight gave me chills. I thought, "What if he's right? Is there ever a limit we cap ourselves at being great enough?"

Later, I spoke with another leader in the group, William. We shared our backgrounds, and as we sought guidance from a spiritual advisor, I asked him how he felt about the message he received. He admitted, "I doubt myself and my purpose often." The message I got was loud and clear. Here was someone who had been a consistent leader, gathering people from all walks of life, creating community events to inspire connection and service. Yet, even he wrestled with self-doubt.

In that moment, I realized something profound. I was hearing the same message over and over again: *doubt*—doubt in purpose, in ourselves, in what we have to offer. And I had to ask myself: What is the mirror showing me? Am I still doubting my own belief in myself?

This was such a beautiful question to ponder in my thirties, a time when I am finally starting to understand who I am as a woman, as a person in this world. But it also challenged me to transcend those old limiting beliefs. If I want others to follow me, to believe in my vision, then I must first believe in it wholeheartedly myself. If I don't back myself, how can I expect anyone else to? I need to be so sure of who I am, what I stand for, and what I believe in, that doubt has no place in my life.

The lesson here was clear: *Unconditional love starts with loving and trusting yourself first.* When we hold unwavering belief in our own worth and purpose, we can begin to show up fully for others. The doubts and fears may always try to creep in, but I now know that it's up to me to stand tall, rooted in love, in my own power. The universe mirrors back to us what we project—and I'm choosing to project belief, love, and strength.

Self-Actualization and Personal Empowerment:

The realization that it is time to stop "waiting for things to fall into place" and instead *take the bull by the horns* speaks directly to the concept of "*self-actualization*—the "psychological theory" proposed by Abraham Maslow, which suggests that the ultimate goal of human development is to become the best version of oneself, fulfilling one's potential. This moment marked a key shift in my consciousness, from passively wishing for change to actively creating it. The desire to "make things happen" represents an internal decision to claim one's own agency and power in shaping their life.

This is also a form of *self-empowerment*, no longer waiting for external circumstances to change, but taking control of the journey. This decision to act aligns with *unconditional self-love*, which requires a deep acceptance and trust in one's abilities to affect change in their own life, without needing external validation.

Recognition of the mirror of doubt. These "coincidences" are not merely chance encounters but are signs from the universe that reflect my inner conflict. This idea aligns with the *law of attraction*, a psychological concept suggesting that the energy we project outward is mirrored back to us by the world.

The mirror is reflecting self-doubt, a common human experience, and it prompts us to consider how these external reflections speak to the internal belief system.

This question—"Am I still doubting my own belief in myself?"—is at the heart of this chapter's exploration of *unconditional love*. Unconditional love for oneself means overcoming self-doubt and the limiting beliefs that prevent us from fully stepping into our own worth. It is a call to transcend those old, familiar insecurities that have held us back, and to fully embrace their power and potential. The lesson is clear: the moment I learned to trust myself, *doubt had no place* in my life. This marks a psychological shift from self-doubt to self-empowerment.

Dancing Into My Own Light

I felt something beautiful: my mind, body, and spirit came together in a dance of their own. It's the kind of feeling where you just know things are aligning, where every movement feels like a release, a reminder of who I'm becoming. It's funny because I pulled an affirmation card that was all about dancing, and honestly, it couldn't have been more perfect. The synchronicity made me smile, knowing that this journey I'm on isn't just about pushing limits—it's about exploring the parts of myself I'm still discovering.

Dancing has always been an outlet for me, a way to express what words sometimes can't capture. But let's be clear, I don't dream of becoming a professional dancer. What I want is to be an artist—someone who sings, writes, and dances, and lets the creativity flow in whatever form feels right. The freedom of expression is what matters to me. I don't need to fit into someone else's mold of what it means to "make it." Dancing isn't about perfection; it's a channel for energy.

CHAPTER TWENTY TWO

NOURISHING THE BODY.

Sara called me out of the blue, as she often does, on our off and on again "fake marriage" and we quickly fell into our routine of brainstorming ideas—this time, our conversation centered around our usual ideas of "world domination" through the lens of food. We both share a passion for exploring how food shapes our lives, and how society's relationship with it is often misunderstood.

For me, this conversation felt especially significant because of my own long journey with food. When I moved to North Carolina 12 years ago, I looked as though I was three months pregnant—not because of pregnancy, but because of the way the food I was consuming was affecting my body. It was eye-opening, and I've been on a healing journey ever since, learning what my body actually needs and desires, rather than following trends.

Sara, with her background in nutrition, explained the process of digestion and how it takes years for our bodies to truly develop the muscle memory needed for proper digestion. We even dove into the topic of true nutrition for babies and the struggles new mothers face. She mentioned that she wanted to market her business to support mothers in their nutrition journey, which got me thinking about how we often find ourselves overwhelmed by choices. I've worked with clients in the past who made excuses about not wanting to cook multiple meals for their families or who were confused about which products to buy, often feeling pressured by the ever-changing consumer culture driven by capitalism.

That's when it hit me—why do we keep buying into the next "best thing" when it comes to food, especially when it's not necessarily the healthiest option? We're bombarded by advertisements and trends, but the truth is, we need to shift our focus to what's actually good for us. It's time to stop letting ourselves be brainwashed by the system and start taking action. We can begin by educating ourselves on holistic practices and learning to nourish our bodies with real, whole foods. This isn't just about following fads; it's about making mindful choices that will genuinely benefit our health.

The lesson here is that we need to be intentional about what we put into our bodies and take responsibility for our choices. Instead of feeling overwhelmed by the pressures of the next big trend, we can simplify our approach to nutrition by going back to the basics—learning what's actually healthy and sustainable. I'm committed to this process of continuous learning and action, and I encourage others to join me in prioritizing their health in a more conscious, educated way.

Which I took to a whole new example with the Blood Type Diet:

Blood Type Diet:

Have you ever heard of this? Well in my years of nursing and watching as my mother went in and out through years of diets because of her "autoimmune diseases", guess what, mother like daughter. If your mother is going through pain, sickness, or trauma during pregnancy you better recognize that's most likely where your pain is nurtured from, in some sort of sense, and was created while being in the womb. Whether genetically, energetically, or a body frequency, it's where it all comes from.

I started to notice, between high school & college years, I seemed to always feel or look three months pregnant in my stomach area, like my mother, based on foods my body *"wasn't supposed"* to eat. I went down this deep, dark, rabbit hole to find any research central on this topic.

Thanks to the study of cells, I wanted to know more about our blood. Curiously trying to make sense of science, I found all the information I could on the importance of our blood. It's the main fluid of life. In essence it keeps us alive. She creates magic throughout our bodies to give our systems life. Ever hear the expression, "Gotta keep the blood moving?" I discovered the importance of different blood types:

-Quirky joke I use: **"I'm just like my blood type : B Positive"** :)

"There are four main blood types, which are determined by the presence or absence of specific antigens on the surface of red blood cells. The four blood types are:

A – Has A antigens on red blood cells and anti-B antibodies in the plasma.

B – Has B antigens on red blood cells and anti-A antibodies in the plasma.

AB – Has both A and B antigens on red blood cells and no anti-A or anti-B antibodies in the plasma. This is known as the universal plasma recipient.

O – Has no A or B antigens on red blood cells but has both anti-A and anti-B antibodies in the plasma. This is known as the universal blood donor.

In addition to the A, B, AB, and O blood types, there is the **Rh factor**, which can either be positive (+) or negative (-). This means each blood type can be either Rh-positive or Rh-negative, resulting in eight possible blood types:"

A+, A-
B+, B-
AB+, AB-

O+, O-

According to "Cleveland Clinic" myclevelandclinic.org

What is the rarest blood type?

What are the different blood types?		
Blood type	Approximate percentage of U.S. population	Percentage of U.S. population, broken down by ethnicity
A positive A+	33%	White: 33% Black: 24% Asian: 27% Latino: 29%
A negative A-	6%	White: 7% Black: 2% Asian: .5% Latino: 2%
B positive B+	9%	White: 9% Black: 18% Asian: 25% Latino: 9%
B negative B-	Less than 2%	White: 2% Black: 1% Asian: .4% Latino: 1%
AB positive AB+	Less than 4%	White: 3% Black: 4% Asian: 7% Latino: 2%
AB negative AB-	Least common blood type in the U.S. Less than 1%	White: 1% Black: .3% Asian: .1% Latino: .2%
O positive O+	Most common blood type in the U.S. 38%	White: 37% Black: 47% Asian: 39% Latino: 53%
O negative O-	7%	White: 8% Black: 4% Asian: 1% Latino: 4%

Cleveland Clinic

"One of the world's rarest blood types is Rh-null. Fewer than 50 people in the world have this blood type. It's so rare that it's sometimes called "golden blood."

If you want to dig deeper into more knowledge about this topic, I suggest you get the book:

"Eat Right 4 Your Type: The Individualized Blood Type Diet Solution"
by Catherine Whitney, Peter J. D'Adamo, Dr.Peter J. D'Adamo

It really got me reflecting on the deeper currents of life. I found myself immersed in a world of knowledge, uncovering how exercises can be tailored to your blood type, and exploring insights on relationships and raising children. It even suggested that sometimes our blood types just don't mesh well with others, offering a surprising perspective on why certain connections, like the one with a partner, might feel off—perhaps it's the cause of that "mischarge" or misfire of energy between us, where the positive and negative cells clash.

The idea of "mischarge" in blood cells is more than just a physical concept—it speaks to the imbalance that can disrupt the natural flow of life. Blood cells, each with their own electric charge, dance in harmony, their interactions guiding the rhythm of our bodies. When that balance falters, when the charges are off, the smooth flow of life is altered, and we feel that disconnect.

The blood cells themselves, in their delicate roles, are no different. Red blood cells, tirelessly carrying life-sustaining oxygen, work in a quiet, coordinated flow. White blood cells, like guardians of the body, stand watch, always ready to defend against unseen threats. Platelets, like diligent repairmen, rush to stop any bleeding when injury strikes. Together, they create a beautiful, complex system—a reminder that everything in us is interconnected, fluid, and ever-moving.

Learning about my blood type diet felt like discovering a new piece of the puzzle—another thread to weave into the fabric of self-awareness. It's like reading a daily horoscope, or diving into the wisdom of the Enneagram, Human Design, or your life path number. Each of these tools offers a glimpse into understanding who you truly are. In this phase of my life, I was driven by a need to understand myself more fully—to examine my rhythms, my cycles, my quirks—and how I could harness them to evolve, to become a better human, a better entrepreneur, and a more connected soul.

MENSTRUAL CYCLES: aka Shark Week —*The Period* 🩸

She comes and goes, like a secret guest at a party, sometimes heavy, sometimes light, but sometimes... uninvited. The more I ventured into the world of nursing, the more I realized I had unintentionally become my own science experiment. I spent so much time charting every little detail about my patients' health that I started keeping track of my own—a little obsessive? Maybe, but it helped me spot patterns in the magical mystery of *her* arrival.

Enter technology, stage right. As apps became everyone's new best friend, I found one that helped track my menstrual cycle—*perfect*! And while most women use these apps to predict when they're ovulating, I was taking a different approach: reverse engineering. While they were tracking when to conceive, I was looking for the exact opposite—*timing* when to steer clear of my sexual partners (science to the rescue!). And yes, you still need extra protection, but honestly, understanding my body better felt like a superpower.

What really struck me was noticing how each phase affected me. As a fledgling entrepreneur, I began to pinpoint which parts of my cycle aligned with my most productive moments. Best decision I ever made. However, *of course*, life had its little ways of throwing curveballs. Stress, for instance, could mess with my cycle, or in my case, I spent a whole decade sans-period less thanks to the depo shot.

At the time, I thought this was the greatest blessing the universe could offer. No bleeding? Yes, please! I was young, forgetful, and missing pills left and right—perfect for me! But what I didn't realize was that 10 years of no bleeding wasn't exactly a "gift from the heavens" as I thought it was back then. The body needs to flow and create naturally, and now I'm just crossing my fingers that it won't come back to bite me—*looking at you, menopause*. (Praying, and affirming i'm safe and took the proper protocols)

But you know what? Through it all, I've learned to love this body of mine in the most profound, unconditional way. Getting my period was like a monthly reminder that my body was working *for me*, not against me. It was proof that I wasn't pregnant (thank you, period, for being the ultimate non-pregnancy reminder!). As much as I enjoy the idea of having "the littles" one day, right now that's not on my vision board. I see a vision more of *adopting* rather than anything, but I'm not *rushing* into anything.

The most beautiful part of this journey has been understanding how each phase of my cycle affects me. It's where I truly became a woman—learning to love myself unconditionally, *in all phases*, especially in the intricacies of my period. When we get to know ourselves, inside and out, we understand just how incredible, unique, and complex we truly are.

So, I highly recommend that you take the time to really understand your body—know which phase of the cycle you're in and how to care for yourself accordingly. After all, this beautiful body of yours deserves all the love and attention you can give. Trust me, it's worth it. Below I've laid out some ground rules on menstrual cycles and all of the wonderful phases, and even how to collide with moon cycles.

MENSTRUAL CYCLE PHASES:

Menstruation: (The "Oops, Here We Go" Phase)

Ah yes, the first day of your period, *cue the dramatic music*. The uterus decides it's time to shed its inner lining like it's throwing the most chaotic party in town. You look down, and it's like, "Wait, is that... *yikes*?" It's as if Mother Nature sent you a reminder: "Don't forget, you're *still* a woman!" During this phase, you feel like you could nap for 14 hours straight, but also like you've been hit by a bus. So, what do you do? You go through the motions, power through the discomfort, and pray you're not the only one who suddenly becomes a human sprinkler."

Follicular Phase: (The "I Am Ready to Write a Novel" Phase)

"This is when your body starts to shake off the chaos of menstruation and moves into preparation mode. The uterus is like, "Alright, I'm cleaning up the mess, and we're getting ready to potentially grow a new human!" Meanwhile, your mind has decided to start writing a *4000-page novel* of all the things you could do with your life now that you're free of cramps. You're sharp, you're *almost* optimistic, and for some reason, you're thinking you could conquer the world—if only the world would stop throwing unnecessary tasks your way. You get things done during this phase, but let's be real, half of it is about reorganizing your closet for no reason at all."

Ovulation: (The "I'm Ready to Party" Phase)

"Ah, the glorious ovulation phase. You're feeling *frisky* (yes, you read that right) and suddenly you're the most confident, charming version of yourself. You've got the energy, the glow, and the boob situation? Let's just say your shirts aren't doing them justice. Hormones are running wild, and all your instincts are screaming "Procreate! Now!" Even if you're happily single and *not* looking to make babies, your body is all like, "You know, now's a great time to meet someone, wink wink." Let's just say, if this phase were a dating app, you'd be swiping *right* on everything. Let's dance ;)"

Luteal Phase: (The "Give Me Chocolate and Let Me Nap" Phase)

"And then... the crash." The luteal phase arrives, and suddenly, you're not the confident queen you were a few days ago. Now, all you want is to curl up in your pajamas with a pint of chocolate ice cream, a fuzzy blanket, and your *very best friend*—your pillow. Your uterus is still doing its prep work, but your energy levels have plummeted, and your body is like, "I think it's time for a nap... or 12." It's not quite the full-on "pregnancy prep" vibe, but you're certainly not prepared to run a marathon either. Your emotional range has become *incredibly* wide, and your cravings are as unpredictable as your Netflix algorithm. But hey, the chocolate makes it better, right?"

"So, there you have it: the four phases of the menstrual cycle, each with its own flair, fun, and chaotic energy. Embrace the ride, because even though it can get a little nuts, it's all part of what makes you *you*. You're a powerhouse of hormones, humor, and heart, and don't let anyone forget it."

Moon Cycles:

Menstrual Phase & New Moon:

Ah, **menstruation**—that time when your body sheds what it no longer needs, and you're left with a mixture of emotions and perhaps a mild desire to hibernate under a blanket for the next five days. This phase is often seen as a time of release, renewal, and quiet introspection. In some traditions, this corresponds with the **new moon**, when the moon hides her face in the sky, quietly gathering energy for what's to come. Much like the new moon, **menstruation** invites you to slow down, rest, and reflect. It's a time to pause—take a break, maybe even call in sick to life for a day or two. It's your chance to reset, recharge, and give yourself the space to rest and reset."

Menstrual Phase & Full Moon:

"The **menstrual phase** and the **full moon** share a profound connection, both representing times of intense energy—albeit of different kinds. When your period arrives, it's like the body's invitation to slow down, let go, and reflect. It's the shedding phase, when your body releases what it no longer needs, physically and emotionally. It's also when you might feel more inward-focused, a time for deep reflection and resetting."

"But here's the twist: while menstruation is often seen as a time for release and introspection, it can also have an emotional intensity, much like the **full moon**. The full moon is all about peak energy—she's radiant, she's powerful, and she demands attention. Similarly, menstruation, while a time to release, can feel overwhelming, intense, and even full of emotion. For some, it's a time of heightened awareness, clarity, and insight. You may find that during this phase, you're more intuitive, perhaps tapping into deeper emotions or truths, similar to how the **full moon** brings everything out into the open, illuminating what's hidden in the shadows."

Menstrual Cycle & Waning Moon:

"**Waning moon** and the **menstrual cycle's luteal phase** mirror each other in profound ways, serving as a time for release, introspection, and personal renewal. The waning moon, as it gradually loses its light, is a symbol of surrender, rest, and the completion of a cycle. This phase calls us to slow down, to reflect on the past, and to let go of what no longer serves us, making space for new energy to emerge when the cycle begins again with the new moon. Similarly, the **luteal phase** of your menstrual cycle represents a time when your body and spirit prepare to release—be it a physical shedding of the uterine lining or an emotional and energetic release of what you've outgrown."

Menstrual Cycle & Waxing Moon

"The waxing moon spiritually represents the cycle of manifestation— it's the time to plant seeds, both figuratively and literally, for what you want to bring into your life. It's about setting intentions and nurturing them with care and patience, just as the body is preparing for ovulation, gathering energy and vitality. In this phase, you may feel a deep sense of personal empowerment, as if you're capable of achieving anything. Your confidence and motivation are heightened, and the world feels full of potential, just as the moon's light increases and illuminates the night sky."

"In the **waxing phase** of the moon, there is an emphasis on expansion and growth. It's the time to take inspired action, to start new projects, and to allow yourself to step into the fullness of who you are becoming. Similarly, in the **follicular phase**, your body is preparing to release an egg, signaling that you're in a fertile time—energetically, creatively, and physically. This phase is marked by optimism, renewal, and the exciting feeling that something wonderful is on the horizon. Like the waxing moon's increase in light, your inner light starts to shine brighter as you align with your higher self and your dreams."

Parasite Cleanse:

If you haven't figured it out by now, health is a HUGE priority in my life. Honestly, if there's any way to prove you have unconditional love for yourself, it's by showing love for your body. You *should* do everything you can to take the best care of it. People often tell me, "You look great," or "I can't believe how young you look for your age," they always guess I'm much younger than I am, and my response is always the same: "It's because **I am** my most important investment. I'll spend whatever it takes to ensure I'm in the best health possible. What's the point of being alive if you're not healthy? To me, existing without health is just, well, existing—and I'm sure that's not a pleasant experience. Am I right?"

Chris, called me to do a couple month check in, recently brought up something I hadn't considered: a parasite cleanse. Funny enough, this was something that kept cycling around me for years, but I blocked it out thinking it was "too extreme" and at those times previous years before, it was. I wasn't mentally or physically ready for that step. We were chatting during one of our regular phone calls when he mentioned he was looking into it. Apparently, you're supposed to do it around a full moon since that's when parasites are most active. According to Chris, these little guys come out of the woodwork when the moon is full, like some sort of bizarre full-moon ritual. He joked that they "do all the thinking for you," meaning old habits, and bad belief systems, they also crave sugar because they feed off of it. *Everyone* has them. He even pointed out that if you've ever eaten sushi, you've probably got them— lucky for me, I'm not a big sushi fan, despite living by the ocean in Wilmington where it was easy to get hooked on it.

So, I decided to take the plunge. It starts with preparing your body— getting it ready to detox. Then comes the cleanse itself: no solid foods for a week, a lot of fasting, eating microgreens, taking probiotics, using a binder to help with detoxification, and yes, even doing a daily enema. If you don't know what an enema is, I'd suggest a quick Google search (but I'll give you a crash course in layman's terms). You insert a tube into your rectum that's connected to a bag of warm water, then lie down and let the water flow into your intestines. You hold it in for about 20 minutes (if you can manage), then stand up and release it. The result is, well, a visual of everything that's been hiding in your gut, including parasites and other unwanted nasties. It's pretty intense, absolutely disgusting, and a little *glaringly* eye-opening—but it works. Personally, I refused to peer around and examine my own "output" like some of the others in the chatroom were doing. There were a bunch of people joining together on zoom as a support crew. No thank you!

But then, something bizarre happened. My cat, Cleo, popped around a few times while I was doing my thing in the bathroom, and I noticed she had "worms" too. I thought to myself, "*What the Fu*k?* She has parasites as well? Seriously, what are the chances?!" So, of course, I had to take her to the vet. I couldn't help but laugh, thinking, "*You've got to be shi**ing* *me"*—literally! (Haha.) You just can't make this sh*t up. I hear that all of the time from people. It's so funny, honestly.

I'm not going to lie, it wasn't glamorous. But after a week of affirmations, detoxing, and releasing those toxic habits, I felt incredible. I lost weight that wasn't really mine to begin with, and my skin was glowing. My body was finally repairing and healing itself. It was like I gave my system the chance to reset and re-calibrate.

In the end, the experience taught me something powerful: taking time to care for your body—mentally, physically, and spiritually—is an act of self-love. It's an investment in your health that pays off in ways you may not even expect. When you treat your body right, it shows. While the process may seem a little daunting at first (hello, enemas), the results are totally worth it. So, whether it's a cleanse, a new routine, or simply prioritizing your health in whatever way works for you, remember: you're worth the investment.

Diving deep into the Healing era, I thought "What would a monk do"?

SILENT ZONE:

There was a time in my life when I decided I needed to hit pause and set aside an entire day just for myself. I made Mondays my "day of silence." I wanted to focus on practicing good breathing, self-discipline, and thinking carefully before I spoke—especially since I had a tendency to blurt out whatever was on my mind. This practice helped me become more present and manage disagreements with my employees and in relationships with more insight and understanding. I spent the whole day in nature, flying solo. Of course, work eventually called for me to break my alone time, but I made sure everyone knew about my vow. If it was absolutely necessary, like attending an event or sharing my opinion, I'd handle it via email, a written note, or a quick text. This way,

I stayed true to my commitment while still keeping the lines of communication open and effective. I trusted myself to maintain this practice without letting it slip.

One time, I got into a disagreement with an employee who had overstepped his boundaries. With our crazy schedules and the chaos of stage production, he thought he was just helping out as usual. However, he went out of his way to ask for information that didn't really pertain to him, even though he thought it was necessary for the show's success (which, in the grand scheme, wasn't a big deal).

This situation struck a nerve with me. It made me realize that I was still using some outdated management skills from my earlier days. I remembered a time when I ran my holistic store and made my staff uncomfortable with a poor decision of my own. I was trying to be more open to constructive criticism so I could see my own flaws more clearly. It reminded me of a moment when John Maxwell asked his assistant for feedback. Instead of getting defensive, he handled it with thoughtfulness and maturity, showing what true leadership is all about.

I came to the realization that I needed to take responsibility for my actions and not react harshly to what I saw as his "wrongdoing." At that moment, I understood that my reactions were just as important as his actions. It was a humbling experience that taught me some valuable lessons.

First, I remembered that I'm human, and like everyone else, I make mistakes. It's easy to forget that when we're upset, but recognizing our own humanity helps us approach situations with more empathy. I also had to remind myself that the people around me are human too, with their own flaws, imperfections, and struggles. This was overall why I practiced silence: to be aware of my words and actions.

The most important lesson for me, however, was about the tone of my delivery. This one really hit home. I realized that the way I express myself has a huge impact on how others perceive and respond to me. It's not just about what I say, but how I say it. I understood that I needed to be more mindful of my tone, striving to be calm and collected, especially in moments when emotions run high. I learned that taking a moment to think before I speak, instead of letting my thoughts spill out unfiltered, could make a world of difference in how my message is received.

Also, if you can lead your team up a mountain and keep their energy and momentum high, you're doing something right. This made me reflect on how my team sometimes doesn't listen, and it's a reminder that leadership is about guiding and inspiring, not just directing.

Self-Reflection and Awareness:

The practice of self-reflection, such as setting aside "**a day of silence,**" helps the individual build awareness of their own thoughts, emotions, and reactions. This awareness is the foundation of emotional intelligence.

Emotional Regulation:

"The practice of silence and thoughtfulness before speaking is a strategy for managing emotional responses. Emotional regulation helps prevent impulsive reactions, leading to more constructive and measured responses in difficult situations."

Connection to Unconditional Love:

"Unconditional love often requires managing strong emotions (anger, frustration, disappointment) without allowing them to dictate one's behavior toward others. Just as the individual takes a pause to ensure their tone and words are measured and respectful, unconditional love involves controlling emotional impulses to respond in a way that nurtures relationships rather than damaging them. The ability to regulate emotions allows for more genuine, loving, and patient responses."

Leadership as a Form of Care and Guidance:

The reflection on leadership emphasizes the importance of guiding and inspiring a team rather than simply directing them. Effective leaders build trust and maintain positive momentum, which requires empathy, respect, and an understanding of the team's needs.

Connection to Unconditional Love:

The concept of leadership in this scenario mirrors how unconditional love is expressed in guiding others through life's challenges. Unconditional love doesn't just involve providing care when it's easy but also helping others grow, succeed, and thrive even in difficult times. It's about lifting others up, providing encouragement, and demonstrating love through actions, much like how effective leadership involves guiding people with a sense of purpose and motivation.

Throughout this chapter, we've discovered that understanding your health and wellness is a unique and personal journey. It demands patience, introspection, and a dedication to nurturing both your mind and body. Keep in mind that real transformation starts with recognizing your current state and taking deliberate steps toward the future you envision.

For further insights into analyzing your health and wellness, visit my website at <u>Contact - Aire Stillman Lifestyle</u>. There, you'll find helpful resources to support you in your pursuit of improved health and a more balanced life.

CHAPTER TWENTY THREE

THE IN'S AND OUT'S.

African Diaspora:

Landing this job seemed to just be a dream. At the beginning I was so grateful for the kids. Especially, considering the year I had previous just to get here. The job included a dance program that taught children the early history of where different dance cultures and styles were created, focusing on childhood development through social and emotional learning.

I'll admit, originally, I didn't understand what that meant, even with all of our training because it was hard to understand the cause and effect. Until I could physically see the changes in the children's behaviors. These situations teach kids through daily life skills and help them understand the ins-and-outs of how our environment shapes us. I became a manager quickly, by my persistence. Becoming a stage manager for the Assembly programs, I was able to see that things weren't so clear. In other words, "corporate propaganda." I started to learn all of the growing pains of working inside big business, and the parallels they have. Realizing and learning all of the mistakes that are made, I took note. I needed a new route to continue my plans for non-profit, but I was thankful for the opportunity to spend that time with children.

"A smart person learns from his mistakes, but a truly wise person learns from the mistakes of others."
—Ken Schramm, The Compleat Meadmaker : Home Production of Honey Wine From Your First Batch to Award-winning Fruit and Herb Variations

The Song That Chose Us:

34.1458° N, 118.1489° W

Maggie was a vision of beauty, with her dark hair and sun-kissed bronze skin that spoke of her Colombian roots. She had recently joined the non-profit I was managing, stepping in during a busy transition period. It was the last month of the year, and her role was to fill a gap left by the changing tides of our staff. But what Maggie brought to the table was more than just her presence. She was a bombshell in every sense of the word.

Her vocal range blew us away, but what truly stood out was her musical ear, her dance ability, and the warmth of her stage performance. Even though she had only one rehearsal with the band and a handful of shows under her belt, she stepped into the role like a true performer. She'd record videos, go home, practice, and come back with a polish that could only be described as professional. Her first show was an absolute success, but it was our second show that gave me the chance to sit down with her and learn more about her story.

I asked her about her home-life, her passions, and what brought her to LA. Maggie had been living here for four years, far away from her family and the country she loved, Colombia. She'd recently made a trip home for the first time since she moved, and I could see the emotions it stirred within her. "Are you homesick?" I asked, wondering if the distance had been hard on her. She paused for a moment, then with a gentle smile, replied, "Yes, and no. Being home was a very kind reminder of why I'm out here."

She continued, "At home, I can't exactly be who I want to be or express myself and do what is calling for me. I've been singing my whole life," she said, her face lighting up as she spoke. There was a kind of innocence in the way she shyly pulled back her hair, blushing at the mention of her gift. "Back home, there aren't many options for me to follow that path. The music chose me."

As she spoke, I felt a deep sense of recognition. Her words echoed a familiar truth that I had also discovered in my own life. It's funny how many of us discredit ourselves, downplay our gifts, and let doubt cloud our path. It doesn't matter how long we've been at something or how much talent we have—the mind often tries to convince us we're not enough, that we don't deserve to follow our passion.

I smiled and laughed softly, sharing a piece of my own journey with Maggie. "That's funny you say that," I told her. "I had an ex who once told me the exact same thing. He helped me realize that music was my future too." I paused, letting the memory wash over me. "When he said that, everything in my life suddenly clicked. It became so clear to me. All the signs had always been around me, but I had suppressed them— thinking I didn't deserve to follow them. But when I really looked back, I realized music was the driving force in my life all along. I didn't choose music—music chose me."

As we sat there, talking about our love for music, we shared stories of our childhood, of how the love of music had always been with us, even when we didn't fully understand its significance. Our connection, our shared understanding of how music had chosen us, felt like a sacred bond. Music had always been more than just a hobby or a passion—it was a calling, a force that guided us through life.

Maggie's words reminded me of the beauty in following what calls us, even if the path is unclear. It was a lesson I had learned and one I hoped she would carry with her as she continued to grow in her artistry. Music wasn't just something we did—it was something we were meant to be.

Nasty Girl:

34.1395° N, 118.3830° W

JoJo Gomez was the best choreographer I'd seen in a while. I had such a blast at her other dance class rounds! Her choreography was a mix of fast-paced jazz, pop, and a whole lot of sexy girl energy. I loved the way I felt in her classes—pumped up, moving with purpose, and getting better every week. As soon as I heard she was coming back to LA, I was ready to sign up.

I kept an eye on her marketing and social media. She posted a little teaser of the song and some moves from the upcoming class. Now, as a good student, I always do my research. So, when the day finally came and we started dancing to "Nasty," by Tinashe I was READY. Armed with knowledge of the song, I knew the class was about to be a blast.

5, 6, 7, 8, 9—up, down, ooo, cat, cat, whip, and clip. "Get there, snatch, smile, get there!" The language of dance creation is *hilarious*, but everyone falls in line, sharp and precise with their movements. Suddenly, a loud roar echoed across the room. There's probably 65+ people in the class, so it's hard to see much. It's a fight to get a good view of the moves. Most are uncomfortable being close to the front, but feeling my courage, I wasn't scared. I wanted to be front and center, soaking in all the moves, tempo, and energy. That's how you get better. Everything starts with the energy from the front. But the other side of the room? A blur.

Then, as if the Red Sea parted, out pops none other than the pop star herself—Tinashe.

Now, let me be clear: this NEVER happens. Artists don't just casually show up to dance classes unannounced. They have busy schedules with their own training, singing, promo—whatever it is that makes them *them*. Sure, it happens at tryouts or specialized training sessions, but that's a known thing. This? This was a surprise.

JoJo always says, "Go full out. Fail in class, learn, and get better with action. That's why there's class. Don't waste your money if you're not going to do the work." (**The Teacher**)

I've always said I'm not the type to put celebrities on pedestals. They're just people, just like us—bombarded by people watching every little move they make. They're hardworking and usually at the top of their game, which is why they're there. So, I'm not usually star-struck when I see someone famous out here in LA. Everyone's a star in this town. But Tinashe? She's been in the industry for over 10 years, with multiple hits under her belt, and she blessed us by dancing in class with us.

JoJo created that choreography specifically for Tinashe to use in her promos, music videos, TV shows, and even award ceremonies. So, when Tinashe showed up, she didn't waste any time. We all got to dance for her. And get this—she picked new spicy dancers out of the class for her upcoming shoots. Lesson learned: Always come prepared and on your A-game.

Then, the best part: No warm-up—just jumped right in to dance with us, ready to slay. Her energy? Off the charts. The room was filled with laughter and fun, and we were all completely *vibing*.

Little did we know, that song became the number one track of the summer. It was everywhere—mainstream radio, Instagram, TikTok, you name it. Even other languages were playing it. It was huge. So, to share that experience with Tinashe and my classmates was a massive highlight of my dancing career up to that point.

PRO TIP: Go hard from the start so your body can learn the move and know how to backtrack and correct later if needed. Don't start slow and try to build energy. Get it in your body right away. Understand your staging and always pay attention to your surroundings.

Mutual Respect:

When Tinashe arrives and chooses new dancers for her upcoming shoots, it highlights a moment of mutual respect and recognition. The class's hard work and preparation are acknowledged, and they are given the opportunity to shine. This reinforces the idea of a supportive community where effort and dedication are celebrated. It's about acknowledging people's unique contributions and embracing them without conditions. Unconditional love encourages individuals to recognize and uplift others based on their inherent worth, not just their external achievements.

CHAPTER TWENTY FOUR

GRIEF.

The Weight of Grief and the Power of Forgiveness:

37.8307° N, 122.1659° W

I met Ben, a tall, blonde German man from Berlin who shared a story that shifted something deep inside me. He told me about his spiritual journey and the longing he'd felt for true faith—a Christian community with the kind of "band of brothers" he'd been searching for. Ben had traveled the world, seeking connection and healing, attending various coaching programs put on by Pastor Erwin. But it wasn't until he spoke of his mother that I truly began to understand the depth of his experience.

Ben shared that his mother had instilled in him a love for Jesus, a faith he had always carried. But their relationship was difficult, filled with tension and misunderstandings, until the moment his mother was diagnosed with cancer. It was in her final years that Ben made a commitment to care for her, and through this act of love, he found healing. His faith gave him the strength to forgive many of the wounds he carried, and through the pain of watching her decline, he was able to let go of his bitterness. The relief and solace he found were remarkable— he had been able to heal a part of himself he hadn't known needed healing.

However, even after all this, his relationship with his brother was still broken. Ben shared that he was working on forgiving his brother, but the pain was still raw, and he was struggling to move past it. The topic of grief and loss, forgiveness, and healing came up in our conversation, and he asked me about my own experiences with grief.

I admitted to him that I wasn't sure I had truly grieved some of the losses in my life. As a nurse, I had been numb to the pain of losing patients— I had been so focused on doing my job that I never allowed myself to feel the weight of the grief. But when it came to the loss of my brother, and the loss of friends and family, I felt that pain deeply. I shared stories of my grief over Ben and Miller, two people I had lost in different ways. As I spoke, I felt the heaviness of their absence in my words.

The hike came to an end, and as we reached the top, I walked up to Ben and hugged him. It was then that I shared something I hadn't mentioned before. "You know, Ben," I said, "the name of my deceased brother is Ben." It felt like a full-circle moment—like my brother was somehow reaching out to me through this encounter, reminding me of the power of forgiveness, the depth of grief, and the importance of surrendering to life's pain. It was a profound reminder that life is too short to hold grudges. We must let go of the past, release the trauma in our bodies, and move forward. (**The Teacher**)

The thought lingered with me: "*Why hold on to anger? You might never see that person again. What would you say to the dead?*" For me, the answer is simple: Live fully. Live with love. Live without regrets. The people we've lost cannot be brought back, but they leave us with a precious reminder—to live our lives to the fullest while we still have time.

Later, I came across a sign that read, "We cannot bury the past." It struck me in a way that felt almost eerie. The past, like a buried file, can be hidden away, but it's never truly gone. We can't delete it or burn it, no matter how hard we try. It's a rabbit hole to consider, but the message was clear: We must face our past, not bury it, if we want to heal.

In the book *Illuminate*, I read about the tough decisions that Howard Schultz, the CEO of Starbucks, had to make in 2008, when the company closed 600 stores and laid off thousands of employees. As a leader, he had to bear the weight of decisions that affected thousands of lives, all in the hopes of saving the company. It made me reflect on how one decision, one choice, can ripple through so many lives, and how even in times of loss, there is a chance for new life and new beginnings.

I thought about how this is the cycle of life—death and loss giving birth to new opportunities, new paths. In fact, for every new life that begins, there are many deaths. *Every second, a baby is born, and four people die.* The balance of life and death is constant, and it's in the space between that we are called to live fully.

This lesson is also true within the self. The death of the ego can be the most healing experience we can undergo. My own ego has caused me so much pain and difficulty, but it has also led to the most pivotal moments in my life. It's through the death of that old self that I've been able to unlock new layers of who I truly am. The process is not easy, but it's necessary for growth.

Grief, in its many forms, teaches us to release, to forgive, and to live in a way that honors the precious time we have. In the end, it's forgiveness that heals us—not just others. Forgiveness allows us to move forward, to stop carrying the weight of the past, and to embrace the future with open arms.

VALENTINES: A TALE OF UNEXPECTED LOVE:

During a season of grief, when I needed a victory more than anything, life gave me an unexpected twist. After all the long, sweated-out days of work and training, I was hosting a production for *Life Transitions*, a show about butterflies with 13 acts of all sky apparatus. It was beautiful and symbolic, but somewhere between the high-flying performances, I was still grieving from LA's rough lessons. Still lost in the heavy shadows of loss.

At the same time, I found myself briefly caught up in a situationship with a guy I'd been seeing on and off since performing in Las Vegas. Our relationship was like a puzzle with missing pieces—fitting together only in brief moments, until suddenly, everything shifted. One day, I found myself feeling real feelings, and he was showing up in all the right places, like some sort of serendipitous sign. He was ready to commit to me, and that scared me in the best way possible.

There was just one thing that seemed to weigh on him. He didn't like the fact that I didn't have an animal at home to protect me. *"What are you going to do if something happens?"* he asked one night. In our usual playful banter, we jokingly talked about getting a kitten. It was just a thought—something to pass the time as we laughed about our futures. But somehow, in his determination, he took it seriously.

Before I knew it, there was a kitten ready for me to pick up. And honestly? I didn't feel ready. I was exhausted from work, still processing grief from Miller, and just not sure I could handle one more responsibility. But he begged, and after enough coaxing, I finally agreed, and let me tell you, it wasn't because I was 100% convinced. It was because this kitten was *adorable*. She was everything I imagined: all black with jade-green eyes that captivated anyone who dared to look, with little paws that couldn't have been more precious.

He came to my show to support me, and the next day, he brought her over. For the first week, she was terrified—scared of the new place, hiding in corners, unsure of everything. But then, one morning, I woke up to find her sitting on my chest, staring at me while I slept. It was one of those moments where time stood still, and suddenly, I knew that this little creature was meant to be with me.

I named her "Cleo"—a mix of Cleopatra, the Queen, and Clozee, my favorite EDM DJ, the "Queen of the Jungle." Both were royalty in their own right, ready to rule the house.

Two weeks later, he disappeared. Just like that. Gone. He had been so persistent in his pursuit, and then, just like that, backed away. He *gave* me a kitten and then *bounced*. I remember thinking, "*What the hell? Who does that?*" You can't just drop an animal into someone's life and then vanish! (**The Runner**)

But here's the crazy part—Cleo was exactly what I needed. In my search for unconditional love, she gave it to me tenfold. She followed me around the house, waited for me to get home, curling up with me whenever she could. She loved me in her own way, just like Miller did before. The way she waited for me, the way she made sure I knew I wasn't alone— it was the kind of love I didn't realize I was yearning for.

I'm so grateful for her. Things would have been so much tougher without this little cuddle bug by my side. So here's to Cleo, my unexpected Valentine, who showed up in my life and reminded me what it feels like to be loved, just as I am.(**THE REMINDER**)

CHAPTER TWENTY FIVE

GUARDIANS OF CONNECTION & BOUNDARIES.

The Super Couple:

33.9792° N, 118.4138° W

I had the most incredible experience meeting Michelle **(THE TEACHER)** at the gym. She had this glowing energy about her—matching gym fit, gold accessories, Apple AirPods firmly attached to her ears, brown hair slicked into a ponytail, and a giant rock on her finger. When she turned around with weights on her shoulders, I was immediately struck by this beautiful smile that stretched from ear to ear. I decided I had to introduce myself.

We both had the same energy drink in hand, so I went for it: "Hey, who are you? You're literally the only other person in here smiling as big as I am. I can *kindly* tell you that's impressive." We both burst into laughter, and just like that, we exchanged numbers.

After a few coffee dates, I left feeling so full and inspired. At the time, I was in a bit of a low moment, living at the beach and feeling like I was stuck in a dull routine. Meeting someone with such a bright light felt like a spark I desperately needed. And lucky for me, she invited me over to meet her husband, who was just as incredible as she was.

I had the chance to sit down at their kitchen table in a sleek, modern condo. The light poured through their massive windows, casting a warm glow on the white walls, which felt inviting and serene—like a church with stained glass windows. It truly felt like a blessing to be in their company; they had invited me over out of sheer generosity.

As we chatted, the conversation shifted to a deeper discussion about the importance of various aspects of life: spiritual, romantic, physical, financial, and mental. These were areas I had been helping others with for years, but little did I know, they were about to challenge my own thinking.

Adam, her husband, shared some eye-opening insights about women and our love languages, highlighting how significant they are. But what really resonated with me was his point about how men prioritize **respect** _above love_ or anything else. He explained that men don't want to be made a fool of in public, and that it's important to agree with them when it's appropriate. Larger issues, he said, should be addressed privately. He also talked about treating men like leaders, allowing them to take charge and not nagging them like they're children. And while men are fully capable of picking out their own clothes, above all, they need the space to ask for help when they truly need it.

This perspective led me to reflect deeply on my own life. I began analyzing the people and situations that had been frustrating me. At the time, my roommate was eating all of my food, offering to pay me back later, but then texting me passive-aggressive notes. When I returned home, he'd act as if nothing was wrong. He'd even enter my room without asking, or go through my things when I wasn't around.

Then there was another friend who ghosted me, only to act like everything was fine when we met in person. And one of my best friends had told me he was coming to my event, texting me that morning to confirm, but then didn't show up—no call, no text, just complete radio silence. He acted like it wasn't a big deal.

That's when it hit me. I wasn't so much angry about their actions; I was frustrated by the lack of **respect** they had for me. That made me stop and ask myself, where might I be disrespecting others in my life?

The bigger realization came when I realized I was disrespecting myself. I had been lying to myself, making excuses, and pushing aside my own priorities—whether it was self-care, finances, or fitness. I had been avoiding things that truly mattered to me. But now, I was ready to face them head-on.

I was so grateful for Adam's insight, as it helped me connect the dots—not only in my relationships with others but also in my relationship with myself. It was time for a change. **(THE TEACHER)**

Let's dive into how to be the kind of person you want to hang out with—without getting too heavy about it. First off, **being a good listener** is key. It's not about waiting for your turn to talk (we've all been guilty of that), but really tuning in to what others are saying. So, next time someone is pouring their heart out, try not to interrupt with your "perfect solution" right away. Instead, just nod, maybe toss in a "that sounds rough" and let them know they're heard. It's a game-changer.

Next up: **being thoughtful**. This one's pretty simple. It's like giving someone a mental high-five when they least expect it. It's about noticing others' feelings and taking them into account before you say something. A little kindness and courtesy can go a long way, even if it's just holding the door open for someone or complimenting their shoes.

Then there's **consideration**, which is all about making sure you're not the person who interrupts in the middle of a story or blasts music at 2 AM. Respect people's personal space, tone down the gossip, and remember that just because something seems like a great idea to you, it doesn't mean it is to everyone. We all have different levels of "personal space"—honor them.

Now, **being responsible**: When you mess up (and trust me, we all do), own it. Apologize without trying to turn it into a giant drama show. A simple "Hey, my bad." can do wonders. It's not about perfection; it's about being honest and making things right.

Then there's the whole idea of **being open-minded**. It's easy to get stuck in your own bubble, but sometimes it's good to pop that bubble and let in some fresh perspectives. People have different views, and that's okay. Listen to them, even if they make you scratch your head. You don't have to agree with everyone, but respecting those differences can make life a whole lot more interesting.

And when it comes to **being helpful**, remember this: you don't always have to save the day with a cape and a dramatic rescue. Sometimes just offering a listening ear or helping someone carry groceries can mean the world. Acknowledge what others are doing well, too—it's like throwing little confetti of positivity wherever you go.

Speaking of communication, **being clear** is crucial. If you want something, say it directly. If you need help, ask for it. No need for mind games or cryptic hints. Speak your truth, but do it calmly and with a sprinkle of confidence.

When it comes to handling tough situations, **being prepared** makes all the difference. Nobody likes a conflict, but being ready to face one with a level head and an open mind is key. Being able to find solutions instead of just complaining about problems is a skill that'll make you stand out in the best way.

Finally, **being willing to change**. This is the magic ingredient. If you mess up or learn something new, don't be afraid to admit it. Growth happens when you're open to making changes, whether it's how you approach people or how you see the world. Nobody's perfect (except maybe your grandma, but she's been perfecting that for decades).

So, there you go. It's about being kind, thoughtful, and open, while also owning your actions and being ready to grow. You don't need to do it all at once—just take it one step at a time and be the person everyone's happy to share space with.

These points hit home for me in a big way. The answer became crystal clear: If I wasn't even being respectful to myself, how could I expect to be respectful to others and receive that in return? Perhaps, I was meant to learn those lessons, to realize that I wasn't meant to be in those environments, and they just weren't right for me. It became obvious that these experiences were just mirrors, reflecting my own issues—lessons I needed to learn from and take responsibility for.

Spilling the tea on Body Language:

Is the body, bodying?

Body language is an extraordinary topic that surfaces in many scenarios. Imagine if you could realize that the tools in your life are here to serve you, not the other way around.

Hey Sis, Let's Talk About Your Posture:

Are you slouching over your laptop at overpriced coffee shops? Hunching over your iPhone or straining to uncap your water bottle? Are you giving more attention to your chai latte than to your BFF?

These things should serve you, not distract you. Are you being intentional with how you interact with your environment? For example, how do you hold your purse—does it hold you back?

Posture Matters:

In the gym, your posture is crucial. Poor form can lead to injuries or disrupt your body's balance. I once had a dramatic incident where my ankle got caught in a car's muffler, causing months of pain and a long recovery. The imbalance and chronic issues taught me a valuable lesson about the importance of proper posture and balance.

Body Language Signals:

Your body communicates like a symphony. We constantly send non-verbal signals through our movements, facial expressions, and eye contact. Here's how to make sure your body language is sending the right messages:

Positive/Open Body Language: Face the person you're talking to, use open gestures, and show engagement.

Negative/Closed Body Language: Avoid crossing arms, turning away, or being physically distant. These cues can create a sense of unfriendliness or disinterest.

As I sat there reflecting on all the things I had learned, I realized that the key to building better relationships—whether with others or myself—was about more than just good intentions. It's the little things that make a big difference. For example, I noticed that constantly checking my phone during conversations wasn't just a habit; it was downright disrespectful. I'd catch myself scrolling through messages while someone was speaking, and I could see the disappointment in their eyes. So, I made a pact with myself: put the phone away, make eye contact, and actually *listen*. It was a game changer.

Speaking of self-respect, I couldn't ignore the importance of basic hygiene. It's not about being fancy; it's about showing that you care about yourself and those around you. So, I started brushing my hair, using deodorant, and dressing appropriately for the occasion. It sounds simple, but it made me feel more confident and, frankly, more respectful of the people I was interacting with.

I also had to reevaluate how I dressed for different situations. Whether it was work, a gym session, or just a casual meet-up, I realized that dressing for the occasion mattered. I didn't want to be the person showing up underdressed or looking out of place. A little thought about the setting went a long way.

One of the most enlightening lessons was learning not to interrupt. I've been guilty of cutting people off mid-sentence, thinking I knew what they were going to say. But I soon realized that it was not only rude but it also undermined the flow of conversation, I decided to just listen, let others finish their thoughts, and wait my turn.

On the lighter side, I also became more conscious of my smile. I'm pretty sure my "forced smile" was more creepy than friendly. So, I made an effort to smile genuinely. It's amazing how much more connected you feel when your smile is authentic.

And let's not forget the handshake—something I never really thought about until someone pointed out that my handshake was... well, weak. After hearing that, I focused on giving a firm, confident handshake, because, let's be honest, nobody likes a limp handshake. It's all about showing enthusiasm and respect.

Another big one: eye contact. I realized that avoiding eye contact made me seem disinterested or insecure. So, I made it a point to maintain eye contact during conversations. It's not about staring people down; it's about building trust and connection.

Then there's speaking clearly. For the longest time, I had a habit of mumbling or speaking too softly, which led to a lot of miscommunication. So I worked on projecting my voice and articulating my words, which made conversations much smoother.

Respecting personal space also became a priority. I was guilty of standing too close to people at times, unaware that I was invading their personal space. I made a conscious effort to step back and give people the room they needed, and surprisingly, the conversations felt less tense.

Finally, I became more self-aware of my own body language. I practiced in front of the mirror and asked for feedback from trusted friends. Sometimes, you don't realize the signals you're sending out, but being mindful of my posture, facial expressions, and gestures helped me project more confidence and respect in all my interactions.

It was like a switch had flipped—little adjustments in how I communicated and carried myself were making a big impact. And the more I practiced, the easier it became to show up as my best, most respectful self in every situation.

You always gain by giving love
—Reese Witherspoon

Boundaries:

Love, in its infinite capacity, has the power to both illuminate and bewilder. It can inspire us to reach for the stars, yet at times, it entices us to lose ourselves in its fervent grip. If you're anything like me—a so-called "**hopeful romantic**"—you've likely surrendered pieces of yourself to someone else, convinced that this sacrifice was the price of love. Perhaps, like me, you've mistaken infatuation or longing for love's truest form. Over time, I've learned that love given freely, without expectation or condition, holds the most profound beauty. When we act from a place of love—not to receive love, but because our hearts overflow—we transcend the transactional and embrace the divine.

This realization demands self-awareness. It requires us to untangle ourselves from the habits and patterns that no longer serve us and break us free from the reflexive need to please or to prove ourselves. Even now, I catch myself wrestling with the echoes of old behaviors, questioning whether my actions stem from genuine care or the shadow of insecurity. The lesson is clear: love must never be a chain that binds, but a gift that liberates.

Too often, we fear that withholding an action or a word will create distance, that in doing less, we risk losing someone we hold dear. Our minds slip into scarcity, painting vivid fears of abandonment. Yet, true love does not thrive in the soil of guilt or obligation. It blossoms in freedom, where acts of service stem not from fear, but from an unshakable desire to uplift and nurture.

Still, amidst these reflections, I invite you to pause and wonder: have you ever considered who might be afraid to lose you? In the quiet moments when doubt creeps in, remember that you, too, are a vessel of love—worthy, cherished, and irreplaceable. When you love yourself as deeply as you hope to be loved, the boundaries you create will no longer be barriers, but bridges to authentic connection and understanding.

The Importance of Boundaries:

Boundary- Setting:

The reflection highlights the significance of boundaries, describing them not as walls but as shields that protect individuality. Boundaries allow individuals to maintain their integrity and ensure that relationships remain balanced.

Relevance to Unconditional Love:

Healthy boundaries enable unconditional love by fostering mutual respect and ensuring that neither partner feels overextended, dependent, or manipulated. Boundaries are the foundation of self-respect, and without them, love can become conditional or transactional.

Reflection 101: Mr. Killa:

When I started caring more about him than myself, he stopped choosing me. It was like I lost sight of who I was in the hopes of becoming who he wanted me to be.

In my pursuit to make him choose me, I was losing myself. I kept thinking that if I just did more for him, showed him I could fit into his life seamlessly, he would want me more. But what he loved about me was my independence—my ability to stand strong on my own. He knew I didn't need him, but I felt like I did. I started bending and changing for him, infiltrating his world in ways I thought would make him love me more. But instead of bringing us closer, it created distance. I wasn't fitting into his life the way I thought I should, and he wasn't ready for a partner like me—a wife.

This experience taught me something vital: I need to stay strong in my boundaries, no matter how tempting it is to bend when things get tough or convenient. I don't need to drop everything for someone else just to prove I'm worthy. I need to honor my own space, my own needs, and stay true to myself.

I can't let the desire to be chosen make me forget that I'm already whole. I need to choose myself first, always. Boundaries aren't walls; they're shields that protect what makes me who I am. The right person will appreciate that strength, not be threatened by it.

Loss of Self in Relationships:

Codependency: A common dynamic in relationships where one partner becomes overly focused on meeting the needs or expectations of the other, often to their own detriment. This is a hallmark of codependency, where one's self-worth becomes enmeshed in how much they can give or sacrifice for their partner.

Relevance to Unconditional Love: True unconditional love requires maintaining a sense of self while loving another. It's about giving freely, not out of need or desperation, but from a place of abundance and self-fulfillment.

Theory and Self-Validation: The desire to be chosen reflects an externalized need for validation, rooted in insecure attachment patterns. This behavior often stems from a fear of rejection or abandonment, causing individuals to overcompensate by trying to prove their worthiness of love.

Non-Negotiables of RELATIONSHIPS:

After years of dating, dodging a divorce, dealing with artists, actors, athletes, celebs, and navigating a series of "f**k boys," I've learned a few crucial lessons. Each relationship has taught me something valuable: what I've learned and will carry into the next, and what I won't tolerate again.

Of course, each relationship is unique, shaped by the partner, the environment, and the goals involved. But if you haven't learned the lessons you were meant to, you might end up in a relationship that feels eerily similar to your past ones. Ever noticed those people who date a version of their ex? It's like they're going for a clone. I did that once, whoops! We all might have a "type," but the reality is they keep finding themselves in the same situations. The common factor here ? Hate to break it to you, but the issues might be within **you.**

Let's get real: it's time to make a list of your non-negotiables. You're not just looking for a playmate; you're looking for a life partner. The best advice I've heard is: "**stop dating for a boyfriend, start dating for a husband.**" Focus on the qualities you really want in a partner and stop falling for potential. Look for someone who embodies the qualities you'd want in your future spouse, not just someone you hope will change into that person.

First off, stop saying you're looking for a "boyfriend." That language is cringy and sounds childish and might leave you struggling with what to call your new partner. "He's my man." It sounds like you own them (are they your dog?). "My partner" can also sound like you're in a lesbian couple (which might not fit your social setting). Maybe "I'm dating" is simpler. Or, if you're feeling old-school, "significant other" also works. If you're feeling adventurous and you're in the U.S., you might use "lover," which suggests a hot and steamy affair. In other parts of the world, "lover" just means someone sweet. Funny how language can vary so much!

Choosing based on criteria like these might seem superficial, but it actually helps you avoid future problems. Life is tough enough without adding relationship drama. Instead of ghosting, be honest about your values. If your values don't align, let them know—don't just disappear.

Attempting to build a life together with separate foundations will only lead to problems. Relationships thrive on unity. In the midst of this whirlwind, I had to pause and ask myself: *What truly matters to me? What values and beliefs do I refuse to compromise on?* It wasn't just about finding love or success; it was about finding alignment with someone whose worldview matched my own.So, here's a solid start for your success below.

Create Your List of Non-Negotiables:

Values:

One of the first things I came to realize was just how essential my values were—especially the ones rooted in my spiritual foundation. I've always felt a deep connection to my faith, and in a relationship, it became abundantly clear that a shared sense of faith wasn't just a bonus—it was non-negotiable. It wasn't about simply sitting side by side in a pew on Sundays; it was about how we saw the world, how we treated others, and how we faced the storms that life inevitably throws our way.

Then, one day, a lightbulb moment hit: I needed someone who not only respected my beliefs about human rights and equality, but who also showed that respect through action. It wasn't enough for someone to just nod along; they had to live it, breathe it, be it.

This also led me to confront some harder questions within myself, like, *"How do I really feel about politics?"* Ah yes, the never-ending debate of modern times. In a world where everything seems so polarized, I realized I couldn't afford to sweep my partner's views under the rug, especially if they were worlds apart from mine. I distinctly remember a conversation about politics that opened my eyes wider than I expected. It made me see just how aligned—or *not*—we truly were. At that moment, I discovered what I truly needed in a relationship. A connection that runs deeper than words—one built on shared values, respect, and a mutual understanding of what it means to be human.

Lifestyle:

Then came the moment of reflection—the gentle but persistent nudge to think about lifestyle choices. It wasn't just about how I wanted to live my day-to-day life, but how those habits would weave into a shared future. I've always treated my health like a sacred treasure—eating well, working out, and keeping my body as strong as a fortress. Mentally, I was all about growth—feeding my mind, spirit, and finances with the same care I give my body. So when it came to a potential partner, I knew I couldn't just settle for someone whose habits were as opposite to mine as night and day. I didn't need a workout buddy who could bench press a truck (though, you know, that would be nice), but I did need someone who understood the importance of being mentally and physically healthy. A partner who enjoys an adventurous spirit, a good hike, or spontaneous dance-offs in the kitchen was ideal. Movement was key.

Then there's the whole social habit thing. It dawned on me that, at my core, I'm an introvert with an extroverted twist. I crave my quiet time, but I also adore meaningful social connections. I realized I needed someone who respected my need for personal space, but who could also join me for an occasional dinner with friends—or a full-on karaoke battle with people we barely know. A balance between solitude and socializing became an essential must-have in my partner checklist.

And then, of course, came the delicate topic of drinking and smoking. Let's just say, I wasn't about to dive into a relationship where habits like those would overshadow the kind of health-focused life I wanted to build. It wasn't about being a health-snob (though, let's be real, I do love a good smoothie), it was just about knowing what made me feel my absolute best. When it came to living a vibrant life, I needed someone who'd be right there with me, choosing water over whiskey when the moment called for it—and who'd understand that some days, a solid nap beats a night out. Priorities, my friends, priorities.

Views on Sex and Relationships:

Then came a conversation that truly rocked my world: "What do I believe sex is really about? Is it pleasure? Intimacy? Procreation?" Is it pleasure? Intimacy? Procreation? Or, is it something even deeper, something that touches the soul? For me, it's all of the above, wrapped in a beautiful, complicated bow. I wanted a partner who could not only appreciate the sacred dance of intimacy but who also understood the difference between a fleeting encounter and a deep, emotional connection.

But, of course, the real juicy questions came next. "*How often is enough? Daily? Weekly?*" The never-ending debate! And then the real kicker—*Do you find sex to be part of who you are?* Well, let's just say, I have a bit of a *large appetite*. Like Tinashe says, I need a partner who can match my "freak." We're talking a lifetime commitment of fun, laughter, romance, spice, and tenderness. A perfect balance of being able to change things up, keep it playful, but also have those moments of sweetness.

So yes, let's agree to a lifetime of joy, passion, and the freedom to be as *freaky* and *loving* as we want. Who says you can't have both?

Future Goals:

As I ventured deeper into the wild and wondrous terrain of my life's journey, I couldn't help but confront the bigger picture—"What did I want my future to look like?" It was like sitting down to design my own personal masterpiece. Did I want kids? If so, how many? How would we parent them, discipline them, and make sure they knew the difference between a good taco and a bad taco? (Very important, obviously). These weren't just questions about biology or even bedtime stories; they were tied to my deepest values about family, legacy, and the kind of world I wanted to create. The idea of raising children with someone who shared my vision—values that ran as deep as roots in the ground—became a non-negotiable. Parenting with the right partner felt like a life-altering decision, one that required more than just a strong partnership, but a shared sense of purpose.

And, naturally, the conversation shifted to business. As someone with entrepreneurial dreams larger than my caffeine intake, I realized that owning a business wasn't just a passion—it was an entire lifestyle. I needed a partner who didn't just support my ambition, but who could see our future painted with the same entrepreneurial brush. Was building something together, co-owning a business, even a possibility? The thought of not just sharing a life, but sharing a legacy, of building something meaningful and lasting together became one of my ultimate goals. If we could build an empire side-by-side—now, that would be the ultimate testament to our alignment. A kingdom, a business, a family... I could see it all in my head. I'd even imagine a little victory dance when we crossed the finish line (a little dancing never hurt anyone).

Once you've defined your values and what you really want, hold on to them with the fierceness of a toddler clutching a cookie. Trust me, it's easy to get swept up in charm or be distracted by a pretty checklist, but those deeper issues? They don't just vanish. I've made that mistake more times than I care to admit. And let me tell you, there's nothing quite like the moment of realizing that charm doesn't pay the bills or raise children who know the difference between a good egg and a bad egg. Keep your boundaries strong and your vision clearer than ever—it's the best thing you'll do for yourself.

"YOU WON'T FIND PEACE IN THINGS THAT AREN'T MEANT FOR YOU"
—Michael Bliss

I once dated this amazing guy who was basically the poster child for everything you'd think I'd want. He was soft-spoken (so mysterious, right?), owned nightclubs (hello, VIP life), and had a heart so big it could probably house an entire orphanage. He was the kind of guy who would give you the shirt off his back—assuming he wasn't too busy wearing his all-black extension of his personality. He had a lot of things I *desired*—like a future car (matte black Range Rover, check) and casting projects for the homeless (check, humanitarian vibes), but there was just one little *tiny* issue: our values were completely misaligned.

Here's where things got tricky. He wanted a basketball team's worth of kids—six or more. I wasn't even sure if I wanted *one* child of my own, let alone six! He loved staying up late, binge-watching movies and TV shows, which is a lifestyle choice I will forever admire—if I was, say, 22 and living on caffeine and Red Bull. But here's the catch: I'm in my 30's, I love reading (not the same as watching TV, FYI), going to bed at a reasonable hour (9 PM, to be exact), unless I'm up writing or creating art, and plotting my next business venture before I even thought about how to make it to the end of a movie without falling asleep.

We were like two puzzle pieces that looked similar but just couldn't connect—kind of like trying to jam a square peg into a round hole, but fancier.

Now, here's the kicker: my non-negotiables? *Great communication* and a *health-conscious lifestyle*. So, while he was jetting off to his next event opening, I was over here working on my business goals, reflecting on my wellness routine, and literally looking up "best green smoothies" on Instagram while reading self-help books. We tried. Oh, we tried. But no matter how much we pretended to be into each other's worlds, the reality hit: we just weren't a match.

It was like the universe had put this shiny object in front of me—he was everything *on paper*—but as I took a closer look, it wasn't quite *right*. It was like Goldilocks and the Three Bears—only, instead of the porridge being too hot or too cold, it was a misaligned future. And let's be honest, who's going to live with a basketball team in a Range Rover when they'd rather curl up with a book at 9 PM?

So, lesson learned: alignment of values and goals? *Super* important. Don't fall for the shiny stuff—check the foundations first. It's all about compatibility, folks. Keep your standards high and your values even higher. And if the Range Rover's black, but it's missing the communication, you might want to think twice.

CHAPTER TWENTY SIX

CYCLES OF LOVE: BREAKING PATTERNS, INNER STRENGTH.

Deserve: The Cycle Continues:

I'm reflecting on healing my heart. I remember a time when I felt totally lost—swamped by the overwhelming weight of my fears. I would lie awake at night, my mind racing, unable to shut off the thoughts of all my failures. It was like this endless loop of self-doubt. One evening, after another restless night, I realized something needed to change. I had to confront those fears head-on. But to do that, I had to first acknowledge them. I closed my eyes and thought about people who have hurt me, and once again, MK came to mind. It felt like this situation was meant to be a lesson for me. I had a similar realization when my uncle passed away and I couldn't attend the funeral. I felt guilty, like I "should" feel worse. Fawn once told me she felt abandoned when I moved away, and I was shocked. I had no idea I made such an impact on her life. Over the years, other friends have shared similar feelings since I left home. It made me realize that was also how Mr. J might have felt when I packed up the house and dipped. I just vanished in a matter of a day.

While processing these emotions, something unexpected happened: CHI reappeared out of nowhere. My phone ran early in the morning before work. His number popped up on the screen, like a ghost from the past. I thought it was a butt dial. Excited, I answered, he reached out to tell me he hit all his goals of buying a truck and serving the country on the road, and was coming back to town, we chatted for a while. He suggested I wear "something special." He wanted to take me to dinner. Waiting for his call hours later, he ghosted me, disappearing like a magician.

Thankfully, I stuck to my original plan of working out and spending time on myself. But, oh, it still stung. I couldn't help but think, "Really? *Seriously*?" It felt like he had vanished into thin air, like one of those magic tricks, you know—David Copperfield-style. Gone, without a trace.

A few weekends later, the phone rang again. His number popped up on the screen, this time I let it ring. A couple of hours later, it rang again. I stared at the phone, feeling like I was watching a rerun of a bad movie. "Two strikes, you're out," I thought. The first time? Sure, maybe I could chalk it up to bad luck—shame on me. But the second round? A no-show, no explanation, just *poof*, gone again. (**The Runner**)

Nope, third time's not the charm. I'm no one's comeback story, especially not for someone who's already played me once. I've got boundaries, respect, and a little thing called self-worth. I'm not in the business of running in circles or revisiting exes. I'm moving forward, not backward.

Another realization: I also made plans to dance with my dear friend KLur. We were going to do some dance choreography together. We checked in a few times during the week, but on Saturday morning, she didn't reply to my text. When I followed up later, utter silence, she still blew me off. Another ghost in the wind. I started to reflect on these experiences and realized that I couldn't hide from this pattern any longer. It was clear that the universe was trying to connect the dots for me. (**The Reminder**)

So, I began a practice of self-reflection. It wasn't easy, and it wasn't pretty. I'd sit down and ask myself the hard questions: Why was I so afraid? Where did these thoughts come from? It took patience and a lot of self-compassion, but it was the key to unlocking my growth. The feeling of abandonment I was experiencing seemed to be mirrored back to me by others, but I began to wonder if it was more about my relationship with myself. Was my little self—the one that has been suppressed—feeling abandoned? It seemed I was projecting these feelings onto others and getting them reflected back to me. It was time to heal.

Dictionary: *"Abandonment: The act of leaving someone or something, or ending or stopping something, usually forever. Abandonment issues can stem from abuse, neglect, or other stressful experiences during childhood, such as divorce, death, or illness. These traumatic experiences can impact brain development and lead to depression or substance abuse (which, truth be told, I have definitely struggled with)."*

I used to think I wasn't "addicted" because I didn't have that personality type, but the truth is, I'm addicted to love. I'm a "hopeless romantic."

There was a time when I thought I could go through everything alone—work, heartbreak, stress—I kept it all to myself. But after a particularly tough week, where everything seemed to fall apart, I realized how isolated I felt. So, I took a leap and reached out to a friend. I needed someone to talk to, someone who would listen, without judgment.

That conversation was the turning point for me. It reminded me that I didn't have to carry the weight alone. Slowly, I began to build my support system—friends, family, mentors—people who I could count on to remind me of my strength and guide me when I felt lost.

There was a period when I was so focused on pleasing others and being there for everyone around me, that I neglected myself. It wasn't until I reached a breaking point that I realized—*if I wasn't taking care of myself, how could I truly help anyone else?* So, I started working on myself, setting boundaries, and focusing on my own mental health. As I began to do this, I noticed that the right people started showing up in my life—people who encouraged my growth, and who were on a similar journey."

The work I did on myself became the foundation for a support system that truly nurtured me. I learned that leading yourself is the first step to attracting the right kind of people into your life.

Looking back, I can see how crucial it was for me to embrace that fear and push through it. That moment wasn't just about overcoming a challenge; it was about realizing my own strength and resilience. I had to acknowledge my fear before I could move past it. And now, when I face a similar situation, I remember how that feeling of discomfort led to growth. So, I urge you—if you're stuck, take a moment to face those fears. Acknowledge them. Only then can you start to move forward.

Okay, let's talk about self-care. I know, I know—you've heard it a thousand times. But I'm serious. I was the worst at this. I thought self-care meant a bubble bath, but it's more than that. For me, it was saying **"no"** when I wanted to say **"yes"**, taking a walk when I felt overwhelmed, and just being kind to myself when things weren't going perfectly. Trust me, I get it, we all think we can power through. But you need to listen to your body and mind—they're telling you something.

Fear of Abandonment:

Abandonment Anxiety, Attachment Theory: My reflection repeatedly highlighted feelings of being left behind—whether by romantic partners, friends, or family. These experiences suggest unresolved abandonment issues, possibly rooted in early-life experiences.

Addiction to Love:

Love Addiction, Dependency, Emotional Regulation: By identifying as a "hopeless romantic," I acknowledge a potential dependency on love as a coping mechanism. Love addiction can arise from an attempt to fill emotional voids or escape feelings of inadequacy.

Relevance to Unconditional Love: Love given from a place of addiction or need often comes with expectations or conditions. True unconditional love emerges when love is shared freely, without the expectation of it being a solution to one's inner struggles.

My story offers a powerful journey of self-discovery, resilience, and healing. By acknowledging my fears, breaking patterns, and setting boundaries, I shifted towards a healthier, more unconditional love—both for myself and others. This path reflects the essence of unconditional love: it begins within and radiates outward, grounded in strength, authenticity, and self-respect.

CHAPTER TWENTY SEVEN

Dissolving Your Nature.

STARS CAN'T SHINE WITHOUT DARKNESS:

I've found that the darkness can be pretty fun when you learn to dance with it instead of constantly shaming it. Instead of keeping our shadows locked up in chains of sadness, let's embrace them. I had this revelation the other night while I was showering. I noticed this dark glow around the curtain, and for a moment, I thought it might be Cleo, my ever-present little shadow kitten who's always up in my business. (Kind of like a pesky younger sibling). But when I pulled back the curtain, she wasn't there. That's when I realized that it was my own shadow playing in the light, dancing along with me as I sang and danced under the shower. The water felt like a loving embrace, showering me with joy and laughter.

So, what is self-love anyway? It feels like a lesson that's never really over.

Driver's License:

Lately, I keep hearing people talk about life as if it's all about choosing the right vehicle to reach your goals and dreams. It's a metaphor that makes sense, but honestly, it got really frustrating when I realized I had to retake my driver's test here in California. Obviously annoyed, as I've had my license then for about 15, give or take, years it felt almost insulting. It feels like every state has its own set of rules, and California is like its own country with its own quirky regulations. The government here moves at its own pace, which can be pretty annoying.

Anyway, I've been wrestling with the idea of going back to the basics of studying for this test. Tests have always been my weak spot, but I'm determined to tackle this one since it's my goal for the month, and I'm determined to get it done before my birthday. A nice present to myself: happy "California resident." Everything around me is screaming that it doesn't have to be perfect, I just need the courage to try. So, I'm diving in this week, because more doors will open if I do, right?

Reflecting on this, I thought about how I used to study and practice driving. I remembered the weekly driving school sessions I'd taken when I was younger and all those hours spent practicing with my parents. They were so nervous every time I got behind the wheel. I even have this vivid memory of driving into the other lane to pass a car, thinking we had plenty of time, while there was oncoming traffic heading in our direction. My mom nearly had a meltdown. It was like she was a hairless cat leaping out of its skin! She couldn't believe I was in such a hurry that I'd endanger both of us just to cut this slow driver in front of us. It was reckless, I understand that now.

The point is, driving requires tons of practice before you're considered "qualified." You spend days honing your skills before finally passing the test and getting your license. And then you're thrilled to get that photo taken, trying to look your best as they snap the picture.

The whole process is a bit like life. You're given a "government number" (your Social Security number) that marks your progress on the metaphorical monopoly board of life, isn't this Matrix fun? But if you didn't practice and learn the rules, you wouldn't pass the test. It's funny to think I've been driving with old Wisconsin plates for years, trying to get settled in California, and now I'm back to square one with new ones.

But let's talk about relearning. It's something we all roll our eyes at, but the truth is, we need to learn, unlearn, and relearn throughout our lives. It's about healing from old patterns and gaining new knowledge. For me, studying for this exam has been a way to refresh outdated skills and recognize bad habits. I've lived in several states, each with its own set of rules, and it's almost like every street has its own unique traffic laws.

In Hollywood, for instance, people just sit at intersections until the light finally turns red, and if you don't go, you'll be waiting forever. So, even though retaking this test has been frustrating, it's also given me a fresh perspective. It's a reminder that we all need to revisit and renew our skills regularly. And if I have to take this test again, I'm taking it as an opportunity to reassess other areas in my life that might need a new perspective.

CHAPTER TWENTY EIGHT

IT TAKES A VILLAGE.

What Does It Mean to Cultivate Community:

Let's be real—community is something we all crave, even if we're too scared to admit it. We want to feel accepted, validated, and, let's face it, included in the group chat. But instead of sitting on the sidelines waiting for someone to invite you in, here's an idea: what if you made the first move?

I learned this the hard way—quickly and awkwardly, as most lessons go. Like many of us, I wanted to be part of a community but was terrified to step up and say, "Hey, can I join in?" I'd overthink everything. *"What if they think I'm weird? What if I'm rejected?"* Spoiler alert: none of that mattered. The magic happened when I decided to invest myself.

Instead of waiting for someone to notice me, I started saying hello first. I introduced myself to people in groups I admired. I made connections over shared interests, cracked a joke or two, and kept showing up. The truth is, cultivating community is a lot like planting a garden. You've got to water it, check the pH levels (metaphorically speaking, of course), and keep showing up with your seeds of effort.

And guess what? One interaction isn't enough. In sales, they call this "touches"—the more meaningful interactions you have with someone, the more trust and rapport you build. So, I didn't stop at saying hello. I followed up, stayed consistent, and kept showing up. Slowly but surely, the invitations started rolling in, opportunities opened up, and friendships blossomed.

For instance, when I wanted to be involved in Insomnia Productions, I joined a couple of departments. Not only did I meet new people, but I made myself indispensable by being flexible and willing to help. When I moved to California and started attending church, I decided to treat it like my home. My "toxic trait" is making my house look like no one lives there (seriously, I clean *too* much), so I brought that same energy to my church family. I joined the serving team, cleaned, organized, and helped wherever I could. Before I knew it, I had a circle of friends and a real sense of belonging.

Here's the kicker: by committing myself fully, I created ripples I never anticipated. Over nine months, those small steps led to friendships, job opportunities, and events that enriched my life beyond measure. One small decision to get plugged in turned into a beautiful, life-changing experience.

There's a phrase I hear in my team that always sticks: *"I'm all in."* Not just dipping my toes in lukewarm water, but diving headfirst. When you're all in, you hit your goals faster—obviously. But let's be honest, being "all in" depends on your season of life.

Building a community is about showing up consistently and authentically, even during hard seasons. People can't read your mind, so communicate. If you're struggling, let your community know what's going on instead of assuming they'll figure it out. Great communication builds trust and intimacy, and trust is the foundation of every strong community.

As Erwin McManus said, "Language is our vehicle, and communication is our oxygen." The deeper our communication, the stronger our sense of community. When we cultivate community, we're not just building friendships—we're creating a support system, a family, and a home.

So, take the plunge. Dive in. Be all in. Your future self—and your future friendships—will thank you.

BUILDING YOUR OWN LOVE CLUB:

Picture this: you're walking into a room full of strangers, but somehow, it feels like home. There's this warmth in the air, the kind that wraps around you like a cozy blanket you didn't know you needed. Welcome to the "*Love Club.*" It's not some exclusive, velvet-rope society, oh no. This club is open to anyone who believes in unconditional love—like the kind that doesn't come with strings attached, no expiration date, and definitely no judgment. You don't need a special handshake or a secret password—just the desire to show up as your real, messy, beautiful self.

Now, how do you create such a magical space? Well, it all starts with one simple thing: vulnerability. Yep, that's right. Throw those walls down like confetti at a New Year's party. Let people see your quirks, your scars, and those moments when you trip over your own feet in front of everyone (who hasn't been there?). Vulnerability is what gives love room to grow. It's the fertile soil in which compassion, empathy, and connection bloom.

Next, you've got to nurture it. Picture love as a garden, and you're the gardener. Every act of kindness you give is like watering a flower—whether it's sending a text just to check in, offering a word of encouragement when someone's feeling down, or making your famous mac and cheese for a friend going through a tough time (because let's be honest, food is a love language). And just like plants, the people in your *Love Club* need space to grow. Let them be who they are, without pushing them to change or fit a mold. You've got to embrace their roots, even if they're a little different from your own.

The beauty of this club? It's not about perfection. It's about showing up, showing love, and letting yourself be loved back. You don't have to have it all figured out. In fact, some of the best moments are the ones that happen when everything is a little messy—like laughing so hard at inside jokes that tears stream down your face or comforting someone with the perfect "it's okay to cry" hug. Love is imperfect, and that's what makes it real.

And, of course, you've got to celebrate it. Don't just sit around talking about love, go out there and *do* it. Organize spontaneous dance parties in the living room, start a kindness challenge, or create a tradition of random acts of love. A love club thrives on its energy. The more you give, the more it multiplies, like an infinite supply of good vibes.

In the end, it's not just about creating a support system—it's about creating a movement. When you build a community rooted in unconditional love, you don't just change lives, you change the world, one act of kindness at a time. So, get out there, find your people, and watch how love can build a tribe stronger than anything else in this world.

Another Author:

Well, here I am, pen in hand, realizing what unconditional love truly means—especially when it comes to this book. I've been dreaming of writing this for over twelve years, and let me tell you, it hasn't come without a whole lot of thoughts and doubts swirling around in my head. What should I teach the world? What lessons are worth sharing? And which parts of myself do I expose without feeling that nagging shame creeping in?

I'll be honest, there are still bits of me I'm not completely comfortable with, pieces of my story that I'm not yet fully ready to share. But I've been vulnerable enough to surrender the pain I've carried, to let go of all the things I once thought defined me. It's taken me a while to get here, but I now know that those experiences, the ones that used to haunt me, no longer have the power to shape who I'm becoming. I've healed, and that's the gift I'm giving to myself.

But you know what? The most extraordinary, unconditional love I've received during this entire journey? It came from something I didn't expect at all—the writing of this book. I am proud of this journey I've been on, and now it was time to create my own community.

Enter Haley. **(THE EMPOWERER)**

I'm lucky enough to have been chosen to work with an amazing women's publishing company, and through that experience, I met Haley. Now, we didn't exactly meet the way you might think. I had been bouncing around our community groups inside the publishing company, trying to connect with others who might be going through the same experience I was. I found Haley, and we started messaging, all excited because we were about to work on a content day in Las Vegas but we were both from Los Angeles. Women from all over the world were flying in and shockingly to me only a few from LA were writing books for our **"Voice's of 100"** women project. They created a docu-series on each woman to express self-empowerment. Each author has their own book published, and voices spread to the world to create inspiration for generations to come.

But then, as life does, it threw us a curveball. Haley got sick on the day we were supposed to meet, and we missed each other completely. We even ended up standing in line next to each other, completely unaware. She had given me a funny description of her outfit (blue), and I told her I'd be wearing purple. But when it came down to it? Neither of us was wearing what we'd described. She thought I was wearing pink—I was wearing light lavender, and I thought she was going to be in royal blue, but it seemed more like a floral dress. Classic, right? It was as if the universe was playing its own little game of hide and seek with us.

Fast forward a few weeks, and we finally meet—at a coffee shop, no less. We realized that we had *almost* met that day, but we both had our blinders on, thinking we knew what the other looked like. Typical, right? But, oh, when we did finally meet, everything clicked. Haley is this radiant, athletic redhead with a heart as big as her spirit. And she's got an incredible support system—her pup Mocha. Her vibe is contagious, and you can't help but want to be around her.

It's been almost a year since then, and what a ride it's been. We've been through so much together, both of us in the middle of huge transitions in our lives. She was stepping into a new chapter in her own story, and I was just trying to figure out what the heck I was doing in the world of PR and publishing (and I still can't quite believe I'm here).

Haley has her own book coming out, too, and I can't wait for you all to read it—it's a powerful reflection of her life, her experiences, and her journey. I encourage you to keep an eye out for it.

But the thing is, when you're navigating through life's roller coasters, everything is easier when you have a partner in crime. Someone who holds you accountable, who reminds you why you're doing this, who helps you wade through the highs and lows. Trust me, it hasn't always been smooth sailing, but it's been *so* worth it. We've spent hours in coffee shops, at fashion shows, on long walks, and everywhere in between, finding inspiration, sharing ideas, and supporting each other.

Having a friend like Haley during this whole book-writing journey has been nothing short of a blessing. I'm so incredibly grateful for her, for her friendship, and for the unconditional love we've given each other along the way. This whole process has been transformative—not just for my book, but for me as a person.

Haley and I are so in sync that it's almost eerie. I mean, when it comes to the ups and downs of love, we've both been riding the same emotional rollercoaster. Picture this: we were each entangled in these love stories, with all the longing, the desires, the drama—and—plot twist—we were both dating guys whose names just *happened* to start with the letter D. Not only that, but when it came time to write our books, we both spontaneously decided to change the names of the men in our stories. And guess what? Out of the blue, we ended up picking the exact same "disguise" name for our characters.

We laughed so hard at each other in disbelief over the phone when we realized. It was one of those moments where you just can't help but laugh and say, "You can't make this sh*t up." It was like the universe was having its own little joke at our expense, knitting our tangled love lives together with an extra dash of irony.

But the real kicker? Our relationships were like these twisted spider webs, beautifully complex but a little too messy for comfort. We had both found ourselves longing for deep love, craving healthier connections, but still tangled up in the remnants of our toxic pasts. It was as if we were both writing our own love stories, but stuck in the same chapter of confusion and yearning.

But here we are, two women turning over new leaves, stepping into the new year with fresh intentions and hearts open to love that's healthy and real. No more twisted webs. No more repeating the same old patterns. Just two friends, ready to embrace a new beginning—and who knows, maybe a new "D" in the future—but this time, it'll be a whole different kind of love story.

This is my first book, the end of a chapter in my life, and the beginning of another one. I'm thankful for the community we created, and have to rely on if we need resources. As I close the book on this experience, I carry all my gratitude with me, not just for the book, but for the journey itself. The journey of unconditional love, of healing, of friendship, and of new beginnings. I'm excited for the next chapter—both in life and in the books to come.

So here's to love, to friendship, and to the beautiful, messy, perfect journey ahead. With all my love and gratitude, bring on the next chapters.

Psychological Healing:

Healing and no longer allowing past experiences to define who I am or become. Releasing trauma, letting go of painful experiences, and moving forward with a renewed sense of self.

Healthy Attachment:

The relationship is built on mutual support, empathy, and shared vulnerability. They both go through personal transitions and challenges, yet they serve as pillars for each other, providing emotional validation, accountability, and encouragement, emotional resilience, and social support.

Reflections of Purpose:

"I love the way you blush, when I tell you, you shine,"
—**unknown**

It's the kind of moment that stays with me, a small spark of recognition that you are exactly who you're meant to be. I've always believed that my fulfillment in life comes from seeing the highest version of someone's self-expression, the way it radiates when they finally realize their own potential. It's like catching a glimpse of someone's soul, their truest form, and seeing the way it lights up the world.

Years ago, I used to ask my clients and students, "If you could have any superpower, what would it be?" Their answers were always fun—flight, x-ray vision, telepathy, super speed. But for me, my answer was always the same: I would want to be a reflection in the mirror, showing them the greatness I see in them. I would be their biggest cheerleader, their mirror, reminding them of how far they can go. (**The Learner**)

One of my favorite things in life is getting to witness those moments when people I love and care about step into their greatness. It's like watching a light bulb go off in real time. I'll never forget these moments:

Alisha, holding her camera, capturing the sexual beauty in women who've long hidden it. She unlocks the power of self-love and empowerment through her lens. Watching her work has been like witnessing a quiet revolution, one click at a time. Working on projects with her brought out so much joy for everyone.- I was blessed to do our self–love portraits for my Seven Deadly Sins project.

Mr. Killa, pouring his heart and soul into his music—whether he's writing, producing, singing, or DJing—(DJ LOVER BOY,) each beat and lyric is a piece of his heart laid bare for the world. Watching him create is like watching a poet breathe life into sound. The way his eyes widened and a smile from ear to ear always brought happiness to my soul.

Andrea, would handcraft beautiful dainty jewelry. She works tirelessly to meet her deadlines, piece by piece with intention and care. I was so honored when she gifted me a half sun from her collection when I was moving away. We were always on the same wavelength, living life very parallel. Her gift was in the spiral of her whole experience; she was a gift.

Astro, sharing his art graphics in the form of a book, showing off the seasons of creation he's molded with his own hands. He was so proud, I admired that. There's something so profound in seeing someone give the world pieces of themselves, and Nate does this with such raw, unapologetic grace. He's a really hard worker.

Rachel, she literally created an entire container (literally) of creations. From jewelry to painting, her skills were endless, but the most profound moments were watching her be a teacher/mentor/mom, she lit up to see others grow, and be in their childlike energy. She gave them the gift of openness to create. Beautiful soul.

Kelly had a way of loving through words and the artistry of aesthetics—her creativity flowed effortlessly into skincare and self-care, turning the ordinary into something enchanting. She could conjure magic on the tiniest canvas, transforming a simple nail bed into a masterpiece. Every time she painted my nails, I felt not just adorned, but deeply appreciated, wrapped in the beauty of her craft.

And then, there was my friend Marseilles. Watching her walk in her first fashion show and then perform her own music, it was like seeing her step into her true self. The joy that filled my heart was overwhelming, and yes, it brought tears to my eyes. But it was what happened next that really took me by surprise: she sang to her boyfriend next to me, and I saw him blush. That was the moment. That sweet moment where someone, in all their brilliance, chooses to share their love and their light with the world. It's the kind of love that fills up the space around them, lighting up everything.

These are the moments when you know you're not just existing—you're thriving. You're supported by a community that sees you, loves you, and roots for your success. That's what I live for: helping people step into the light of their own greatness.

Another friend: Romane, directing the room during a music video shoot. His vision for film is extraordinary, but what's even more fascinating is the way he weaves his theories of life and existence into every frame. To watch him work is to see someone completely in their element, shaping the world around them with his creative power. The vision he has inside his mind is nothing sort of magic. His direction is wise, and humble.

Each of these moments—the blushing, the singing, the creating—is a reflection of love. Love for one another, love for the craft, and ultimately, love for ourselves. When you step into your purpose, when you fully embrace your gifts, you not only shine—you light up the world around you.

"We create the life we desire through the choices we make, the sacrifices we endure, and by choosing not to search for someone who will love us unconditionally, but by making the decision to love them unconditionally."

Witnessing Growth as Fulfillment:

Altruism, Vicarious Growth: By fulfillment in seeing others grow and succeed you align yourself with the psychological concept of altruism—deriving joy from helping others without expecting anything in return."

Community and Interdependence:

Social Support, Collective Efficacy, Interdependence: My experience underscores the power of community—a network of people who uplift and support each other. Each example is a testament to my role in fostering collective growth and mutual inspiration.

Key Themes and Insights on Unconditional Love:

Unconditional Support: The role as a "cheerleader" mirrors the essence of unconditional love—being present for others and rooting for their success, without imposing personal desires or agendas.

Celebrating Individuality: Each person's story underscores the value of embracing your unique talents and perspectives. Unconditional love honors individuality, recognizing that everyone's light shines differently.

Creating Space for Growth: By fostering an environment where others can thrive I was able to show unconditional love and create safe, nurturing spaces that encourage exploration, growth, and self-expression.

The Ripple Effect of Love: When we step into our purpose, we don't only fulfill ourselves as individuals, but we also inspire and uplift others. Unconditional love has this ripple effect, spreading light and positivity far beyond the immediate relationship.

How to Have a Clear and Healthy Breakup (And Why You Need It)

Alright, let's get into it. Breakups. They're like pizza—some are good, some are not, but you're usually just hoping for an easy one. And trust me, you deserve that. But what happens when you've had the *perfect* breakup? Like, it was loving, it was passionate, maybe even a little beautiful? I know, sounds like a unicorn in the breakup world, right?

But then, here's where the plot twist happens. You try to keep it friendly. You try to hold those boundaries like a pro, but it's *so* easy to fall into the comfort of old habits. The texting. The late-night chats. You're trying to be supportive, but, come on—*it's time to stop!* Cut the strings. Let go of those invisible cords. Seriously, even when you're in a new romantic relationship, don't let the past take the wheel. There's no room for three people in a two-person romantic relationship, even if it's playing out on a subconscious level. If you haven't cut your cords, and you're still texting your ex or "friends" —it can be damaging for the new relationship to develop.

Sometimes breakups aren't even romantic. Maybe it's a friend. Like, take my friend Whitney. (*"**The Runner.**"*) We met in our nursing unit back when I worked in the ICU. She was a blonde bombshell. We became fast friends. She'd come in hot, outta nowhere, and before I knew it, she'd be gone, leaving me chasing her. Talk about *seriously confusing*. At the time of our friendship she was getting married, and at her wedding Mr. J and I weren't coupling very well. I had a bit too much to drink, and he made some comment about not wanting to get married or some nonsense. I vaguely remember it, but being harsh, with even our friends next to us making disgusted faces, it was a big scene. Whitney decided she didn't want to be a part of our story anymore, embarrassed. When she decided to cut the cord on our friendship I was deeply hurt. I knew I had been the one to mess up, but a lot of my own wrong doings were my fear and my body projecting from other hurtful relationships I was in at the same time. I felt heartbroken when she stopped speaking to me. She took a part of my heart, I was literally heartbroken. We had become fast friends, working together, working out together, soon inseparable, then suddenly gone as fast as the wind. Leaving a hue over me I could not ignore:

Seia (THE HEARTBREAKER) -- We bonded quickly, like two kindred souls drawn together by proximity and circumstance, becoming inseparable for a time. Over four years, our friendship was a tapestry woven with shared experiences and deep connection. But amidst the beauty of our bond, there were threads of discord that began to fray.

In the turmoil of our friendship, it seemed I was unwittingly confirming the fears she had long harbored—that women could be unreliable, even harmful as friends. My own insecurities within my relationship with Mr. J led me to choices that hurt her deeply, tarnishing the trust we had built. Our paths began to clash, the harmony of our friendship unraveling into discord.

When her relationship with Lucia came to an end, so too did her presence in our lives. I spent countless moments wishing for her forgiveness, hoping one day we might find our way back to one another. But the wounds were too deep, and for her own peace and healing, she needed to move forward.

Some bonds are not meant to last forever, but that doesn't diminish their beauty. We were both deeply hurt by the break of our friendship. Seia's presence in my life was a fleeting but powerful reminder of connection, and though we've parted ways, I carry the lessons of our time together in my heart.

Or **Mo** — The "bestie replacement." During COVID she was the one who somehow showed me how to love fiercely, how to be supportive, and how to embrace the art of mentoring. But here's the thing: you can't lead someone to become the person you envision for them. They have to want it for themselves, to grow into their best self—maybe the one you see in your head, but it's their journey, their decision.

I was so eager to help her, to guide her through the maze of business development, helping her build her fitness empire. But it turned out, she wasn't ready to climb that ladder of success just yet. I admit, I rushed her process—out of love, of course—but it wasn't what was meant for her at that time.

Somewhere in the mix, I even played matchmaker, pulling the strings of a chess game to get her and Mr. J's best friend together. She became the "replacement for the friend before her." Trading spaces, hoping to see the queen win the match. *Checkmate.* But as time passed, leaving my relationship with Mr. J it was clear: our friendship had run its course. It was time for me to step away from the "couple lives" chapter and let the dynamics shift so I could grow into my next adventure.

I thank God for Mo, for all the lessons she taught me—especially about how to handle breakups like a pro. Sometimes, though, the universe has a way of nudging you where you need to go, even if it's not what you'd planned. **(THE TEACHER/LEARNER)**

One of the most heart-wrenching breakups was when Caroline (**THE ETERNAL**) and I decided to part ways. We were *inseparable* for years—partners in crime, co-adventurers. Oh, the memories. When we "broke up," I didn't want it, not really. But sometimes, life has other plans. Too many issues had piled up over time, and even though we'd moved across the country together, found new places to call home, and even adopted Miller as our fur baby, something shifted. One Christmas break, she went home to visit her family for a month I spent all my time with Isaiah cooking, cleaning, and going to the gym. The dynamic of our friend group changed. The space between us grew too wide

Afterward, I moved in with Isaiah **(THE REMINDER)**, and we divided our lives like a long-overdue yard sale—splitting assets, dividing up the bits and pieces. I took Miller, of course, my constant companion. But for a while, it felt like we might never repair our friendship. I wasn't sure we'd ever find our way back to each other.

Then, out of nowhere, my brother Ben passed away. Caroline, as if by fate, showed up to support me. That moment of unexpected tenderness between us began to heal what we thought was broken beyond repair. If she hadn't shown up when she did, I'm not sure we'd ever have found our way back.

Who knew that death could turn into such a sweet memory? If that's not a plot twist, I don't know what is. Life sure does have a way of surprising you when you least expect it.

Ah, **Mari**. Let's talk about her. Our girl group slowly drifted apart over the years in Wilmington, swept away by the tide of life events. But one year, Mari was going through a tough time with her roommate, and I thought, *"why not invite her to live with me and Mr. J?"* She graciously accepted, bringing her dog, Spaghetti, who, let's be real, was basically a VIP guest in my guest room.

For a while, everything felt cozy—until it didn't. Our energies started to clash, like two instruments out of tune. If I remember correctly, I was a bit *too* overbearing? When she settled back into a new home she bought eventually, she had to break up with me. And honestly, I needed the space, too. There was so much happening in my life at the time. I was in the middle of a growth spurt (the emotional kind), and needed time for reflection and recalibration.

But surprise—it wasn't the end of us. Life had its way of working things out. Over time, we healed. About a year later (thanks, life experiences!) we started to reconnect, slowly rebuilding our bond. I was preparing for my move to California going through everything in my house. We'd meet for coffee dates to return the things we'd left behind during our time together, and check in on each other's lives. Becca's business had taken off in different directions in the meantime, and she even started a podcast! One of her episodes was about rebuilding, letting go, releasing, and creating something new in a friendship. It was beautifully done.

Over the years, we've kept in touch—almost monthly, like clockwork. The split hurt, but looking back, it was the kind of pain that gave birth to something even more meaningful. In the end, we came out stronger. **(THE TEACHER)**

And then you go back to the lovers: let's not forget Damon. You'll get to know more of that later:

Oh, Damon- **(THE REMINDER)**. I'm not the type to break up and get back together and keep the cycle going on and off, but him? He was *different*. Fast forward to us doing the break-up dance—seven times. Yes, seven. By the fifth time, we thought, *this is it, the grand finale*, after a week of space and some soul-searching. Our situation was unique. Ours wasn't just a love story—it was a series of circumstances stacked so high, you'd think fate was playing some twisted game with us.

The night before, I'd overreacted. I just wanted it to be over, but I wanted to be respectful, at least do it face-to-face. Then he called in the morning to make plans, but I had to follow up to confirm, and instead, he texted me. "I don't think so, it's been enough time apart, we have too much at stake. When can I come get my things?" And I thought, *"Alright, okay, I'm going to need a backup plan... because this is going to be one wild ride."*

Cue the weirdest emotional rollercoaster you could imagine. We said goodbye in the most unexpected way, love making. And then—oh yes— there was me, asking him to stay just a little longer until my heart finally let go. A physical release. (No biggie, right?)

The next day? He was texting me again, and I'm like, "NOPE." But hey, that was it, right? I had to finally cut that cord. For real.

We broke up, two more times until the ground breaking moment when I was done, but GOD- *LITERALLY PUT ME IN HIS HANDS.*

In the end, here's what you need to remember: breakups are hard, but sometimes they're the clean breaks that help you grow. You don't need to drag the past along with you. You deserve the release and more importantly, you deserve the peace that comes from letting go. And hey, when you finally break free, you'll have your own bouquet of sunflowers waiting. 🌻

CHAPTER TWENTY NINE

THREADS OF IDENTITY.

Why Do Women Wear Mismatched Socks?

I often ponder why mismatched socks seem to be a common choice among women. As I can say for myself, I do this without even thinking or caring. But like everything about me there's depth to it. Personally, I don't fuss over matching socks when I put them on, and it appears many other women share this indifference. Yet, men often seem to prioritize matching their socks meticulously.

In hindsight, this raises an intriguing question: why do women spend so much time perfecting their outfits? It might take hours to choose an outfit that fits well, reflects the right style, or captures the desired essence. But when it comes to socks, many of us are surprisingly nonchalant. Our feet, which support and balance us, seem to get overlooked in favor of more visible aspects of our appearance.

Growing up in America, we're bombarded with messages telling us we're not "perfect" enough. Amid these pressures, perhaps mismatched socks represent a small, deliberate act of rebellion—a way to defy the obsession with flawless appearances and embrace a bit of imperfection. It's a subtle reminder that while we may obsess over every detail of our outward appearance, sometimes it's okay to let the small things, like our socks, be just a bit imperfect.

In the grand scheme of things, maybe it's about finding a balance—recognizing that while we care deeply about the clothes that shape our outward persona, it's perfectly fine to let go of minor details and embrace our individuality in small ways.

Name Basis:

I met a girl at the LA Fitness in Playa Vista. *The girl.* **(THE TEACHER)** Absolutely gorgeous. You know the type—long, dark hair cascading down her back like she's stepped out of a shampoo commercial. Her skin? Glowing. Like, she had the perfect sun-kissed glow even though we were indoors. I was immediately like, "Okay, I'm practicing being intentional and memory strength, I need to talk to her." Her name was AJA, taking initiative. I was curious about the origin of her name and asked her about it. She told me that her parents named her after a term from the Muslim tradition, which means "the perfect woman." Just think about that for a second—what a huge expectation to place on a little girl in a world that constantly reminds us of our imperfections. We got to chatting, and the more she talked, the more I realized—this girl was *not* just a pretty face. She had this energy about her, this natural confidence that wasn't trying too hard.

She shared that this has been a lifelong lesson for her. As she's grown older, she's come to understand and embrace the meaning of her name, gradually learning to embody that essence with confidence. She wore her confidence very well I might add. Through her I was able to learn that we must embody all of our essence.

Unconditional Positive Regard: This concept, introduced by Carl Rogers, refers to accepting and valuing a person without conditions or expectations. Aja's name, meaning "the perfect woman," suggests a societal expectation that might feel conditional. However, her journey to embody that essence reflects a deeper understanding of self-worth that transcends external validation. When we practice unconditional love, we appreciate the inherent worth of a person without imposing unrealistic standards.

Embracing the Makeup Mask:

The realization hit me while I was on the phone with my current "flavor of the month", (that's a man I was having "relations" with in my situationship) applying my daily makeup while contouring. I had learned the art of makeup at a young age through dance shows, pom squads, and just growing up as a girl. Applying it always took time, but as I got older and trends shifted, I found myself increasingly frustrated.

Living in North Carolina, my best friend, Caroline landed a job at Sephora and became a true perfectionist with makeup. She was incredibly talented, but the process seemed overly elaborate to me— contouring and highlighting felt like it took forever. Over the years, makeup evolved into a billion-dollar industry, and it wasn't until my 30s that I decided to take it more seriously. I really didn't believe it should take longer than 15 mins to apply makeup, in my opinion. But I also know better, that art takes a long time, and multiple settings to apply.

I'd heard from mentors around my age who shared similar sentiments— having "tomboy vibes" and not feeling the need to wear makeup to feel good. Then it dawned on me: if I was leaning too much into my masculine side, maybe it was time to embrace my feminine side and apply that concept to my life overall. It struck me that makeup could be a way to reconnect with my feminine energy.

As I painted spots, contouring dots, and lines on my face, I had an epiphany: makeup is a lot like war paint. It's preparation for the daily battles we all face—whether it's navigating traffic, dealing with the pressure of celebrity culture, managing the chaos of motherhood, or even surviving the intensity of instagram/tik-tok shoots. We put on these masks to help us face the world and fight our personal battles, emerging victorious in our own unique way.

There's no judgment here for those who love makeup, for anyone who chooses to use it to cover up or alter their appearance. But it's important to remember that makeup is just one tool. The real strength comes from knowing who you are without it. True victory comes when you work on conquering your self-esteem, when you realize you're worthy and capable without the layers. You can still fight the battles and win, whether you have makeup on or not. It's about embracing your true self and finding strength from within.

CHAPTER THIRTY

PROFOUND STRANGERS.

Third Time's a Charm:

Have you ever had one of those moments when you run into the same person over and over again, and you start to wonder if the universe is playing some weird game with you? That's exactly how it went when I met Tommy **(THE REMINDER)** at my gym.

I had never seen him before, but there he was—a tall, lean, and handsome Chinese guy (not typically my type, but hey, we're not picky, right?). He was decked out in all black: a cut-off shirt that showed off his toned muscles, black shorts that gave off the "I mean business" vibe. Basically, he looked like he walked straight out of a fitness magazine.

We struck up a brief conversation, and when I introduced myself, he mentioned that he'd seen me around. I laughed and said, "Yeah, I don't wear my contacts at the gym, so I have no idea who anyone is. I'm just here, staying focused and not paying attention to distractions."

Because, let's be real—the gym is my sanctuary. It's my place to clear my head, get out of my own thoughts, and just push my limits without worrying about what anyone else is doing. But still, there was something about Tommy. It wasn't just the fact that he was hot and had muscles that could make any personal trainer proud (which, let's be honest, definitely helped). It was that small exchange and the feeling that maybe, just maybe, this wasn't going to be the last time we ran into each other.

It was like one of those weird coincidences where paths cross at just the right moment. Little did I know, this seemingly random gym encounter would turn into something much more than I expected.

To my surprise, I bumped into him again at my church. He was friends with one of the singers on the worship team and I was amazed by the singer's incredible voice. It shouldn't have been so shocking, though, living in LA, even with 18+ million people, we end up in our social circles. I'm starting to realize how small the world can be much like it was back in Wilmington.

Curious, I decided to dive deeper into our conversation. It turned out he was leading a double life in finance because that's what society—and his family back in China—had expected of him. His whole life had been mapped out according to these expectations. But after a near-death experience (NDE), he decided he was done running from his true passion. He chose to follow a new path and become a music producer, driven by his love for how music can connect with and move the heart.

I admired his shift from a predetermined path to pursuing his dream. His insights on sound waves, emotions, and the power of music were inspiring. When he showed me some of his music, my heart was on fire. It's incredible how a life-altering event can completely redirect our paths, isn't it?

Everyday Desires:

In some way, we all want our everyday experiences to matter. Author and former marriage and family counselor John Eldredge asks, "What if those deepest desires in our hearts are telling us the truth, revealing the life we were meant to live?"

As idealists at heart, we often prefer to present ourselves in the best light, crafting motives that sound good. And when we create space for others to do the same, we foster connection.

We all crave transcendence—to be part of something bigger than ourselves, to find meaning in the world and the people around us. We want to be the ones who rise above, take a stand, and do what is right, honorable, and true.

When we share our stories, others feel encouraged to share theirs. Together, we can create a powerful community. When your journey becomes our journey, we're both compelled to see where it leads.

As I reflect on the journey of my book, I've come to realize that each soul we meet is not by accident, but rather part of a cosmic design. Every person we cross paths with, whether a lifelong companion or a fleeting moment, holds a purpose we may not always see. In the grand play of life, we are all actors, stepping onto the stage to fulfill roles we agreed to long before our first breath. These encounters, both gentle and intense, are the lessons we promised ourselves we would learn—each person a teacher, a guide, or a mirror.

I believe that beneath it all, we come from the purest essence of love, an infinite well that connects us all. And through the many faces we meet— **THE ETERNALS** souls, **THE HEARTBREAKERS, THE EMPOWERERS, THE REMINDERS** and so many others—we move closer to understanding that love. I've made sure to add each character connection by each character in the book as reference. It is a journey that is messy, beautiful, and transformative, weaving us into the beings we are meant to become. In this sacred dance, we find that each encounter, no matter how fleeting or profound, is a piece of the puzzle that reveals the true essence of unconditional love. Perhaps, as we walk this path, we start to understand that we are all here to fulfill a role, one that carries us back to love itself.

Stranger With Her Art:

34.0915° N, 118.3508° W

Enjoying the swing sets after a long day at the music store, this sweet little gem of a park fills me with the gentle embrace of a place that truly holds my heart. Closing my eyes under the golden sunshine, I let the moment linger before opening them again. That's when I noticed something unexpected—handwritten chalk arrows pointing towards a little building I'd never really paid attention to before. To my surprise, it was an art gallery. Full-on rooms dedicated to showcasing art! Who would've thought?

Hollywood always has its surprises. Everywhere you go in LA, you expect to run into people—and not just any people. Everyone here has a story. Some are celebrities, others immigrants; some are both. Wherever they're from, each person carries a lifetime of journeys and dreams. I try to always be the best version of myself, treating everyone with kindness. Holding doors open, offering a hand, or just sharing a warm smile—simple acts of kindness that ripple outward. I don't put people on pedestals; I treat everyone the same. But it's always funny to realize later that the stranger I held a door for was a billionaire or someone with an incredible story I'd only learn about afterward.

There's something magical about this city—the energy you put out has a way of returning to you. Good things, bad things, all of it circles back. And so, I've learned to savor the surprises, to revel in the chance encounters that make life feel like a treasure hunt. Sometimes, it's a billionaire. Other times, it's someone from halfway across the world who barely speaks English but smiles as though they've won the lottery of life just by being here. Gratefulness radiates from them, untainted by entitlement of others here. Many prayed for the chance to escape their circumstances, to find freedom here. In America, we have this incredible gift called **free enterprise**—the freedom to dream, to create, to be our own bosses. It's a privilege we often take for granted.

And that's when I bumped into her, Siyowin. **(THE REMINDER)**

She was stunning—tall and slender, with jet-black hair that cascaded like a river of ink. Her Native American heritage was unmistakable, woven into her presence like threads in a tapestry. She could have been a supermodel, but there was something far deeper in her eyes. They glowed with a quiet intensity, yet beneath that light was a shadow—a sadness that flickered like embers of a dying fire. My gaze followed hers to the artwork on display—human-sized paintings that seemed to pulse with life. They depicted her people dancing, surrounded by an aura of fire and shadows. The pain radiated from the canvas, raw and unfiltered, as if the art itself was alive, breathing, and burning.

"Is this your work?" I asked, my voice soft with reverence. She hesitated, shy yet proud. "Yes, it is," she replied. "I was just sitting in my room one day, feeling overwhelmed with emotions, and I started to create—anywhere I could. On cardboard, walls, street signs, wood... whatever I could find. It's the trauma I feel, passed down through my family and our land for generations. I needed a way to release it."

"Incredible," I said, awestruck. "Can you tell me more about yourself?"

She smiled faintly, the kind of smile that holds both pride and pain. "I grew up not knowing my gifts, not knowing what I was good at. One day, I started experimenting with different mediums. Over time, I realized I had a talent for art and illustration. It became my way of self-discovery, a way to express my pain and the pain that had enslaved me. As I grow, I've come to understand that releasing these emotions through art transforms them. The grief blooms into something beautiful, something I can hold and understand."

Her words lingered in the air, as poetic as the art that surrounded us. The paintings spoke a language of their own, one of resilience and rebirth. I looked back at her, deeply moved. "You have truly touched my soul today," I said. "Your art, and the love you've poured into it, radiates with a beauty that is both profound and transformative. Thank you for sharing this with me."

She nodded, her glowing eyes reflecting both gratitude and hope. In that moment, I felt the unmistakable power of art—to heal, to connect, and to remind us of the beauty that can emerge from even the deepest wounds.

She felt a deep sense of pride and gratitude for the opportunity to share her art with others. To her surprise, when she first began showcasing her creations, people connected with them on a profound level, praising her work and eagerly asking to purchase anything she made. Overwhelmed with joy and encouragement, she decided to start a small business, fueled by the hope of giving back to her family—a family that had long felt the weight of loss and despair. Through her art, she found not only a purpose but also a way to restore what they thought was gone forever.

CHAPTER THIRTY ONE

MAKING ANOTHER LOOP.

RING THE ALARM: Here We Go Again

In Case of an Emergency pt2.

Walking across Larchmont in LA, there are two possibilities: either you'll be fine, or you're going to get hit. That's it. People here rarely pay attention, and it's made me hyper-aware of my surroundings. In other towns, you can count on **no one** waiting at the crosswalk, but in LA, always assume a pedestrian is there.

On this fateful day, it was me. I got run over by a young Chinese guy in a white BMW. At first, I thought it was a joke, like Ashton Kutcher was about to pop out with a camera crew for a new episode of *PUNK'D*. I mean, that show had long since ended, but living in Hollywood, I still wouldn't have been surprised. I figured maybe he was a New Yorker, and he was just trying to scare me with a warning sign telling me to hurry up, but then the car rolled back, and forth. Startled, I thought, "Surely, this car wouldn't actually run me over."

But then, it came at me again, and this time, I felt it—my ankle was caught under the muffler. Panic surged through me as I banged on the windshield, screaming bloody murder, "What the hell? STOP!" It wasn't until that moment that the driver realized what was happening— he was running over a person. I was in shock, my mind spinning, adrenaline flooding my system. I didn't know what to feel. All I could do was react, trying to process what was happening, but in that moment, it was as if time slowed down and the world around me went into a blur.

So, here I was again, needing care. I needed an emergency contact or at least someone to help me. Hobbling home to ice my foot, it became clear

I needed to go to the ER. With no insurance, I had to call an Uber. My best friend Daniel, at the time, was hours away, deep in his own depression. I didn't bother to call him—how could he help me when he wasn't taking care of himself? When he found out later, he was crushed. I didn't reach out. He would've sprung into action, but he also knew his mental state. It's crazy how we self-sabotage for love.

Hobbling around, I felt the stares of pity from passersby, and I wanted to disappear. There are so many people worse off than me. I saw a whole family of homeless people begging outside Rite Aid while I limped to the pharmacy for some meds. All I could think was, I'm tired and wrecked. I was in uncharted territory, but at least I was better off than most. Thank God for that.

Ubering home was a struggle on a Saturday in peak summer in LA. Forget about it. Finding parking is a headache, and my driver couldn't even locate me. But what's a girl to do when she can't walk? How can you take care of yourself when you feel like damaged goods? I felt my fight for independence slipping away. I even looked up the spiritual meaning of an ankle injury—lack of support. Damn, that hit hard.

Months later, I stubbornly pushed through, but the lack of support led to another nightmare. I developed pain on my other side—my hip, which then seeped down to my knee. Lots of swelling. During Bible study, the pain was throbbing. The pastor asked us to gather in groups, listening to what God had to say. I started crying, realizing He was guiding me to find my support system. I needed to feel safe and have others to lean on—physically and emotionally. It was a reminder to run to Him... or in my case, to hobble toward Him. With all of this, I needed to find a good support system. One, love myself and relax. Two, there are many others that are here and want to love and support me. Three, keep looking for those in the community, because it takes a village to care!

Healing Era: A Little Less Control, A Lot More Jesus:

Let me just say it: the idea of facing California solo? Terrifying. It started off as a tiny little pain in my hip—no biggie, right? I thought a good stretch and a little time with my trusty foam roller would be enough to shake it off. But surprise! Suddenly I'm in an MRI machine, X-rays on deck, hobbling around in crutches, popping pain meds that only offer the illusion of relief. Turns out, my body was hosting its own private pity party. The meds wore off, and the pain cranked up tenfold. Oh, the agony—ready to scream bloody murder.

And after the recent on-and-off circus with my rock-solid significant other, I found myself needing another crutch. So, I turned to the only place left I could—back to Jesus for some divine healing. He was now officially my emergency contact.

A weekend in bed followed. Ah, rest. How underrated it is...until you're *forced* into it. Suddenly, the world outside feels like a distant memory, and all you're left with is your own personal pain-fest.

And let me tell you—healing? Not for the faint of heart. I can barely put the agony into words. It was like the universe took all the discomforts of life, packaged them into one excruciating experience, and handed them to me with a big ol' bow on top. My heart was shattering, my body screaming in agony—honestly, it felt like I was giving birth (yes, I went there—graphic, I know). All I could think was, "God, please be with me, because I'm pretty sure my body is falling apart."

I wasn't drinking, I wasn't smoking, and let's be real, I wasn't "fuc*ing the pain away" like I used to. Nope, it was just me, prayer, and some serious receiving from the Big Guy upstairs. Honestly, I couldn't have made it through without my church family. Huge shout-out to Tessa and Damon—thank you for being my rocks during this time. Months before, I was Googling what was causing my ankle pain, and surprise! It was a "total lack of support." But months later, I was *literally* lifted up by the support of my church community, and trust me, that difference was life-changing. They literally held me up, as I almost fell down in agony, crying.

So, the lesson here? Why was I ignoring my body? It was literally trying to tell me something, like a check engine light flashing on my dashboard. And me? I just kept hitting the "ignore" button. "Ah, I'll be fine," I thought, while running around asking every professional I could find, "Hey, I've got this pain—what do you think it is?" Spoiler: no one could really pinpoint it because, let's face it, we're all juggling work, life, and bills, and who's got time to listen to the body's complaints when we're already stressed enough?

Now, let me tell you, I love the high of a good workout. I'm the girl who thrives on a lean physique—flat stomach, toned arms, nice legs. But, admit it: who doesn't enjoy a little extra attention when you're looking your best? I mean, I won't lie—I like to feel hot. But, as it turns out, there's a price to pay when that "hotness" becomes your currency for getting what you want. And it's exhausting.

The funny thing is, I thought I had it all under control until I realized I was attracting the wrong kind of attention. Sure, I looked great dancing in heels (who doesn't love a little shimmy?), but there's a fine line between confidence and chaos. The sexual energy that came with that lifestyle? Not exactly what I'm going for anymore. Intimacy? Yes, please. Random hookups for the sake of it? No, thanks.

And so, my big realization hit me: I need to stop forcing myself into situations that don't serve me. I thought I could control it, but the results were not what I wanted. What I want is intimacy—the kind of closeness where someone sees me for who I am, not just as someone to fulfill their desires. (Which, by the way, is exactly why I didn't go to King's apartment for our first date in the first place. But that's another story...).

As I heal from this hip injury, I've been asking myself some tough questions about life and what I truly want. The storm is raging, but I won't be blown down.

Now, let's talk about practical stuff. You know me—I'm that girl who always knows a guy for everything. Need a plumber? I got a guy. Need help with an errand or a business connection? Yep, I know exactly who you need. I'm a networking queen, living by the referral system. So if you need something, you know who to call. I'm basically your personal Google for life's problems.

But for now? I'm learning that sometimes, I just need to let go, trust in the universe, and let the right people lift me up. 🌼

Facing Pain and Vulnerability

Physical and Emotional Pain: My hip injury became a metaphor for ignored emotional wounds. Psychologically, this mirrors how individuals often suppress inner struggles until they manifest as physical symptoms such as somatic complaints—where emotional pain finds a voice through the body.

Forced Rest: Being "forced into rest" symbolizes the necessity of slowing down and acknowledging pain to begin healing. It's an uncomfortable but essential step, as avoidance often perpetuates cycles of distress.

Turning to a Higher Power:

Seeking Divine Support: Returning to my faith reflected a psychological shift from self-reliance to surrender. In psychology, this aligns with the concept of *locus of control*. Moving from an internal locus ("I must fix everything") to an external one ("I trust God/others to guide me") can alleviate the overwhelming burden of control.

Community Support: My church family's role underscores the importance of social support systems. Psychologist Abraham Maslow's "hierarchy of needs" highlights belongingness as fundamental to well-being. Feeling seen and supported fosters resilience during hardship.

Finding Clarity in Chaos: My California Experience:

You know that moment when your old shadows start creeping back in, like that last slice of pizza you told yourself you wouldn't eat but can't resist anyway? Yeah, I've been on this "healing journey" for the last three decades, and surprise!—clearly I'm just getting started. Sure, I've learned a ton about myself, but let's be honest: until I can break the cycle, I'm stuck on repeat. It's like the universe is playing the same episode of *Friends* over and over and I'm waiting for a new season to start. I'm really trying to change my narrative, though—just a little rewiring.

So, I had this humbling experience recently that made me question whether I'm even qualified to be excited about a position I was applying for. Spoiler alert: I was.....but we're here for some good laughs, right? Stay tuned: California has its own vibe, and I'm learning it *daily*. Every job I've gotten here has been weirdly magical, like finding a $5 bill in an old jacket pocket—unexpected but not exactly life-changing. At first, I'll be like, "There's no way this could be a real opportunity." And then, like a magic trick, the illusions fade away, and BAM!—there's the dirty grunt work. Surprise!

So, I got a callback for a social media position. Honestly, I felt like I had the credentials to run NASA, but I was in true scarcity-mindset fashion desperate for anything, so I decided to go anyway. When I showed up, what I thought was an interview quickly devolved into something... else. Instead of the usual "tell us about yourself" routine, they handed me a packet of work, gave me access to all their passwords—basically, I was given the keys to the kingdom—and then tossed me a shirt. Oh, and they also asked me to fill out W-4 paperwork, and told me to come back the next day. It felt like an audition for *Survivor*, not a job interview.

I was bewildered. "Oh, okay... California..." I thought. I hadn't even been told what the pay was. During the meeting, one lady sat next to the owner, who was too busy to even glance up from her desk. I wasn't introduced to her, and I had no idea she was important until the last 15 minutes of my two-hour visit. It felt like a bizarre reality show. But hey, who am I to judge?

When I came back the next day, I found another person filling out W-4s. I leaned over and asked, "Did you get the job too?" She looked at me like I was insane and said, "I've never even been here before." As she started filling out her forms, the elusive owner strolled in and asked if she had any questions. The applicant said, "I thought this was an interview? Why am I filling out paperwork if I don't even work here?" The owner just shrugged and said, "Oh, HR will get back to you tomorrow. Sorry, that wasn't clear." Yeah, lady. NOTHING WAS CLEAR. At this point, I was questioning my entire life's purpose.

Then, I was told I needed to fill out a form on my "own time" and do three hours of work. Oh, fun. *Really?* As if on cue, nothing worked. The Wi-Fi, the passwords, even the programs she wanted me to log into—everything froze like a dial-up internet connection in 1999. My computer was slower than a sloth on a caffeine detox. So, we're clearly not on the same page. I tried to explain, but she cut me off, saying, "I don't want to hear it." Well, excuse me, I'm just trying to get on your chaotic train. She responded, "I don't need a tutorial; I just need it done." Great! So do I, but I need a working internet to pull that off.

After three hours of nonsense, she was visibly frustrated. "So let me get this straight: in three hours, you haven't completed anything?" As if I were some lazy slug. Um, no. It wasn't my fault that the whole thing felt like a game of *Whack-a-Mole*, where every problem popped up just as fast as I could fix one. She wanted things done her way or no way at all. Fair enough. It's her business. But expecting me to work for five hours without pay? C'mon, lady. And asking me to sign W-4 forms without actually hiring me? That's some next-level trickery right there.

I was getting anxious with imaginary deadlines and tasks I had no access to. My old thought pattern kicked in: "Wow, I'm obviously not qualified. Maybe I'm just dumb." But then I remembered, *nope*, not today. This is literally my first day. It's okay to struggle, to not have everything figured out. There were zero clear expectations, aside from the random packet they handed me. The whole thing was a circus, and I didn't even get to ride the Ferris wheel.

Looking back, it's almost hilarious. In fact, I'm glad nothing worked out, because let's be real: we were not vibing. That's like trying to squeeze into a pair of jeans you wore in high school—sometimes, it just isn't meant to fit. And that's totally fine.

Ironically, I'm writing a book on communication, and here I am, unable to communicate with a person who doesn't even make eye contact. Sometimes, even with all the tools in my toolkit, there's just a stubborn apple that refuses to be picked. Not everyone is meant to vibe, and that's okay. I'm learning to embrace these lessons, trusting that the right opportunities are out there, just waiting for me to walk in.

After two days of witnessing the *ultimate* business model of chaos, and wasting my time and energy (not to mention getting no pay), they casually mentioned they'd call me the next day. Spoiler alert: they didn't. And I wasn't exactly planning to answer the phone if they did. We were not a good match.

As I continue navigating this journey, I'm learning to redefine my narrative and embrace the beautiful mess of growth. Because hey, every experience teaches us something—even when it feels like a dumpster fire.

Trust the Timing, Embrace the Process:

Soaking up some sunshine, playing volleyball with my church friends (because, you know, I'm a wholesome human who still enjoys some good clean fun). We were laughing, running around, and just enjoying the moment. Suddenly, one of the new teammates, Heff (**THE EMPOWERER**), dropped a little nugget of information that sent me into *shock*.

He casually mentioned he had just moved from Wilmington, NC. *Wilmington?* As in *my* Wilmington, the place that used to hold my heart and probably the last place I thought anyone would randomly move from to end up playing volleyball on a Saturday afternoon in, I don't know, a town that was *nowhere near Wilmington.* I literally froze mid-air, probably looking like a confused volleyball player who had just been hit in the face by fate. Thank goodness my BFF Daniel was there to witness it. Otherwise, I'd probably be questioning my own sanity right now.

It's funny how life works, isn't it? Here I was, in a completely different state, doing completely different things, and *bam*, life sends me a reminder of "home." This wasn't just any ordinary meeting either. Heff—tall, fashionable, sweet, and full of good vibes—was exactly the type of person you feel better after meeting. You know the kind: the ones who walk into a room and the whole place just lights up. If you don't have those people in your life, you're doing it wrong. Find them, keep them, and trust me, you'll feel better every time you see them.

We immediately started bonding over all things small-town life, Wilmington, and just laughing about the randomness of it all. We clicked, effortlessly. The universe—God, life, whatever you want to call it—has a way of tossing these synchronicities our way. And for a brief moment, I couldn't help but wonder: *"Why did we meet? Is this a long-term thing? A friendship? Or is he just here for a season to teach me something?"*

A few weeks later, I bumped into Heff at another church event. Same energy, same high vibes. It felt like electricity—every time we saw each other, it was like a mini lightning bolt of joy sparked between us. I'm not saying I believe in soulmates, but the universe definitely has its ways of bringing the right people into your life at the *right* time. You don't always get to pick who enters your world, but sometimes, you meet someone and just know they're a gift—temporary or not.

Here's the thing, yall, Life has a funny way of *exactly* putting people and experiences in front of you when you need them. Jeff wasn't someone I expected to meet that day. But he was there, teaching me that not every person in your life is meant to stay forever—but some of them can leave a lasting impression.

Action: Trust the timing. Embrace the people who bring light to your life, even if their presence is only temporary. If you meet someone who lights you up, don't question it. Just *feel* it. Sometimes, those fleeting moments will shape your future in unexpected ways. And remember, the goodbye process is made with love *for you*, even if you don't fully understand it at the time.

So next time you feel a *spark* or meet someone that *just clicks*, don't overthink it. Just enjoy the ride, let the energy flow, and trust that the universe knows what it's doing. You're in good hands.

CHAPTER THIRTY TWO

CHAOS OF SEASONAL PERSUASION.

Embrace the Shadows, Celebrate the Growth

In September 2024 on a random day I decided to start doing a little spring cleaning in my cozy townhouse (yes, in September, because who says you can't have a fresh start just because it's fall?). I was elbow-deep in a sea of clutter, sorting through papers when—*BAM*—I stumbled upon an old letter I'd written to myself. The kind of letter you pen when your mind is doing a full-on spiraling routine. You know the one: you're anxious, replaying every little situation in your head, convinced that if you just think about it enough, the answer will magically appear. Spoiler alert: It won't.

I read the letter, and my heart sank. It was from August 2023, and it was a reminder of a time when I was really struggling. The letter read:

"You demonstrate love by giving unconditionally to yourself. As you do, you attract love from others who can love you without conditions." —**Paul Ferrini**

"Today, I experienced a newfound feeling of love. I didn't let my monkey mind pull me backward. Instead, I focused on the graceful path ahead. I took a deep breath, stepped outside for some fresh air, and cleaned my space. I was remembering my own power and the strength of my thoughts. I've reached a new level. I'm walking alongside my shadows and clearing out my heart."

Oh, the irony. It was like a message from the *past me* (who probably needed a hug) to the *present me* (who really just wanted to eat an entire pizza and bottle of wine while binge-watching Netflix). But there it was: a reminder that even in my most uncertain moments, I had the tools to rise above. It was like finding a note from a friend who *knew* you would need it later.

September Reflections: The Struggle Is Real:

Now, if you've ever had a month that feels like it just *sucks*, you know what I'm talking about. September has always been my toughest month in my book every year. It's the month where I tend to reflect too much. A little too much, actually. And let's just say I've got a track record of relationship heartbreaks that seem to sync up with the changing weather. This year, I was once again riding the wave of "**why do all my relationships seem to end when the leaves start falling**?" *Cue: The Green Day song* "Wake Me Up When September Ends." That song hits me in the feels, every. single. time.

As the weather gets colder, I've learned that I'm highly susceptible to something we call "seasonal depression." Yep, it's real, and it's not just about the weather. It's like the world shifts into cozy mode and, suddenly, my cute summer fling is nothing more than a sad memory that fizzles out quicker than the last few rays of sunshine. So, naturally, I want to hibernate. I've become a master at putting on my comfy sweatpants, shutting myself off from the world, and pretending I'm totally fine, while secretly plotting my emotional comeback.

The last few relationships? Well, they've been... *complicated*. Two were true love (or so I thought), and losing them made me feel like my heart was in a blender set on "puree." The other two were more like detours—tests to help me unlearn old patterns. But here's the kicker: I still felt like I was in turmoil. It was as if I was stuck on a merry-go-round of *emotional drama*, with no "stop" button in sight.

But as the month drew to a close, I noticed something—*a shift*.

Action: Embrace the Growth, Even in the Toughest Seasons

So here's the thing: I realized that all this reflecting, this emotional rollercoaster, it wasn't for nothing. Life's challenges, the heartbreaks, the emotional breakdowns—they were helping me grow. I wasn't staying stuck in the same patterns. I was evolving.

Sure, I was still a little messy in the process (aren't we all?), but the more I embraced my own shadows, the more I learned to walk alongside them, not fight them. I started to shift my focus from my pain to my power. And honestly, once I stopped resisting, I could *finally* feel that new wave of growth coming.

So, lesson learned: Don't fight the tough seasons. Let them teach you something. The cold weather, the loneliness, the heartbreak—it's all part of your journey. Trust that even when things seem bleak, there's always a shift around the corner. You're not spiraling forever. You're just finding your next level. And remember, when life hands you a tough September, *grab a pumpkin spice latte*, cozy up in your favorite blanket, and *trust the process*.

The bottom line? Growth isn't always glamorous, but it's always worth it. So, embrace your shadows, learn from them, and keep marching forward. Because, trust me, the best chapters are always written in the most unexpected seasons.

BUT IN CASE YOU DIDN'T LEARN THE LESSON AND WANT TO SWALLOW A BIT MORE...

Dancing with Depression:

Days I Don't Want to Exist Anymore

What do you do on the days when you just can't handle it anymore? I was feeling sick of my own thoughts and this place we call home—Earth.

There are so many problems here, and it's overwhelming to figure out where to start. Everything feels intertwined, caught in some endless cycle.

You just stop. Stand still.

Today, the air felt different. Standing in the sunlight, I felt the gust of cold, brisk air—like the whisper of the wind rustling through the leaves. Cars rushed past, but the pain inside me didn't seem to fade. It lingered, a heavy weight that overshadowed the warmth around me. The world moved on, but I felt stuck, caught between the beauty of the moment and the ache in my heart.

I woke up with a heaviness, like I'd drunk poison the night before and absorbed someone else's pain. I did drink, and I hooked up with an old friend, but it got me nowhere. I thought I'd head to the music studio, but it was a bust. I went from two encounters in one day to feeling utterly depressed. It feels like all the good serotonin was drained away in those hours of escapades.

Honestly, I'm tired of the world. The politics are disheartening, homelessness is rampant, and the systems—schools, jobs—feel like modern-day slavery. Applying for jobs is a joke. You can apply forty a day and hear nothing, or see no results. I heard a disturbing statistic that some companies post jobs that aren't even open, just to create the illusion of growth. It's a vicious cycle of disappointment.

Moral of the story: today felt like one of those days, battling my old thoughts and dehydration. I slipped down that familiar rabbit hole, but managed to pull myself back with my coping tools: hydrate, go for a walk, do my physical therapy, bike ride, and hit a coffee shop just to be around other people. But of course, my tech died, and it felt like I accomplished nothing.

As I walked, my knee throbbed with discomfort, and I found myself stopping in my tracks, taking slow breaths and looking into the sun for a sign.

I cried out, wondering if anyone noticed and if they'd stop to check on me. Of course, in LA, people only focus on themselves. I said a little prayer in my head: "Help. Send me something good, please. I'm really hurting." This summer has felt painfully slow, and as the next season approaches, I'm still jobless. Thank goodness for my backup cushion.

I'm doing my best to avoid a pity party, but my body is overworked, which frustrates me because feeling strong usually helps clear my mind. Yet here I am, stuck in pain, lacking work, and financially strained.

I paused for a moment, letting the weight of the day settle. My thoughts were racing in a hundred different directions, and I couldn't help but feel a little lost. Why wasn't anything working out? I thought about the 18 million people in this city—each one of us hustling, trying to make better decisions, to find jobs, to find purpose. In a sea of so many, why did it feel like I was stuck?

As I walked through the motions, it hit me: **maybe these jobs, these opportunities, they weren't right for me.** Maybe God (or the universe, or whatever higher power you believe in) had other plans. I mean, if these jobs were the ones for me, they'd be here by now, right?

But as much as I wanted to place blame elsewhere, the truth was, I was in a season of growth, and growth doesn't always feel comfortable. It wasn't the right time yet. I was still healing from past pain, still untangling the mess in my heart, trying to make sense of it all.

The people I came into contact with each day were a reminder of how busy the world is. They were running around, consumed by their own chaotic to-do lists, barely able to think or breathe. It made me wonder, what would happen if I stopped? What if I allowed myself to just *be* for a moment, instead of constantly pushing forward?

Asking for help had always felt like a battle. It was like waving a white flag, but not knowing if anyone would come to your rescue. There were times when I felt like I was the only one who understood what I was going through, and that made it hard to ask for support. How do you even find the balance between staying strong and knowing when to lean on others?

And then, I had a realization: without a purpose to wake up for, we risk losing the will to wake up at all. That thought hit me hard. The past week had felt... aimless. I found myself questioning everything. Was I still in a season of solitude, trying to figure out these challenges, or was this just a phase I needed to push through?

As I sat with that question, I realized something crucial: Sometimes, you have to let yourself sit in the uncertainty. Because in that uncertainty, you find clarity. I didn't have all the answers yet, but maybe that was okay. Maybe I just needed to trust the process, even when it felt like I was standing still.

Then the best and most unexpected gift came when a beautiful brown and spotted dog started barking at me from across the street. Her owner quickly tried to apologize, but the dog remained focused on me, waiting patiently. I decided to approach her; I needed to walk that way to get home. As I neared, I gently held out my hand, and she immediately came to my side.

She licked me and snuggled against my legs, and in that moment, I realized this was a message from God—a sign that He was listening. He didn't send a human to check on me. He had sent this loving creature, the type I cherish most. Her owner, noticing her excitement, said he didn't know why she was barking. I told him "she sensed my pain." He assumed I meant some dark shadow over me, which might be true, but really, she recognized that I needed love.

She noticed my discomfort and communicated with her gentle presence: "It's okay, I'm here." Dogs convey so much without words, and that's exactly the kind of communication I needed. Sometimes, it's not about spoken words, but about the safe embrace that reassures us we're not alone.

I felt tears welling up as my prayers were answered in mere moments. This encounter was a reminder that God is present in our struggles, encouraging us to transform our pain into something greater. Use that art. Use that pain. Let it become lessons and love for others.

CHAPTER THIRTY THREE

REKINDLEING.

Hello, Old Friend:

Reconnecting with friends and sharing unconditional love can be one of the most fulfilling things in life. Sometimes, we get so caught up in the hustle that we forget to reach out to the people who matter. So, when you decide to reconnect, why not make it light and easy? A quick message can do wonders, but it's all about the vibe you send.

Try something like this: "Hey! I just wanted to say hi and reconnect. No rush to reply if you're busy, just thought I'd reach out!" A simple text that says you care, without putting pressure on the other person. It's like giving a little gift of space and kindness, allowing the friendship to grow back naturally, no strings attached.

Remember, it's all about the thought behind it. Whether it's a "just thinking of you" message or a "hope you're doing well" check-in, that sweet note can go a long way. Plus, when you share that little spark of unconditional love, you're not just rekindling a friendship, you're reminding both of you that life's better when we've got people to lean on, laugh with, and share moments of joy.

I've always carried with me the peace of mind and heart that comes from never burning bridges with people. You just never know what life has in store for you, or who those people might bring you toward down the road. The connections we make, even the ones that seem fleeting or distant at the time, can sometimes lead to unexpected miracles.

People change, circumstances shift, and paths cross again in the most surprising ways. That's why I believe it's important to leave things on good terms, even if you're not sure what's ahead. You never know when someone who once seemed distant might come back into your life, offering you opportunities, wisdom, or even friendship when you least expect it. Life has a funny way of weaving things together, and the relationships you nurture today might be the ones that carry you to new heights tomorrow. So, with that in mind, I always aim to keep things positive, knowing that what goes around has a funny way of coming back around.

FLASHBACK REFLECTIONS:

It was one of my first dates with Mr. J. He brought me to this cute "Paint and Play" place and told me to pick out a piece and go to town. I wanted to create a masterpiece.

I had a flashback to all the times I was with my old girlfriends. We could all be creating the same piece of art but I'll be comparing myself thinking, "I should be way more advanced" and I place this expectation on myself that my art should be better than theirs. So suddenly their art is a way to boost mine into better detail.

It all became clear to me while it was my "wife's" (Sara) birthday.

I had an injury, so we did our usual date— "sushi"--- but then came home to paint. As we were talking about our emotional instability it occurred to me that even when creating art, I have to compete. I can't seem to just enjoy the nature of creation. Just doing something for enjoyment, I'm always trying to make it look better than others. It all came to me when I'd bring my friends to wine and design.

The last time we had painted a couple of weeks before, we painted at her house and we had little "boxes" to paint. She stated this beautiful creation of colors and I was trying to think of a deep "rooted" idea. I ended up painting this beautiful heart piece box into the universe, "The heart of the sky". But, as we sat to paint in my bedroom, drinking cacao,

I was so happy to make creations on canvas look completely different. She created this beautiful butterfly box.

My memory suddenly hit me: to Caroline, her husband was a fantastic artist. He made this beautiful painting of an atomic heart, but one day when they were on the brink of divorce, he broke the painting in half. A typical dramatic display of emotional turmoil. She was devastated to see the painting wrecked. Later they ended up reconciling their issues and staying together, but that memory and story always stayed in my heart. I once had another friend explain to me that I was always dealing with other people's experiences. That their stories became my own burdens, because I always wanted to take someone else's pain away. But all of that pain and secrets had to go somewhere and I felt it was my duty to absorb them. This act of mine was also noticed by a complete stranger I had met. She realized it was a cry for help and asked, "With everyone's burdens and secrets on you, where does it go? And how do you handle all of that information?"

It never dawned on me that I was consuming so much and storing it. It's been a journey of self-discovery over the years to realize I can empathize, but I don't need to consume all of their emotions. Most times, I can just be an observer of other people's emotions. I can allow myself to gain insights based on the information, but I don't need to consume it.

All that to say, why did I consume so much? Why do I take out my own self-doubt in competition? Why do I place these self-imposed expectations on myself that don't need to be there? They don't need to be so serious or so full of worry.

In fact we all have our own art. Our own emotions and ways to store them, suppress them, or release them. Any masterpiece they create is just as beautiful and parallel to mine. I don't need to compete, instead I try to learn from their strokes or tools of creativity.

Painting is my creative catharsis, getting to paint in a room full of my friends was inspiring and loving. Choosing colors that describe me and the essence of the art and getting to sit with my friends and paint was a reminder to my inner child to heal those friendship wounds. That we can all be cute and paint together. We were all healing childhood wounds that day and were able to create, educate, and release. One of my friends brought her niece, and watched her be such a supportive role model and explain the ins and outs of painting. I admired her and I encouraged her niece to use any creative expression she needed, that's the whole point of it.

"The biggest act of self love is to live for yourself and not for others. Do the things you always wanted to do. Even if you have to do them alone. Go to that art class. Listen to your favorite songs on repeat."

Affirming The Little Things:

You can start to feel it in the air, and start to feel the sunshine moving in different directional changes. I was outside one afternoon, just taking a mental clarity walk away from the computer screen where I had been sitting all day. A black man in an all black suit, mustache, dapper sensation, and cigarette attached to his lips, stopped to smile and gesture hello, I smiled, as I was just in awe staring at the sky. He was pleasantly surprised by my response, "Aw, I'm just admiring the earth."

The seasons of change and all September brings to offer. The leaves start to die, hell that morning there was an earthquake. Mother nature is going to make moves whether or not you decide to. She's going to cleanse —and shift.

Mindfulness:

A psychological practice that involves being fully present in the moment, focusing on the sensations around you without judgment. Mindfulness has been shown to reduce stress, enhance emotional well-being, and foster deeper connections with both ourselves and the world around us.

Impermanence:

It's a recognition that change is inevitable and natural, and that embracing this cycle can lead to growth and renewal. Something like an earthquake, an event that signals powerful natural shifts, further emphasizes our need to acknowledge and accept the changes that life brings. The observation of the seasons changing and the awareness of the **earth's cycles** represents an appreciation for **impermanence**.

SIT WITH YOURSELF: GREEN FLAGS

After years of soaking up advice and self-help mantras, I realized that the key to growth wasn't just listening to endless tips—it was about actually taking action. It's funny how much "advice" can pile up like a stack of unread emails, all marked as urgent, but never quite getting opened. You know the ones: *Make time for yourself, Honor your boundaries, Challenge yourself, Take time to know yourself deeper, Calm your nervous system*—I mean, is there a limit to how many times I'm supposed to breathe deeply in a day? At one point, it all started to sound like a playlist on repeat. It's like I was trying to become an expert at life without ever actually living it.

But then, something clicked. I had to actually *do* these things. It wasn't just about writing them in my journal or plastering them on sticky notes around my house. It was about embodying them, making them a part of my daily existence.

So, I started by making time for myself. Simple, right? But if you've ever found yourself saying, "I'll just do this one more thing, then I'll take a break," you know how challenging this is. I finally decided to just sit. No multitasking. No scrolling. Just sitting with my thoughts, my tea, and maybe a good book (or just the silence).

I also realized that growth is not all about being comfortable—it's about challenging myself. I had to push through my comfort zone, even if that meant not getting it "perfect" every time. The truth is, challenges are where the magic happens, and if you're not facing any, you might be stuck in a very cozy, but unproductive, rut.

Next up: calming my nervous system. This one was a toughie, but it's a game-changer. You know that feeling when you're on edge, like you're constantly in "fight or flight" mode? Yeah, I had to learn to let go. Taking a minute to breathe, to just be, to let the anxiety dissipate like a bad Wi-Fi signal—it was like my brain started giving me a high-five.

I also started holding space for my emotions—something I hadn't really done before. It wasn't enough to just push them away with the latest Netflix binge or a dessert (though, let's be honest, cookies are always a temporary fix). I had to sit with them, understand them, and let them pass like clouds instead of storms.

And let's talk about boundaries. Oh, how many times I've let my boundaries be tested, like an overcooked piece of spaghetti being pulled in every direction. I've learned to say "no" with confidence. And, more importantly, I've learned to say "yes" to things that truly align with who I am. No more over-committing out of guilt—life's too short for that.

Through all this, I began to recognize the people in my life who truly *showed up* for me. They weren't just passing through; they were rooting for me, inspiring me, and accepting me as I was. These were the people who wanted to see me succeed, who cheered me on when I made small wins, and who showed me what it means to be loved unconditionally. The people who truly *chose* me, even when I had a messy day or two (or five).

So, as I continue to grow, I've learned that it's not enough to just talk about these lessons. I have to live them, apply them, and surround myself with people who make me feel like I'm on the right path. And maybe—just maybe—I'm finally starting to get the hang of this whole "self-care" thing. Who knew it could be so transformative? The best part of the puzzle is that these same qualities I'm learning to embrace aren't just important for me—they're also green flags in your partners. If you want someone who's supportive, calm, and willing to show up for you, then those qualities should be present in the relationships you choose to invest in.

At the end of the day, I've come to realize that we're all just one relationship away from changing the course of our lives. The right person can help you grow, challenge you, and even help you rediscover yourself in ways you never thought possible. And I think that's the real magic of life: knowing that each relationship has the potential to shift everything—for the better.

CHAPTER THIRTY FOUR

BEING PREPARED FOR DISASTERS.

PLAN B: YOUR DISASTER PLAN?

Alright, let's talk about something not-so-glamorous but incredibly necessary: your disaster plan. Now, I know it might sound a little morbid, planning for the worst, but trust me—sometimes it's best to dig your well before it's full. Planning ahead, especially for the unexpected, can save you from complete chaos later. I've lived in places where natural disasters seemed to hit every year, and the "stop, drop, and roll" drill wasn't just for fire safety—it was for everything! No, I'm not suggesting you expect the world to end tomorrow, but having a backup plan? Always a good idea.

Now, let's address the elephant in the room: who gets all your stuff? Yep, you heard me right. If things go sideways, who gets your favorite mug, your prized collection of comic books, or (more importantly) your extra phone chargers? Just kidding! But seriously, do you have a plan for when disaster strikes? Are you packed and ready to go, or are you planning to wing it when the next apocalypse hits? (We all know someone who's secretly hoping that their life isn't interrupted by a little thing like "being prepared.")

Let's get into the real nitty-gritty. Have you set up an emergency kit in your car or house? I'm talking about the basics—first aid, flashlights, food that doesn't taste like cardboard, and, of course, a good stash of batteries. And hey, if you're feeling a bit more extreme, knives, guns, and all the things that make you feel like a survival expert on a reality show. But, here's the kicker—who's going with you if you need to evacuate? And how are you getting to them? Because let's be real—your GPS might go out when you need it most (and do you really trust the grid anyway?).

I actually have real paper maps of the grids I live in. Sounds a bit old school, but trust me, if the power goes down and that little map app on your phone is just a sad, blank screen, you'll be thanking your past self for planning ahead. I've marked out the escape routes, the nearest safe spots, and even a couple of secret hideaways in case I need to lay low. Not to be paranoid, but... just in case!

Here's how to turn your emergency plan into something practical and, dare I say, a little fun. First up: the Emergency Kit. It's easy to think a couple of granola bars and a bottle of water are enough, but let's kick it up a notch. Think beyond the basics. Imagine having a portable charger, a flashlight, a first aid kit, and a water filter all neatly packed. And here's a pro tip—throw in some cash. Why? Because ATMs might decide to take the day off, and you'll want to be prepared. Oh, and if you can squeeze in a tiny camping stove? You'll be the proud chef of your survival crew. Nothing like whipping up a hot meal in the middle of a crisis.

At the end of the day, Plan B is about giving yourself peace of mind. It's not about expecting doom and gloom, but having a backup plan so you can relax when things get unpredictable. So, take a deep breath, get organized, and maybe even invest in a few ridiculous survival tools that make you feel like you're starring in an action movie. You never know— it might just be your Plan B that saves the day.

Next, let's talk about the map situation. We live in the age of GPS, but what happens if the grid goes down? That's where paper maps come in. Yes, the old-school kind—the ones that make you feel like a true adventurer. Take a good look at your surroundings, figure out your routes to safety, and maybe even memorize a few of them. You never know when you'll need to take the scenic route out of dodge.

And of course, who's on your team? Who are you going to call when everything goes sideways? Make sure you have a solid list of trusted people and emergency contacts. While traveling, I made a backup "emergency list" on paper, just in case phones die and the digital world goes dark. Group chats? Life-saving. They're like modern-day smoke signals, but faster. You'll want to stay in touch when you need it most.

Now, here's the most important part: stay calm, and stay comedic. When everything hits the fan, the last thing you want to do is panic. In times of chaos, a little humor goes a long way. Imagine sitting with your emergency squad, joking about how you're going to survive on granola bars and good vibes. Because let's face it—if you can laugh through a disaster, you're winning at life. So, while the preparations are serious business, don't forget to throw in some fun. It'll make the journey just a bit more bearable, no matter what comes your way.

Hurricane Season:

Here's the reality check: living in a place that's constantly at the mercy of the earth means making decisions that can completely change the course of your life. One day, you're living your best life in paradise, enjoying your peaceful island life, and the next day—boom!—your house and family are in disarray. It really puts a damper on your plans, doesn't it? A situation like this makes you realize how important it is to have a backup plan. What's your fail-safe? What's your Plan B? Are you covering your own... Well, you know what I mean.

Let me ask you this—do you have paper maps for when the GPS goes out? I'm talking both metaphorically and literally. What happens when the world as you know it gets flipped upside down? Are you prepared? I'm not trying to scare you, but we all need to be honest with ourselves— no one's coming to save you.

Take Asheville, NC, for example. That place was demolished in a matter of moments after being hit hard by a hurricane. Where's the fight-or-flight response? Where are the safety resources? It's easy to feel overwhelmed when disaster strikes, but something truly beautiful emerges from the chaos.

While I was living in NC, I witnessed something that changed my perspective. Hurricanes were almost expected, but what I saw in the aftermath was incredible. Through all the disaster and pain, there's a sense of unity that rises above it all. People stop focusing on the petty dramas of their everyday lives and come together to serve others. Neighbors gather supplies, lend a helping hand, and support each other in ways that are nothing short of magical.

Everyone is pitching in—packing food, clothes, tools, and anything else that might help someone in need. It's a reminder that, even in the worst of times, we have the power to come together, rebuild, and find strength in our community. So, while the storm might tear things apart, the bonds we create in its wake are the things that truly keep us going.

There was a year when devastation arose. Hurricane Matthew hit, and it destroyed the city. I was one of the lucky ones who evacuated during the storm, but coming back was a whole different story. The highways that had been open just the day before were now closed, and it took extra days and hours to make it home. When I finally arrived, Wilmington felt like an island, cut off from the world, with supplies being flown in. The government had long declared a state of emergency, but it felt surreal to return and find my home surrounded by debris, downed street signs, and the destruction of surging floodwaters.

What really caused the most damage wasn't even the hurricane itself— it was the tornadoes that came in with it, wreaking havoc in their wake. The aftermath was like nothing I'd ever seen. But what stuck with me, what really shone through, was the response from my church and community leaders. They always rise to the test. Leaders from all across the country and various ministries poured in, ready to divide and conquer. Teams were sent out all over the town, and even though the city was shut down—jobs closed, businesses closed—everyone went to serve. They didn't focus on what they lost, but on how they could help others rebuild.

My team was sent to clean a small neighborhood—shoveling debris, clearing wreckage, helping find shelter and food for families. But there was one house we worked on in particular that left a lasting impression. A giant tree had fallen directly on a large third-story home, splitting it almost completely in half. We spent the entire day cutting up the tree, moving the fallen bark, and clearing debris. Along the way, I met other volunteers, and even though we were strangers then, it felt like fate. Years later, I would cross paths with some of those same people, bringing with it a strange sense of full-circle moments.

Through it all, it became clear: when disaster strikes, it's not the damage that defines us, but how we come together in the aftermath. We rebuild not just our homes, but our sense of community. And that, in the end, is what really helps us weather the storm.

Whether your storm is big or small, or even a natural disaster, it's still a storm. The real question is, how are you preparing yourself—before, during, and after? "Are you digging your well before you're thirsty?"- Harvey Mackay

Most of us live in survival mode, and it's hard to think beyond the immediate. But planning ahead, having a backup plan for every aspect of your life—that's the smartest decision you can make.

Think about it: financially, career-wise, when it comes to car care, and your home. Are you prepared for the unexpected? It's easy to focus on the day-to-day, but when a storm—literal or figurative—hits, it's those who've done the prep work who are the most equipped to weather it.

It's about setting yourself up now, so when life's challenges come your way, you're not scrambling to find a solution. You're ready.

Life Lessons: Embracing the Struggles:

Life is full of obstacles, and navigating them often feels like driving on an open highway with three distinct lanes, each presenting its own challenges.

In the **slow lane**, life feels calm and easy. You're cruising along, going at a comfortable pace, and everything seems under control. But then— *bam*—you hit a speed bump. Suddenly, you're bouncing up and down like a lowrider, feeling the jolt in your bones. It's frustrating, but you get through it. The bumps feel more like hiccups, but they still make you pause, rethink, and re-adjust.

The **middle lane** is where most people spend their time. You're coasting with the crowd, just another car in the sea of others, going with the flow. But when you hit a speed bump here, it's not just a little jolt. You scratch your bumper. The impact is harder, leaving scars and scratches that can take time to heal. The journey feels more challenging here, filled with deep cuts that don't fade quickly. It's the lane where the struggles can leave lasting marks, but they also offer growth.

Then, there's the **fast lane**. You're speeding ahead, full throttle, feeling unstoppable. You're flying through life with adrenaline, but when you hit a speed bump, it hardly even registers. The bump is barely noticeable in the grand scheme of things. You roll right over it, keeping your speed, your momentum intact. The damage is slight, barely felt, and you keep going. The fast lane might feel like the best lane to be in, but even here, there are obstacles to overcome.

Living at the beach, I learned an important lesson from the turtles during hatching season. We were told not to help them, no matter how badly we wanted to. The reason? The struggle to make it from their nest to the ocean was essential to their survival. Most of the little turtles wouldn't make it to the water, not because of predators or dangers, but because they hadn't developed the muscles needed to survive in the open ocean.

The journey from nest to sea was more than just a physical one; it was about building strength, endurance, and resilience. Without that struggle, without those obstacles, they wouldn't be prepared for the life ahead of them.

Just like the turtles, we all have our own version of this journey. We have to go through hard things—challenges that force us to grow and develop the muscles that will help us survive and thrive in life. These struggles aren't just setbacks; they are the very things that build us up, making us stronger, more capable of handling whatever comes next.

We can do hard things. And it's these hard things that prepare us for the next waters we must navigate. So, whether you're in the slow lane, the middle lane, or the fast lane, remember that each bump, each struggle, is shaping you. It's building your muscles, making you ready for the bigger journey ahead.

CHAPTER THIRTY FIVE

WEAKNESSES.

BLIND SPOTS:

There are areas in your life that you just can't see. Sometimes it's because you truly can't see, and other times it's because you're pretending not to.

"I often watch celebrities who wear sunglasses all hours of the day, almost as if they're putting on this persona that "they can't see the haters." It's a funny situation. They think they're so "cool." Sunglasses are worn at photoshoots, at clubs, during brunch, in restaurants, and, believe it or not, even in church services. But the truth is, the act of blocking or covering our own eyes isn't just a fashion statement—it's sending signals to our brains that it's too dark, even when it's not.

Metaphorical blindfolds are the ones I'm still trying to uncover within myself. Over the last 12 years, I've had to start over so many times, sometimes wondering if I'll ever find clarity. In the last four years, since COVID hit, it's been a constant cycle—where I'm living, who my clients are, what I'm working on, what job I have, and what business I'm pouring my energy into. And honestly, it's exhausting. It feels like I've been wandering in the dark, trying to figure it all out, and just when I think I've got one piece in place, something shifts, and I'm back at square one.

The reality is, you're not good at anything when you begin. It's like watching a toddler trying to walk for the first time. They fall, they stumble, but they keep getting back up. And even though they can't see the road ahead, they continue to move forward with determination, unaware of their blindfolds. There's no shame in starting over. The challenge is learning to trust yourself in the process, even when it feels like everything is falling apart.

So, I guess that's what this journey is about—removing the blindfolds, one step at a time. The goal isn't perfection, it's progress. And sometimes, it's okay to fumble in the dark as long as you keep moving.

Emotional Stability:

Picture this: a woman with emotional stability walks into a room. She's the calm in the storm, the eye of the hurricane. She notices everything—the way the air smells, the subtle shift in energy—but remains serene. She gracefully avoids drama like it's an obstacle course and exudes kindness like she has an endless supply of it. When challenges arise, she doesn't panic or melt down. Nope, she faces them with the kind of emotional maturity that we all secretly envy. This lady is so composed, even her shadow stays cool.

Now, I've heard it time and time again, especially from men in my dating life: "I prefer a partner who won't make a scene in public, but can express frustrations in private." This isn't just some throwaway line—there's truth in it. And I had the chance to truly understand it in my late 30s, thanks to my millionaire friends, who taught me this lesson the hard way.

I was on a trip with a couple—Megan and Adam. After enduring over 24 hours of flight delays, they finally arrived at the counter, only to discover that their luggage had been lost, and their flights were canceled for two whole days. Megan was visibly upset, on the verge of tears. But Adam? Adam was the picture of calm. He didn't lose his cool, and his unflappable demeanor worked wonders. The staff, seeing how composed he was, scrambled to find a solution. The moral of the story? Managing your emotional state often leads to a better outcome.

This reminded me of all the times in my life when I did *not* manage my emotional state well. Like, remember those temper tantrums I threw as a young adult? Yeah, those were fun. And during a particularly rough patch when my body was rebelling—hello, toothaches, migraines, joint pain, and popping blood vessels in my eyes—it became clear that stress had taken over. My body was practically waving a red flag, saying, *"Hey! Something's wrong! Pay attention!"*

It's kind of like when your car alerts you that something's up. "WIPER OUT" is clear, but the engine light? That could mean anything. Similarly, my body was giving me signals—limping around, feeling drained, and wishing I could just snap back to normal. But the truth is, I had to listen to my body, take a step back, and allow myself to be patient.

Here's the funny part: I've been so empathetic towards others, but when it comes to myself? Not so much. I was struggling, and all I wanted was to be "normal" again, to run around like I used to. The idea of sharing my struggles made me anxious. I mean, who wants to admit they're struggling, right? Especially when you're in your 30s and everything feels *way* more intense than it used to.

But here's the breakthrough moment: I'm learning to be intentional in how I respond to life. I'm learning to check in with myself and give myself the same patience and grace I so easily give to others. It's a work in progress, but hey, growth doesn't happen overnight.

Reality vs. Fantasy:

Now, on to a different but equally eye-opening topic—crushes. You know how it goes: you meet someone, and suddenly they seem like the hero of a story. Their stories are so charming and grand, and you start thinking, *"Wow, this person is amazing!"* But are they really the hero? Or is there more to the story?

Take, for example, one guy I had a huge crush on. He literally told me, "You don't want to hang out with me." And yet, every time we were together, there was this electric chemistry. We had this magnetic pull, but the reality was that I kept pushing him away. Why? I didn't know. It was like I was playing some weird emotional game with myself.

Then there was this other guy—sweet as pie. He helped me move, carried my stuff, and even got lunch with me. He was going through a tough time with his ex, and he made her out to be the crazy one. And me? I, of course, tried to take on his emotional baggage. Sound familiar? *"I can fix this,"* I thought. But then it hit me: I had to stop trying to carry everyone's crap. You can't fix people who aren't asking for your help— and that's a big lesson in emotional boundaries.

So here's the takeaway, yall: Sometimes, we create characters in our minds based on the stories people tell us. But those stories may not always be the full truth. It's important to take a step back, look at the bigger picture, and recognize that not every person who walks into your life is a knight in shining armor. It's okay to set boundaries, to recognize that not everyone's drama is yours to fix.

Life, love, and crushes are all part of the adventure. The key is to stay grounded, stay real, and most importantly, stay patient—with yourself and others. Trust me, it's a journey worth taking.

FED- CPR:

I was over doing it, life that is. Everyone around me thought I was crazy for going to Vegas, but it wasn't even a thought process. I knew the doctor said one thing and everyone thought I should be taking it easy, but a new character was unlocked. God literally unlocked a new level of the word "patience" for me. I'm always in such a rush, but he wanted me to be still. This is a funny experience, I was learning right before my courageous trip. The reason for the adventures into the land of sunshine for shady people is a leadership convention my business partners put on.

When I tell you this isn't an event I want to miss, it's because I'm surrounded by an arena of 15,0000 people that are loving, kind, supportive, and helpful. It's not just about business, it's about life skills, spiritual, mental, physical, and financial education. Where being supported in life is to be holistically supported in every aspect in life.

Handicapped:

I have a whole new respect for what it means to be unable. When I was in nursing, I learned the gift of patience—everything with the elderly moves at their pace, kind of like island time. When visiting outside the States, things happen when they happen and the concept of "on time" is meaningless to them. In faster-paced places like New York, being "on time" often means you're late. Even in international business, time feels irrelevant, but still manages to keep things on track. In LA, people strive to be "on time," but social settings usually expect them to arrive fashionably late.

The moral of my story is that when you're hobbling everywhere instead of a balanced walking, you have to rely on others to help take care of you. Meaning, you should expect to take a lot of time, and being patient is only where it begins. Caring for another human is incredibly physical, it requires giving all your strength and energy to support someone else—a wild concept when you think about it.

While heading to Las Vegas for a business conference, I had to confront my own reality. At that moment in time, I was injured for a season that felt like infinity. Weeks went by and walking became extremely hard for me. It was so bad, I was using medications just to survive the pain during the day. I was told I needed to use a cane, but it was extremely hard on my mind. It took me months to stop being so stubborn, I needed that tool. At that point I had been in pain for months, not sleeping because I'd wake up with throbbing pains in the middle of the night, and couldn't get comfortable. I had been wearing a stem cell patch, using a 10's unit for electrotherapy, foam rolling, and a massage gun. I'd gone to get a few massages, as well as my daily PT exercises. So traveling was a difficulty. I struggled to sit for long periods of time, and wasn't able to stand past a total of 10 minutes. It was too much pressure on my hips, legs, back, and ankles. Arriving at the arena, I quickly realized this was going to be a bigger hurdle than I could ever have imagined. However, missing the event wasn't an option for me. I take pride in myself, and my future and this conference wasn't one I was going to miss. Arriving there I realized there were just too many steps and stairs to navigate around the arena. Thank goodness a friend suggested I get ADA assistance, which I would have never considered. Even though I was walking slowly, I resisted the idea of needing help. However, I had to realize that having that support was more than necessary.

On day one, I thought I could manage with just my cane, but the waiting was too much on my feet. I couldn't stand on my ankles and hips for long. Walking slowly reminded me of a song my brother used to sing about our grandma—"Grandma Walking Slow." I found myself laughing at the thought of it, realizing that sometimes, we just need to embrace the pace we're at.

The geography was overwhelming, even with the help of my cane and pain medication. I needed extra support because I couldn't stand for very long or sit for too long, so I ended up requiring wheelchair assistance. Each time I needed to go to the bathroom, I had to notify the staff, who would radio for help. I had to wait for them to come and get me in a wheelchair, then navigate the ground floor, up to an elevator, since they had closed all the bathrooms on that level for the "higher elite" since "they were paying more," but not even making a priority for ADA access. "*That's Crazy*," I thought.

Once we reached the elevator, I had to make it through four sets of doors before finally getting to the bathroom. I was helped to stand and hobble into a stall. I realized how much I had undervalued that support. By the time I needed to go, I should have asked at least 20 minutes earlier because the whole process took another 40 to 45 minutes.

Red Zone:

Luckily, everyone was so sweet and eager to help. I really saw the beauty of ADA in those moments, as others in my section were quick to offer assistance. One couple noticed me struggling to walk alone and, without hesitation, Jane kindly offered to give me a ride on her rollator. I sat down, and she wheeled me all the way to the bathroom and back. The whole ADA section felt like a supportive community, with everyone cheering each other on. It was heartwarming to witness how the people around me were so focused on celebrating the small victories.

But this experience also made me realize how much harder it can be for those who rely on ADA. The distances from parking lots, the availability of elevators and ramps, and the number of stairs at different locations are all factors that make mobility so much more difficult. Going to the bathroom, for example, I couldn't help but wonder why the accessible stalls are often the furthest from the sinks or doors. It's not a space issue—the space is there—but it still causes unnecessary complications. One woman shared her own struggle with me: "If I bring my rollator into the bathroom, I have to use the big stall. But one time, I left it outside a smaller stall, and it was stolen while I was inside. Now, I wait for the accessible stall, but nothing frustrates me more than seeing someone who doesn't need it sitting on their phone in the stall, wasting time while I wait."

It was an eye-opening experience for me. And I had a huge revelation— why do I have so much patience for everyone around me, always ready to listen and wait for others, but I struggle so much with being patient with myself? I was shocked! I noticed how anxious it made me when others helped me, or when someone had to wait as I moved slowly. All I wanted was to move quickly, "normally," and get back to my old life, to dance again.

The truth, though, is that I can't return to that old life. Once I'm healed and my body is fully capable again, I'll be stepping into a new and better version of myself—one that knows how to be patient, especially with me. This experience has completely shifted my perspective, giving me a newfound sense of empathy and understanding for both myself and others.

Season "Two" of Cali Chronicles: Vegas Nightmares:

Being in ADA is tough. Sometimes, we sit in our misery and wallow in pity for too long. I don't really know why, but some days when people ask if I'm okay, I can muster a smile, while other days, I can't hold back the tears. One moment, I'm perfectly fine, and the next, I'm on the verge of breaking down. But I'm determined to stop resonating with a frequency I don't want anymore. I refuse to live in pity or sadness, so I've started to politely decline to respond to those feelings. I'm focusing on healing, not dwelling on the past.

God places you in spaces that are meant to build your character for the next phase. I've often wished to be somewhere I'm not quite ready for. I know I need to evolve into that person, I need to grow. It's time to open myself up to building, listening, and—most importantly— stopping my stubbornness. I need to accept constructive criticism and learn the script. Do the hard things.

I have to turn the script around, be a student, and let go of my stubbornness. I need to be open to change and stop explaining who I once was or wasn't. It's time to cut the entitlement and release those old versions of myself. We're not in those life experiences anymore, and they didn't work for a reason. Stop expressing ideals of the past, we're in the NOW. Be more present, this is the only moment that matters, everything else is just of another time in space.

Now, we're in a new "miracle territory". The only time where anything is possible and in creation towards a better tomorrow. Let's use the intentional tools available to us. It's not magical, but it's transformative.

Unexpected Roads:

36.1156° N, 115.1512° W

At the conference in Vegas, I realized that I can't rush the process. I need to be patient with my relationships, my business, and the direction I'm headed. At that moment, I understood that I must take things slow and let them grow naturally. I'll get there, but it doesn't necessarily have to be on my timeline.

Part of me knows that my relationship shouldn't be a secret. I'm trying to be honest with my mentors, but how do we navigate six months with something hidden? Why am I approaching it this way? It feels like a slow burn since we met—couldn't we have just waited? Why am I chasing validation? That's the biggest question. I'm doing it subconsciously in every area of my life: work, church, my business, and my speaking engagements.

I struggled with this "**superiority complex**," tossing out the credentials and status. I can't stand it when people name-drop; that kind of energy feels so thirsty. The real ones don't chase—they attract and say fewer words. That's where I want to be: becoming the best version of myself, especially when the lights are low and no one is watching. I don't need validation. I don't need to be noticed.

I wish things were more open between us, but only time will tell what happens. I like him and want to talk to him. I love that he wants to see me and encourages me. He's genuinely selfless, just wanting to make me happy. He's the sweetest.

I know managing my mind and energy across three different avenues is tough, but I'm not going to let that get in the way of my work credentials. How beautiful it would be if we did this together—a real love story! We could help so many people. He inspires me, and I inspire him.

What's crucial for me is healing my body and spirit. I've realized that God has a funny way of guiding me down unexpected roads. When I thought my biggest dreams were possible, I felt ready for what's coming. But now I see there are so many avenues to explore —and I must avoid distractions.

The real question is: which direction will I choose? Will I listen and be patient with all these elements in my life? All I feel is pressure, but then I remember: pressure cuts diamonds.

Delayed Gratification:

This kind of patience helps with emotional regulation and resilience, especially in the face of uncertainty. It allows us to wait for longer-term rewards instead of seeking immediate results.

Letting Go of Superficiality:

My desire for **authenticity** over appearances shows itself in my discomfort with "**superiority complexes**" and the tendency to seek status or credential for validation.

Self-actualization—becoming the best version of myself—can only occur when we are honest and true to who we are, without the need to impress others or live up to societal expectations.

Unconditional love requires us to love ourselves and others **beyond external accomplishments**. It's not about credentials, status, or what we can offer; it's about accepting and loving what's real and unadorned.

CHAPTER THIRTY SIX

RHYTHM OF REPETITION.

Where Do You See Beyond the Truth? Living Without Fear:

34.1020° N, 118.3458° W

In a small circle of girls I met at church, we started discussing our age groups and the idea of having children. One girl, Hope—a sweet blonde with straight hair—said, "I can't even imagine having kids right now. I can barely get my life together, and I'm 25." Next to her was Grace, a brunette in a bun and an American flag sweater. She echoed the sentiment: "Yeah, there's a lot in my life I need to work on before even considering kids, and I'm 30."

I found myself nodding in agreement. "I feel the same way, and I'm 32. But that's why I work with kids. I get my dose of inspiration from them without having to live with them." We all laughed, appreciating the lighthearted take on a serious topic, especially as we reflected on our friends from home who are already juggling multiple kids. It was striking to see how different our lifestyles were.

As the day went on, I began to reflect on my own journey. I thought about all the career changes I've made and the states I've traveled to or moved between. I've taken my career seriously up to this point, realizing that I'm really just getting started. I've attempted six businesses that didn't pan out, but each one has taught me valuable lessons—lessons that feel like training for the future and for who I'm becoming in my thirties.

When I look at my life as a book, I see how vast my experiences have been. I've never taken the easy path. Each challenge has fueled my desire for exponential growth, and every lesson is shaping me for something bigger than my wildest dreams.

Hyper Independent:

Yeah, I'm talking to all you givers out there, the ones who are *so* used to helping everyone else but have no idea how to let others help you.

This lesson hit me hard, like a surprise plot twist in the middle of a rom-com. I hear it all the time from fellow entrepreneurs—***"I'd rather do everything myself. No one can do it as well as I can, so I'll just take it on."*** Sound familiar? You're so used to carrying the weight of the world on your own shoulders that you don't even know *how* to ask for help. Or worse—***you won't ask,*** because you're convinced you'll be better off doing it yourself.

But here's the thing: that mindset? It's slowly wrecking you. Often, this behavior comes from childhood—when you learned that you weren't safe if others did things for you, so you took over. Maybe, in some cases, you even had to *become* an adult and take care of your parents before your time. So, you skipped adolescence, and suddenly, you're stuck carrying the emotional weight of a lifetime.

But here's the real kicker: when does the realization hit that the road you're on is just... expired? Maybe that door you walked through wasn't even the right one. But *why* would it open, right? Was it just a lesson disguised as a detour?

I can't help but ponder that idea—like I'm standing at the crossroads of my life, holding a cup of coffee, and waiting for the next sign to pop up. Life has a funny way of teaching us, doesn't it?

Healing Era:

Is it just me, or does it feel like healing *never* ends? I swear, each time I think I've reached the finish line, there's another layer of "oh, look—more stuff to unpack!" How deep does this rabbit hole go? Honestly, how many levels can there be before you finally reach the *root* of that eternal pain?

The last few weeks have been nothing but a challenge, testing my patience like a toddler in a candy store. Patience with myself... and others. A little less of the "Don't make me do this!" and a little more of the "Let's all get along."

And then there's the traffic. Oh, the traffic. Is it really road rage, or am I just flustered by my own habits? If I'd only *done it this way,* if I'd only *reacted that way,* life would be so much smoother, right? I can feel the inner control freak kicking in, demanding to steer the ship of LIFE. But hey, I'm not alone in this battle. We're all driving together, right?

But here's the big question: What makes this *story* worth telling? What makes it worth *hearing*? I mean, who's out there just waiting to hear my inner monologue on a Tuesday afternoon? I get it—*everyone's healing,* but how do we even find our way to that magical light? Maybe it's somewhere between the bad coffee and the traffic jams.

So, let's keep this thing rolling. Because in the end, healing's a journey, and maybe it's worth the ride. Or, at least worth the laugh along the way.

Overcoming the Cycle: A Reflection on Growth:

It's hard to admit the moments when you've been hiding from yourself. But sometimes, life has a way of forcing us to see our own faults, to confront the parts of ourselves we've buried deep. Coming home, I felt the weight of everything I had been carrying for years. It was time to take accountability for my past, my struggles, and my own personal growth.

Recently, I watched *Inside Out 2*, a film about emotions, and it hit me on a deep level. The new emotion introduced was anxiety. And that emotion? Well, it felt all too familiar.

Looking back, I can trace the root of that anxiety to years of bottling up my emotions, suppressing them until they manifested as something I couldn't ignore anymore. As a child, I never felt smart enough, good enough, or worthy enough. I was constantly bombarded with feelings of inadequacy. School told me I wasn't smart enough. I struggled with spelling, with math, with basic things that other kids seemed to breeze through. I switched schools mid-year, thinking it would help, but the new support wasn't enough. I was told I'd be held back a grade. I wasn't the youngest anymore; I was either too far ahead or too far behind, and it made me feel like I didn't belong anywhere.

It was always a cycle of comparison. And that's anxiety in a nutshell— always feeling like I wasn't enough, always running a race I never quite understood.

Then came the ego shift. When I was held back a grade, I was suddenly the oldest in the class. It was the first time I felt "power" in a strange way, but it wasn't a healthy kind of power. I didn't feel secure or proud—I felt like I needed to prove something to everyone. I wanted to show that I had something they didn't, even if I didn't know what that "something" was. I started to build walls and project this false sense of superiority. I wasn't just trying to belong; I was trying to dominate. I told myself I knew all the answers, even when I didn't. And when I couldn't find the answers, I made them up.

In truth, I was longing for connection, but I couldn't let myself connect deeply with anyone. I had this ability to get along with everyone, but I never allowed anyone to get close enough to really *know* me. And that's where the anxiety grew—because I was never really myself. I was always a reflection of those around me. It wasn't until later in life that I realized I'd become codependent in my relationships, attaching my identity to others' in order to feel validated. Krystal, Caroline, Issiah, Mr. J, Mr. Killa, Seia, Mo, Daniel, Marseille—they were my mirrors. Who was I without them?

As a kid, I channeled my feelings into sports. If I didn't have a best friend, sports became my new obsession. Some were healthy—like dance and track—but others, like softball, became a toxic crutch. My dad's passion for the sport became a way for him to connect with me, but as the coach's daughter, I often felt the pressure to perform. I wasn't just competing against others—I was competing with the person I thought I had to be. The perfect daughter. The strong, tough girl. I wanted to win his love, to show him that I could be just as good, if not better, than the boys. But when I didn't perform at my best, I tore myself apart. It wasn't about the game; it was about proving I was good enough.

Fast forward to 2022, when I joined a co-ed softball league as an adult. I thought I was ready to get back into the competitive spirit, to feel that rush of being on a winning team. But when the team played poorly, I realized something important: I was still trying to "win" in life. In relationships. In everything. I was focused on proving I was right, trying to score for my own benefit instead of playing for the team. And that's when the light bulb went off. I don't want to be that person anymore. I don't want to play games or manipulate situations to get what I want. I need to focus on my own growth.

It took me a while to recognize the cycle I was stuck in. From the cat-and-mouse games in relationships to the endless pursuit of validation, I had been seeking external approval rather than focusing on my own inner peace. But now, I'm ready to change. I don't need to hunt for love or attention. I don't need to fill my time with distractions. I want to be whole on my own, to be at peace with who I am.

This is the work I need to do. To stop overcompensating. To stop searching for something outside of myself to feel complete. I need to dig deep, ask the hard questions, and face the uncomfortable truths. It's time to grow and mature, to shine a light on the areas I've ignored. I want to become the best version of myself—not for anyone else, but for me.

And so, here I am, reflecting on the path I've walked and the lessons I've learned. It hasn't been easy, and it hasn't always been pretty, but it's been worth it. I've learned that growth isn't linear. It's messy, uncomfortable, and often requires a willingness to let go of old habits, old patterns, and old versions of yourself. But that's how we become who we're meant to be. I'm finally ready to embrace that.

A Moment of Connection:

Have you ever met a stranger, and in an instant, felt a connection that made everything feel lighter? It's like their smile and the way their eyes meet yours somehow make the world seem a little better. I had one of those encounters, again. This "soul" is too familiar.

I stumbled into a crowded coffee shop, fully packed with people. Every table was taken—except for one, where a sweet gentleman sat alone. I hesitated for a moment but decided to sit down. What happened next turned into a surprisingly meaningful hour.

We started talking, and I learned that he owned a cologne company. His passion for scents was evident, but what really captivated me was his storytelling. His words had a way of pulling me in, making each detail feel like a journey.

Curious about how his passion began, I asked, "What was it about your curiosity that led you to take the leap into starting your own business?" Without missing a beat, he dove into an adventure he took to pursue his dream, a decision that changed his life. He spoke about the power of fragrance—how each scent held a story, evoking memories and emotions, sometimes of the past, sometimes of the future.

The most touching part of our conversation came when I asked him what stories his fragrances had evoked in his clients. He smiled and said that some scents reminded people of their grandmothers, of love, of family gatherings. Others brought back memories of quiet moments, of laughter surrounded by balloons. It was amazing to hear how something so simple could carry so much emotion.

As we spoke, time seemed to slow down. I left that coffee shop feeling grateful for the unexpected connections we can make, even with strangers. It was a reminder that life, in its unpredictability, often brings us the most beautiful, authentic encounters when we least expect them.

Psychological Theory of Narrative Identity:

The concept that our identities are shaped by the stories we tell about ourselves. The man's story about how he came to create fragrances, and how others share their emotional connections to the scents, parallels the way unconditional love allows people to narrate their own stories without fear of judgment or rejection. Unconditional love encourages individuals to freely express their own experiences—both the beauty and the pain—knowing that they will be embraced without criticism.

CHAPTER THIRTY SEVEN

UNVEILING NEW HORIZONS: PARADIGM

Lesson in Unison: A Shift in Perspective:

34.0872° N, 118.3430° W

I walked into Sightglass, a coffee shop in the heart of Hollywood, with its massive windows that felt like a distillery, crafting not just coffee but experiences. The space was incredible—open, vibrant, and full of energy. I'd been invited a few times, but today was the day I finally decided to show up. And I'm so glad I did, because I found my new spot—the place where I could just breathe, focus, and get my life together.

I joined a small group of people who were deep in conversation about love. There were three tables of people, and when I sat down, I was hoping to be at the table with my closest friends. But fate had other plans. I was seated with strangers, and initially, I was disappointed. In my head, I felt a little bummed. I wanted to be with the people I already knew, to talk to them, to connect. But the universe, as it always does, had something bigger in mind. It wasn't about what I wanted—it was about what I needed.

As we began talking about love, I started sharing something personal: my experience with a man I was casually dating at the time, Ray **(THE RUNNER)**. I knew in my heart that he wasn't "the one"—not my "husband"—because of where I'm at in life and where I'm growing. We get along well. He has many qualities I've prayed for—he was artistic, grounded, and kind. But there were differences that kept us from truly aligning. For one, I don't drink anymore, and he does. He works in the entertainment industry, around people who live a lifestyle I've chosen to step away from. Our rhythms don't always match, especially when it comes to things like my commitment to the gym, while that's not a priority for him. He slept in during the day to follow his career schedule, which often meant our lives don't line up.

Still, despite all of that, I felt a curious pull—a kind of knocking at my heart. It wasn't about me anymore. Maybe he wasn't Mr. "Right," but he was exactly what I needed right at the moment. He was holding space for me to open my heart and show love in ways I hadn't expected. He did little acts of kindness that I truly appreciated, held my things, led with his heart, and was open and honest. The energy between us was genuine. And as I reflected on it, **I realized that sometimes the people in our lives aren't there to stay forever—they're there to give us something we need in the moment, to teach us something we haven't yet learned. In that moment, I saw that he wasn't just here for me—I was here for him too.**

This was a gift I had to share. Sometimes, when we *block others from our lives, we're also blocking the gift* we have to offer them. They might need us more than we need them. And in those moments, that realization can be a powerful shift in perspective.

I had a similar experience earlier that week, during choir rehearsal. I'd instinctively walked to the left side of the stage, where my friends were lined up, but the leader asked me to move to the other side—based on my energy and height. At first, I was frustrated. I felt like I'd be dimming my light by moving to the other side. It felt like a bit of a punishment (Pure EGO). The other side seemed dull compared to where my friends were, and I didn't want to stand out. I wanted to blend in with them. But then, as I stood there, I had a realization.

It wasn't about me. It was about the unison. Choir is all about blending our voices, not standing out. I was asked to move because my light was needed elsewhere. The others needed my energy, and in that moment, I understood that sometimes our gifts are not just for us—they're for others too.

It's easy to think that everything is about us—our desires, our plans, our comfort. But life has a way of reminding us that it's about the bigger picture, about being in unison with others and knowing when your gifts are meant to shine for someone else.

So, today, I learned a lesson about surrendering my expectations and opening up to the experiences that are meant to teach me. It's not always about getting what we want—it's about receiving what we need. And sometimes, we need to step aside from what feels comfortable and allow the universe to show us the path we're meant to walk.

Love is in the Air: A Lesson from the Mountain:
34.1054° N, 118.3517° W

As I scaled the mountainside with a group from church hiking, a chance encounter with a curious character named "Love" **(THE REMINDER)** stopped me in my tracks. We bumped into each other, and as we exchanged glances, we couldn't help but laugh at the coincidence. Two beings, one called "Love," one called "Aire," meeting high above in the mountains—it seemed like something straight out of a fairytale. We joked that maybe "Love was in the air," as we shared a moment of lightheartedness between the wind and the rugged path.

I was drawn to learn more about him, to uncover the essence of the character that bore such a powerful name. So, I asked, "How did you come by the name 'Love'?"

With a thoughtful smile, Love began to share. "Well, my mom gave me a solid foundation. She taught me the value of love, but she also had the highest expectations. It was as if she showed me what real love was, but never quite gave me the full picture. I never yielded to anything but love. Life, for me, is all about love—it's the conversation in every moment. No matter what happens, I always come back to it. As long as I lead with love, everything else falls into place."

He paused, looking out over the horizon, as if the sun itself had given him clarity. "The sun, you know, is the embodiment of love. I've always felt that I'm on a similar journey, called to spread that same warmth, to help others recognize that love is in everything. In everything they give. It's simple. If I live my life authentically, sharing my experiences with honesty, then I'm giving others the space to feel loved, too. With love, I can connect with anyone—there's no limit."

We spent the afternoon together, and the more Love spoke, the more I felt his presence. His words were simple but profound, and they lingered with me. As the day came to an end, I realized that spending time with Love had touched something deep within me. It wasn't just his words—it was his energy, his ability to be present, and his unwavering belief that love could guide him through life.

The day left me feeling lighter, as though I had been reminded of something essential: the true power of love. Not just the romantic kind, but the love that can transform any situation, the kind that listens, understands, and forgives.

Before parting ways, Love smiled and said, "Keep your eyes out for my song, *Love is in the Air*." He winked, and just like that, we parted at the mountain's peak, each carrying a piece of the other's energy with us.

As I made my way down the mountain, I couldn't help but think: "Love really is in the air." It's in the way we show up for each other, in how we connect, in how we lead with our hearts. Maybe that's the whole point—to share love, to spread it far and wide, and to remember that sometimes, the most unexpected encounters bring us exactly what we need.

Conclusion:

Love isn't just a word or a feeling; it's a force that can guide us through life, shape our experiences, and connect us to others in ways we never imagined. When we lead with love, we're not just giving—it's an energy exchange that has the power to transform. And as we go through our days, if we can carry even a fraction of that love with us, the world becomes a little brighter for everyone we meet.

You Do Deserve Your Own Chapter: DAMON

34.044727, -118.249283

Loving Damon **(THE REMINDER)** was like riding a whirlwind—short, sweet, and a little confusing—but honestly, I've never minded the storm. From the moment I first laid eyes on him, I thought he was cute. But at the time, I was all about that "me, myself, and I" vibe, determined to focus on my own journey.

He walked in, dressed to the nines in your sharp suit, at a banquet party for a sports entertainment event. The place was buzzing with people, the decorations practically everywhere, and yet, he somehow stood out. A little taller than me, with that smooth, chocolate-brown skin, short hair, dimples that could melt the coldest heart, and a smile that could light up the entire room.

I knew right then—things were going to be interesting.

I had this practice, a little self-discipline game, that whenever I saw someone cute, I'd walk away. I'd find a seat on the other side of the room, doing my best to not start a conversation. But of course, the universe had other plans and sat us right next to each other in the same row.

Luckily, there was space between us, with the aisle as a perfect buffer. I also assumed it was better to keep my distance. For months I kept bumping into you at other events, and while it was always fun, I tried to keep it casual. But I was secretly excited each time I saw you. Then, I started dating Mr. "Not Really Right For Me," Ray **(THE RUNNER)** and when our paths crossed you'd ask me about my life. You'd been keeping tabs on me, following closely on social media, you made a comment about our *"matching shoes."* That comment stuck with me, especially since it was tied to a photo from my birthday—when I was all dressed up and genuinely happy. Ironically, I ended up in a horrible fight with Ray that night, a reminder of why I kept finding myself in relationships that were lacking in communication and intimacy. It was really triggering for me.

Meanwhile, I could tell you were interested—your subtle way of watching me from a distance made it obvious. But I was always just out of reach, caught up in my own emotional turmoil. As time passed, we both moved on from the initial flirtation. Then, I began peeling back the layers of past relationships and old heartbreaks I'd been clinging to like a fugitive, unaware that I wasn't giving myself the space to heal. Ending things with Ray was sudden and abrupt, especially after my birthday. The pain and drama of his emotional turmoil became too much. He was going through an extremely complicated time and just shut down, shutting me out. I was realizing I was still heartbroken from years of unresolved wounds—the pain that hadn't healed. Mr. J and Mr. Killa were still jagged shards of broken glass, lingering, and I was aware of them, stuck in that knowing gaze.

One day, at another event while I was struggling with the pain in my leg, I jokingly shared my "fantasies" with my personal trainer about needing someone to nurse me back to health. To my surprise, it sparked something between us. Slowly but surely, our connection deepened, and the quality time we spent together felt both nurturing and comforting.

I craved affection, attention, and love—things I hadn't realized I was missing with Ray. Damon decided to jump in, eyes closed. Our connection hit a remarkable inspiration of life, sexual nurturing, and emotional healing. Then, in true me fashion, I panicked and ended things with you, out of fear. I didn't want to ruin something good, but I was too scared of the circumstances. But, as if the universe was pulling us back together, we found our way to each other again.

Here's the thing: I'm *not* the girl who goes back to an ex. Ever. When I'm done, I'm done. But, somehow, we ended up back together. Weeks passed, and we grew closer. His humor always made me smile, and his intelligence was a huge turn-on. I didn't want a basic conversation with him—I wanted to be challenged, having deep things to talk about. He always actively listened to me. He helped me with chores. He was kind, thoughtful, and helped carry my things. He had the same lifestyle as me, when I wasn't hurt, but you could say we both were a bit "injured," me physically and him mentally—both needing healing.

But then, the space between us started to grow. With Vanessa coming to visit to help take care of me, it was like we had lost our connection. One unexpected night of drinking pushed me over the edge. We broke up, and though I knew it was for the best, I couldn't help but feel **heartbroken** all over again.

Days passed, and I found myself spiraling. He texted me to pick up his things, but instead of just leaving, he showed up with dinner, flowers, and... sex toys. My mind went into a whirlpool. I was initially turned off by the sex toys, despite us talking about them before, but the night we broke up had left me feeling disconnected. It didn't feel like a relationship anymore, more like a "friends with benefits" situation, and that left me with a sick feeling. Truth was that's what the relationship felt like, maybe always. He tried to remind me we were "public" most of the time, and exclusively seeing each other. However, there was a missing piece hidden. We might have only been seeing each other, but the sex was the main course that kept binding us together.

He left his pillow behind, giving me the idea that maybe he wasn't completely done with us. Shortly after, I asked for space—I needed to sort my mind out with God. A week passed, and I knew I needed to see you to finally end things for good. I wanted to get closure. When he didn't respond to my message, I knew it wasn't going to go well.

Then, he didn't text me all night. It felt like he was playing games, and I felt icky about it. But deep down, I was still scared of losing him, like some *"needy cat"* who only wanted affection when it was convenient. My mind played tricks on me, and it was like this tug of war between wanting love and needing space.

Finally, he said he would come to see me the following Monday. Monday arrived, and when he didn't show up, he called telling me that he went to church instead, the anger in me flared up. I hadn't felt that kind of rage in a long time. I hung up on him, only to later apologize for my outburst. I was frustrated, hurt, and so confused. Mad at myself: for being angry with him for taking care of his own priorities, like church. I just felt like he was blowing me off.

The next day, he called. We agreed to get dinner. Later that day I texted "Let's meet at a sushi place." But I looked down at my phone to read his text message reply," I don't think so, I think we just need to end things." It was the very thing I had been dreading over text, but part of me knew it was for the best. I wanted to avoid a cowardly and disrespectful text message breakup. I loved and respected you too much for that. But I was still upset, annoyed, and as I began packing up his things, he came inside. Smiling from ear to ear, he swept me off my feet with a smile so beautiful I could hardly resist. He was so excited to see me, I was in shock. Having no idea what kind of interaction was going to take place between us.

Before I knew it, we were madly making love again. We had "relations" three more times, and in a final moment, I finally let go. My body relaxed, the weight of all the turmoil fell off, and I knew it was time to cut the cord. I felt safe, loved, and happy, and when he left, I knew it was officially done this time.

The next weekend, I cleaned out my whole house—got rid of all your things, washed the sheets, and even the comforter. I needed to clean his scent from my life. He had taken up too much free rent in my head, distracting me, and it was keeping me awake at night. Another week went by, and I knew that if we kept talking, it would only turn toxic again. He was sending me meme's and messages. So, I sent him a message. I told him that I loved him, that everything I wrote in a goodbye letter was true, but I couldn't keep being triggered by our messages. I needed to love him in a healthy manner, and we needed a shift in our relationship.

I ended the text message with, "Let's just let it be in God's hands." He didn't respond, and we hardly spoke. Until, of course, we found ourselves at another event. I saw him across the room, and he was smiling at me. My heart skipped a beat. I couldn't help but smile back. We were sitting far apart, but I felt him looking at me. Suddenly, in a moment of panic the pain from my medication was wearing off, and I needed help.

And then, in a moment of clarity, he did something that left me speechless. When I could barely move, he rushed over and helped me. He literally lifted me up like a baby and carried me to the car. After everything, I found myself "in your hands"—both literally and figuratively. It was like a sign from God, the very thing I had prayed for —"Put it in God's hands, he put me in your hands." You were always there, and you came through. Whenever I needed help, and there you were—my hero.

Emotional Baggage:

Unconditional love, in this case, involves accepting one's imperfections, acknowledging past wounds, and making room for healing. Just as unconditional love means accepting someone despite their flaws or struggles, it also means extending that same grace to ourselves. Without it, we won't allow ourselves to fully engage in new relationships and will struggle to fully "let go" of past traumas.

Cycle of Connection and Disconnection:

My relationship with Damon demonstrates a **repeated cycle** of connection and disconnection. Initially, there's excitement, but due to personal insecurities, fear, and emotional turbulence, our relationship fluctuates between closeness and distance. This mirrors the "**push-pull**" dynamic many individuals experience when they are afraid of being vulnerable or when they've not fully healed from past emotional pain.

Damon's behavior—showing up, offering care, and stepping in to help when I was vulnerable—reflects **unconditional love** in action. It's not about perfection or always getting everything right, but being there when needed, even when things are messy or uncertain.

Emotional Support and Healing

Damon didn't try to fix me or change my situation; he simply offered his assistance when it's needed most. This moment of support highlights a critical part of unconditional love: it isn't about grand gestures or solving each other's problems, but about showing up and being present for each other without judgment. This act of kindness, physically lifting and carrying, symbolizes the idea that love is about helping one another rise above the struggles—literally and metaphorically.

CRUTCHES REQUIRES CHAOS:

It had been months of me in pain, and finally succumbing to walking around with a cane; but the hardest struggles were when I started to graduate to the next level of patience........the one requirement: *Crutches.*

It wasn't while Vanessa was visiting; the biggest realization was that again, "I'm so used to doing everything by myself and I don't want to inconvenience someone else or interrupt what they're doing to add another laundry list of things when I need something done in the same minutes so I just do it myself..."

Can I give myself a break? There's so many things to tend to.

The experience showed us both how funny it is, as recovering "control freaks", to open up and expand... Like just because it's not done the way "I" like the task to be completed, doesn't mean it's wrong. This is a topic I've experienced personally in relationships with significant others and work settings. There are infinite ways to have things done. I needed to be willinging to let go of control. Release the anxiety over the solution.

We could never agree to leave early or on time in Vanessa's world, it didn't bother her. However, it drove me crazy to be late; makes me drive and rush, and I'd been training myself to have better habits. Clean dishes at night, clothes picked out, and leave early enough to start the day. She enjoyed slower mornings; wanted to make breakfast at different times and pushed the time requirements daily. I had no choice to compromise because she was giving me a gift of cooking/cleaning/ and being around.

I wasn't paying her for her acts of service, I could only offer the shelter of a safe home, there was an underlying feeling of guilt and care on my behalf.

So, naturally, I didn't want to keep pushing. I had to focus on making sure I was prepared, in control of myself, and my circumstances. Then, we'd chat about the tough stuff. But I didn't try to coach her or over-explain things like I usually do for others. Instead, I kept the questions thoughtful—just enough to help her wrap her mind around it, but not too deep. Honestly, I was so wrapped up in trying to heal my own situation that I was just so grateful to have someone, *her*, dedicating her time and energy to helping me.

Fast forward to the second-to-last day of her visit. I went to see my PT, and she decided I needed to be completely off weight-bearing on my hip. I was handed crutches to walk out of the hospital. *Oh boy.* It was like a comedy show—me, my purse, and the cane I had come in with, all trying to make a graceful exit. It wasn't pretty. By the time I made it home, I got my ADA sticker and another X-ray. When I came back inside, she could hear the crutches clunking from a mile away. I wasn't used to them at all. Turns out, they weren't even adjusted right for my height! (*Thanks for that, PT.*)

Those crutches? Let me tell you, they're a workout. But, lucky for me, my PT had been making me focus on my core and upper body for weeks. So, for a hot minute, I felt like I was gliding on them—until I lost momentum, that is. You really aren't meant to go full-speed on crutches, but hey, I tried. I'm a force to be reckoned with, after all. But, eventually, I realized—maybe I don't need to be as fast as a race car.

Days went by, and the reactions from people were... *interesting.* At first, everyone was super aware. Doors were held open for me, people offered to carry things, and there were even a few "You got this!" cheers thrown my way. But a couple of days later? It was like I was invisible. People were brushing past me, getting irritated if I was in their way. One time, I was walking next to a doorway, and a lady tried to squeeze through the *inch* of space between me and the wall. I almost lost my cool and gave her a piece of my mind—except, I was at work, so composure was key. Still, I was *furious*.

And then there was the ADA ramp. I was literally at the top, ready to roll down, and these two-footed humans just *blazed* up the ramp like I wasn't standing there with crutches, staring them down with my best "Really?" face. I swear, sometimes it feels like some people don't even *see* their surroundings. It's mind-boggling. I had to resist the urge to shout, "What are you doing? Can't you see I'm crutching here?" But instead, I just shook my head. I was honestly flabbergasted by some of the behavior. It makes you realize how much more we all need to be aware, to be kind, and to care for each other.

This whole experience keeps opening my eyes, shifting my perspective. It's a reminder that kindness is more than just a gesture—it's a way of being. Some people seem oblivious to the world around them, but I'd rather be someone who notices. Because really, life's too short to be anything but kind, especially when it's so easy to make someone's day just a little bit lighter.

Psychological Conclusion:

Think of the crutches as a metaphor *"for the emotional crutches we sometimes need to rely on to grow, heal, and accept love."* The experience of giving and receiving help, and the struggle to release control, are central to understanding unconditional love. It teaches us that love isn't just about "doing things" but about *being with someone*, even in their brokenness, their struggles, and their need for support. True love, whether for ourselves or others, asks us to embrace the chaos of vulnerability and learn that we are worthy of care, without condition.

CHAPTER THIRTY EIGHT

IN GOOD CONSCIOUSNESS.

MY HONESTY:

I want to admit something: sometimes, I doubt my own abilities. Even with years of experience and expertise, I still find myself learning new lessons, gaining new perspectives, and discovering fresh examples of how to approach things. There's always a new variable, a new challenge, a new twist that keeps me on my toes.

But here's the thing: those doubts? They don't stop me. In fact, they've brought me closer to connecting with others. I've learned that the more I embrace my own uncertainties, the more I can be open to understanding people, serving them, and loving them for who they are. It's in those moments of vulnerability, of admitting I don't have all the answers, that the real magic happens. I get to experience life with others in a way that feels truly genuine.

So, while I may sometimes wonder if I'm doing it right, I know one thing for sure: these tools, these lessons, these doubts—they've helped me become a better human, and that's the most important thing.

Against All Odds:

"I see myself in your bad decisions." It's funny how easy it is to get swept up in the chaos of society's distractions. We've all been there—one wrong turn after another, and suddenly, you've fallen into a rabbit hole you didn't even know existed. If you want to change your life, you've got to stop hanging around the people who make it easier to make *bad choices*. The reality? If five of your friends are doing something, chances are, you'll do it too. It starts innocently enough, like a casual hangout

with two friends who want to have a little fun. What starts as harmless can quickly turn into a cycle, and before you know it, you're five days deep into something you didn't even see coming. One decision snowballs into the next, and suddenly, you're deeper than you ever intended. It's like that first drink you thought was "just one," and now you're passing someone's vape pen around like it's a social norm. One late-night "I'll just go out this once" becomes the start of a new pattern—subconsciously seeking trouble, like a moth to the flame.

And let's face it, society is built like a rat race: everything's getting more expensive, work's piling on more stress, and you just want to escape, even for a minute. But here's the truth, as uncomfortable as it may be: *escaping doesn't change a thing.* That weekend you act like a wild animal to free your mind? It's not changing your life in the long run. It's a Band-Aid for a wound that never fully heals. The reality is, the more you give in to these distractions, the more you become a slave to your own self-sufficiency, constantly needing that quick fix.

If you want to *really* feel alive, you've got to take the wheel. Stop following the easy path that everyone else is walking down. It's time to choose YOU. Choose your future. Choose *success*. Choose discipline. Choose a life that *means something*. Because at the end of the day, the best decision you can make is to bet on yourself.

Social Conformity:

Where individuals often adapt their behavior to align with the norms and behaviors of their social circle. If "five of your friends are doing something," it becomes harder to resist. This is a common psychological experience that can be difficult to break free from, especially when the need for social acceptance or belonging is high.

Unconditional love for oneself involves recognizing these influences without being bound by them. It's about making choices that honor your own values and needs, rather than surrendering to external pressures. It's about loving yourself enough to resist unhealthy behaviors, even when everyone around you might be indulging in them.

Self-Sabotage:

Where short-term gratification leads to long-term consequences, often because we fail to pause and reflect before acting.

Unconditional love for oneself means taking responsibility for our **own choices**. It's not about perfection, but about consistently choosing what's best for you. When you find love for yourself unconditionally, you act in ways that nurture and protect your well-being, even when it's hard or uncomfortable.

CHAPTER THIRTY NINE

INTROSPECTION.

SUICIDES:

This topic comes with uncomfortable effects for the people who are left behind. There's no way to control how someone makes that decision, and we may never fully understand the truth of their internal battles. The pain that drives someone to such a devastating choice is often a mix of emotional wreckage—doubt, fear, trauma, and a sense of isolation.

Where do these thoughts emerge from? I started asking myself this question when I was in middle school, after a childhood friend from dance class, Kylie, decided to take her life. Rachel and I were her only friends. I remember going to her house, listening to her frustrations, the tangled mess of teenage angst, and the awkwardness of those years. Kylie wore all black, funky skirts, studded belts, and had short black hair, which she'd dye in crazy colors sometimes. After school at Rachel's house, we'd listen to those emo songs—but with a twist. We listened to Christian artists like Flyleaf and Evanescence. Years later, hearing those songs still gives me chills, especially when I think about how those lyrics captured such deep pain. It's hard to describe, but I felt that little girl's pain—yet I didn't have the words to explain it.

That feeling crept back up many years later when I was in college. A dear friend's brother took his own life. He used to visit us at school often, and we all held a special place in our hearts for him. When we heard the news, the wave of pain hit us all like a tidal wave. It was one of the most uncomfortable funerals I've ever been to, and I've been to many in my life. The pastor, trying to comfort us, spoke of the "darkness" that overtook him. I wasn't sure how to process that. And to be honest, I didn't appreciate him using scriptures to describe our friend's experience.

There's no easy way to explain such a loss, but sometimes we just need to listen and be there for the people we love.

One of the most gut-wrenching thoughts I had when I received the phone call from my mom was when she asked me to sit down. I'll never forget that moment. I told her I was already sitting, and then she told me that Ben had passed away. My first thought was, *this can't be real*. Ben had faced so much in his life. He had a tough childhood with a disability that left one of his legs growing longer than the other. He battled through his own struggles with relationships, and had only a handful of true friends. But what people didn't always see was how deeply he was loved. And I often wonder, did he know that? Did he truly understand how much he meant to the people who cared for him? I pray he knows it now.

He's been on my heart a lot lately, especially as I've been dealing with an injury of my own. I can't walk right now, and the memories of Ben keep flooding back. In a strange way, it's as though I'm walking beside him through his pain, feeling it myself, as I sit with my own limitations. His passing wasn't a result of suicide—though his struggles were certainly deep—it was another extreme health circumstance that took him too soon. But as I reflect during this holiday season, I can't help but think about how tough these times can be for so many people, especially when they feel isolated or alone.

I've experienced this loneliness myself, especially recently when I had to stay on bedrest. Watching everyone else's holiday activities from the sidelines was incredibly hard. I wanted so badly to be part of the world moving around me, but for the sake of my health, I needed to stay in bed. In that stillness, though, I realized something important. I knew I had to use my voice. I had to speak out, share my story, and remind others to reach out—to connect, to check in. There's always someone who needs a little reminder that they're not alone, that someone cares.

I don't know who needs to hear this today, but I know someone does. We all go through seasons of feeling isolated or in pain. But no matter what, you are loved, and there's someone who needs you to reach out, just as you might need someone to reach out to you.

The truth about suicides is this: it's often too late when we understand the depth of someone's pain. We don't always see the signs, and the weight they carry is invisible to the outside world. We have to remember that unconditional love is about being present, even when we don't have the perfect answers. Sometimes, the best thing we can do for someone is just to let them know we see them, we hear them, and we're here. Every day is a chance to show someone they're not alone.

The Man With the Winter Hat and Boots Wearing Shorts:

I walked up to my desk one day to find him pacing around, smiling at me like he'd just seen something amazing. He'd been doing this for days, just grinning and checking in. But today, I wasn't smiling. He noticed right away, and we started talking about life. He mentioned his daughter had come to visit, and I asked how old she was. "17," he said, and I braced myself for the usual "sassy teenage years" talk. But when I asked if she'd gone through that stage, he paused and said, "No, I think she's still in it."

He then went on to explain how his daughter was staying with him, but her mom didn't want to force her to talk to him. I couldn't help but chuckle. I told him I remembered those days—being a teenager, annoyed at my siblings, acting out, and thinking I knew everything. He laughed too. I told him how I regretted it later. You see, I had an older sibling I didn't always appreciate, and we had this huge age gap that made us feel worlds apart. But looking back, I wish I had taken the time to truly understand him, to bridge that gap before it was too late.

And here's the kicker: I never got that chance. My sibling passed away, and it hit me hard that I'd spent too many years being sassy and distant, wishing I'd done more to connect while I still could. That's the thing— regret doesn't come knocking until it's too late, and by then, the opportunity is gone.

The lesson? Don't take your loved ones for granted. Life moves fast, and sometimes, it's only when we lose someone or something that we realize how precious those moments are. So, whether it's a daughter, a sibling, or a friend—love them unconditionally, flaws and all. Cherish the messy, the frustrating, and the sweet. Don't wait until regret hits. Keep the door open for connection. Maybe the next time someone is pacing around your desk with a grin, even if you're not in the mood, you'll smile back. Because you never know how much those small moments might matter later. And that, my friends, is the true lesson in unconditional love.

Anticipatory Grief or Post-loss Regret:

These are emotions that arise when we realize the value of a relationship only after it's been lost. The feeling of not having fully appreciated a loved one before it's too late can create lasting emotional pain.

Need for Connection:

Humans are biologically wired to seek social bonds. However, these bonds are not always easy to navigate, especially when there is emotional distance, misunderstandings, or external pressures. The introspection reveals a longing to have had a closer, more understanding relationship with their sibling—something they can no longer change.

CHAPTER FORTY

THE SYMPHONY OF CONNECTION.

THE GIFT OF SOUND:

I had this conversation with Venessa (Tessa) while she was visiting me in Los Angeles that really stuck with me. I had come to this quirky realization that every relationship, every connection I've ever had, seems to have music at its core. From the playlists we create together to the unspoken harmony we share with others, music is the common thread. Tessa smiled, nodding in agreement, and said, "Of course, music is all about frequency! It's the perfect example of how we bond. When you're on the same wavelength with someone, it's like the BPMs, the frequency, and the electromagnetic fields all align. You vibe together!"

It was one of those "mind blown" moments. I never thought of it quite like that, but it made perfect sense. From there, the conversation evolved into this deep dive into sound theory. It was like we had cracked open a cosmic mystery. Sound is, after all, the foundation of creation, and it wasn't long before I started reflecting on the bigger picture. The first relaxation within my guided meditations on the date of 2-22-22 came to mind. I realized the power of the voice box and how getting my own voice into the perfect frequency could radiate healing sounds. That led me to sound bowls, and right around that same time, I teamed up with CBT Studios to play around in the music studio with microphones, and speakers. Then, when I moved to California, I explained to friends that I had gone down a "musical black hole" to find answers. I started studying sound production. I got together with multiple producer friends to learn what I liked about sound and how I could create it in a song, changing pitches or layering music through sounds and vocals. How powerful sounds are—and then adding words to the mix creates a trifecta of magic.

A couple of weeks after my conversation with Tessa, I found myself deep in a similar talk with Daniel, who was absolutely *amped* about enlightening one of his coworkers on the concept of God. He was practically buzzing with excitement, trying to explain the whole "Big Man Upstairs" theory. Daniel's enthusiasm was contagious, but it made me smile because, well, the way he was talking about sound frequencies and creation felt so similar to the conversation I had just had. It felt like I had somehow tuned into the same cosmic radio station as him.

In religion, we have the concept of God saying, "Let there be light," which, according to Daniel, is not just a metaphor—it's a sound frequency! His voice, His words, created the frequencies that sparked the world into existence. I mean, who knew a divine voice could create so much *bass*?

Then, naturally, I couldn't help but bring up the Big Bang theory. *Literally.* The universe itself is said to have begun with an explosion of sound about 13.8 billion years ago, according to scientists. The soundwaves from that event are still traveling through the universe, creating everything we see. So, here we are, all these years later, still vibing to the echoes of that first cosmic sound. It's like the universe is playing its own eternal playlist, and we're all just trying to find our song in it.

Then, the next day, Dumi and I were talking—he's this amazing friend who has a heart the size of the universe and is on a mission to spread love. He's even started his own foundation called "Love Heals the World." As Dumi talked about his work and passion, it hit me: We were talking about sound again, in a way. Dumi is a beacon of love, and his foundation is all about creating the right frequency of positivity and kindness in the world, while sharing his gifts and talents, but unconditional love to music. I couldn't help but think that our friendship, like the others, was built on the same principle—vibrating at the same frequency of love and understanding. Which is why I believe worship connects so many people. The power of sound with vocals, and lyrics, can just take people *away* into the vastness of space—a healing place for them to release their inner darks.

The beauty of it all is that these deep conversations, whether about sound theory, religion, or love, don't just bring us closer as friends—they expand our view of the world. We start to see life through a different lens, a lens that understands the importance of being vulnerable and open with one another. And the more we learn about each other, the more we realize that we're all really just tuning into the same cosmic frequency, seeking to create harmony in a chaotic world.

Funny how the universe works, right? Four different people, from four different walks of life, all coming together because we're on the same wave—whether we're creating music, talking about God, or spreading love. And at the end of the day, it's all just a reminder that friends find each other on the same frequency, when it comes to sound, love, and everything in between. So, next time you're vibing with someone, just remember: You're probably on the same wavelength—and that's a pretty beautiful thing.

Splice: A Music Memory (Future meets the past.)

Splice is a stranger I met one Sunday afternoon at the music studio. One of the greatest things about connecting with other artists, producers, and engineers is that we all share a deep understanding of our craft. A song's muse is often unpacked during a session, so we're not afraid to dive deep. We only met once, but stayed connected through social media, occasionally popping in and out of each other's lives.

One day, he heard a song playing in the background of a video I posted from a store. He has a keen ear, so I wasn't surprised when he identified the track as Miley Cyrus. He mentioned, somewhat humorously, that he'd been yelled at by a crazy lady on the subway about how important Miley Cryrus's career was. He called it a "coincidence." I knew it was a "god wink," and I mentioned how Miley's albums always send me spiraling through a maze of emotions. The entire *Bangerz* album, in particular, reminds me of a really tough summer.

Intrigued, he asked, "What happened that summer?" I took it as an opportunity to share. That summer was rough because many of my relationships were falling apart, including the one with my best friend, Caroline. The soundtrack of *Bangerz* pulls me back to those moments like they were yesterday. My world was falling apart. Caroline and I were untangling our lives after what felt like a decade together and I took our dog, Miller, to embark on a new path away from her.

Splice asked if Caroline and I were still on different paths. His insight about how friends can drift apart due to natural growth was spot on. I knew this, but I appreciated his wisdom and the space he provided for me to share. I decided to listen to the album again, this time trying to shift my perspective. I wondered if changing my mindset could alter the emotions tied to those memories and create a new experience.

Music has always been an essential part of my life, and I've had this revelation with many other albums and songs. I've come to believe that "I didn't choose music; she chose me."

I often take a trip down memory lane with albums, like when I listened to Fleetwood Mac after leaving Mr. J and our old life behind. The best part of that time was coming home to Caroline and Miller in her new place with her husband. After COVID, being reunited with them felt like a full-circle moment, but I was still dealing with a lot of pain. It was another huge life transition, once again moving away from yet another soulmate.

Splice had a funny way of coming in and out of my life since we met. I suppose I was letting my heart be more open to humans that seemed mysterious. I found them curious and full of intrigue. Splice and I often would engage in each other's life stories. One day we decided to grab lunch, long overdue. He had ate hibachi the night before, and I had been craving it since I left North Carolina. Meeting in downtown LA can always be an experience since that's where the "Zombies" come out to play. We didn't let that stop us from grubbing on some good food together. The moment I smelled the shrimp and steak combination, I was extremely excited! The moment he grabbed our food from the side counter and placed it in front of me, I knew it was going to be a pleasure. "Smells like memories", I stated, and he immediately started laughing. Our conversations were easy. He brought so much light to me that day. He said, "You struggle with being still, but that's literally your last name!" I laughed, and saw the humor immediately. I replied, "Yes, but I'm much more like air,- fluid, and flowing , always in motion."

To my surprise, this revelation was not the only time I heard that. Earlier that week, at a church service, a friend who had been mentally struggling for a couple weeks came up to me and said, "You know, I thought of you today, and it helped me calm down. I said to myself, be like: "Aire Stillman." "Air–take a deep breath, and be Still."

Psychologically:

Humans are inherently social beings and the concept of "vibrating on the same frequency" reflects the idea of **resonance** in relationships. When we are emotionally aligned with others—whether in friendships, family, or romantic relationships—we experience a sense of harmony and **emotional attunement**, similar to how different instruments or voices come together to create a cohesive sound.

Emotionally Focused Therapy (EFT):

Emphasizes the importance of these emotional exchanges in creating strong, loving relationships.

Healing and Sound as a Tool for Transformation:

The reference to sound being a "foundation of creation" ties into the concept of **sound therapy** and the psychological benefits of music. In various therapeutic practices, sound frequencies are used to promote healing and emotional regulation. Music has been shown to activate **mirror neurons**, which help us empathize with others, and it can also trigger the release of dopamine, a neurotransmitter associated with pleasure and motivation. The idea that sound can radiate healing also ties into the **mind-body connection**, which has been explored in various fields of psychology, including **somatic therapy**.

Unconditional Love:

Just as sound has the power to heal and transform, unconditional love offers the same ability to heal emotional wounds. Love, in its purest form, acts as a frequency that helps individuals **regulate their emotions** and feel supported in difficult times. It is through **acceptance and compassion**, key tenets of unconditional love, that we are able to "tune" our hearts and minds to healthier, more harmonious states. Unconditional love, much like healing sound, can create a safe, nurturing environment for personal growth and emotional recovery.

Synchronicity:

Carl Jung —"Synchronicity refers to meaningful coincidences that occur when two or more events are linked by their symbolic significance rather than by direct cause and effect." The concept of shared frequencies between individuals (whether we are discussing God, music, or love) illustrates how people can be drawn together by something beyond mere chance, as if we are "meant" to find each other."

Cognitive Dissonance:

The tension that arises when our perceptions of the world don't match our desires or ideals. People long for harmony and alignment, but life is full of discord. Finding ways to resolve that dissonance—whether through creative endeavors like music, deep conversations, or acts of kindness—helps us feel more at peace. This is an example of **meaning-making**, where we as individuals create purpose and understanding out of life's inherent chaos.

Sound Waves: Music is a Memory

Funny how an old song can hit you like a wave and take you back to a specific time and place where that song just *clicked*. It's like music has this magical ability to press play on the soundtrack of our lives, triggering memories that are sometimes sweet, sometimes messy, but always full of meaning.

I have a playlist in my mind that's made up of these musical time capsules. Take, for instance, the memory of singing *"Jesus Take the Wheel"* with my best friend Krystal. We were probably off-key, but man, we *believed*. There we were, belting out that song into our flip phones at her grandma's house, trying to record ourselves, pretending like we were pop stars. I'm pretty sure no one would ever pay for our album, but we definitely had fun. And let's be honest, in those moments, we were *untouchable*.

Then there's the time I sang *"Red High Heels"* by Kellie Pickler while rocking back and forth in my mom's chair. Emotionally, I was all over the place, but the song was my therapy. Lyrics became my voice when I didn't know how to express my feelings. *"I don't need a man to make me feel pretty,"* I sang, as if Kellie Pickler was my personal pep talk.

Fast forward to a more recent memory. After my injury, Marseli and Classi came over to help me around the house—doing everything from cooking to cleaning. I had made a playlist called *"Holy,"* and Classi, with a smile, said, "You've been a Jesus follower for a long time, huh, Aire?" I shrugged and replied, "Yeah, pretty much my whole life." She grinned, then added, "I can tell, some of these songs are like 15 years old!" But you know what? Hearing us sing together, all of us with our lungs full of praise, in that chaotic moment of life—it felt like pure love.

Speaking of love, there's a tattoo on my side that reminds me of how important it is to open my eyes and my heart. After I split from my ex, I thought about the times I sang *"Amazing Grace"* with my mom. The line *"I once was blind, but now I see"* felt personal. I got that tattoo as a reminder not to be blind to love and to never settle for something that isn't right. My mom's love was always unconditional, and that tattoo is my daily reminder to live up to it.

Growing up, I sang *"Silent Night"* and *"Amazing Grace"* with my mom so often it became almost second nature. We'd sing to calm the bird, sure, but honestly, it was as much for us as it was for him. Those walks down the country roads with the bird in tow—just the three of us and the stars above—were cathartic. Music wasn't just sound. It was a balm for our hearts.

I can still remember belting out *"Bubbly"* by Colbie Caillat in my middle school bedroom, daydreaming about the boy who'd make me feel that spark. I think I was probably trying to get the chords right more than anything else, but I *definitely* wasn't ready to stop singing that song. I mean, who doesn't want that happy-ever-after feeling when you're 13?

Then, there's the moment with my cousins and *Rascal Flatts*—that memory where we all cried together as they told the story of their friend passing away. It was bittersweet, but that song, in that moment, brought us all together in a way words couldn't. We found comfort in the music, a connection that transcended grief.

The funny thing is, music has a way of wrapping all these memories into one beautiful, emotional mixtape of life. And you know what? That's the beauty of unconditional love—it's not just about the big moments. It's in the songs, the little memories, the laughter, and the quiet, shared moments of healing. Music has a funny way of becoming the soundtrack to these kinds of love stories—stories that are woven into the fabric of who we are.

So, next time a song plays and you find yourself smiling, laughing, or tearing up, know that it's not just a tune. It's the pulse of your heart and the echo of love. The kind of love that's unconditional, ever-present, and has a playlist that will play forever.

Dual Process Model of Grief:

It illustrates how individuals experience sorrow and healing in tandem. Love and music both provide continuity and coherence, helping us process and navigate both joy and sorrow.

Music as a Metaphor for Love:

The depth and complexity of love to the variety of songs that represent different phases of life—from joyful moments, like singing "Bubbly" during middle school, to the solemnity of sharing a song with my cousins in grief. We must remember that unconditional love is not only present in the happy moments but also remains steadfast through grief, hardship, and personal growth.

Psychological Insight:

Music taps into the part of the brain that stores emotional memory and sensory experiences. The act of hearing a song from the past connects us to a sense of nostalgia and emotional continuity, just as unconditional love connects us to a consistent sense of belonging and security.

CHAPTER FORTY ONE

UNITED.

The Good Human Guide: Keeping Your Eyes Up

So, here's a life lesson I learned from Bobby **(THE EMPOWERER)**—the most humble, Hawaiian, man at my church Mosaic, by the way. Bobby taught me something that really stuck: *"Keeping your eyes up."* It's not some mystical, philosophical concept, or something out of a self-help book. It's way simpler than that: it means paying attention to the world around you, stepping outside your own bubble, and helping where you're needed. It's about noticing those little things that can make someone else's day better, even if it's as small as a smile or lending a hand.

Let me tell you, Bobby's got the right idea. He's always the guy who notices someone's car in need of a jump, or the one who'll just walk up to a stranger and say, "Hey, how's your day going?" And honestly, it's that kind of awareness that makes him a *really* good human. He's got the right balance of getting his tasks done *and* noticing when there's something else to be done in the bigger picture.

Speaking of noticing things... One of my favorite things is watching people walk by. Not in a creepy, "I'm-gonna-stare-at-you" way, but more like an observation of human nature. There are so many stories unfolding right in front of us, if we just keep our eyes up. It's so easy to get lost in your own world—looking down at your phone, checking your watch, or plotting your next big move—but let me tell you, there's so much more out there if you're willing to look. And those passing strangers? They've got something to teach you. Whether it's their fashion sense, their way of carrying themselves, or even just a small act of kindness, everyone you meet has something to offer.

Now, here's where it gets real. Being a good human isn't about doing the *big* things—it's in the little actions. The things other people won't always notice, but that can still make a huge difference. Like going the extra mile to help your community. Or showing up early to set up, staying late to clean up, and not complaining once about it. It's sending handwritten thank-you notes because you actually care (because who does that anymore?). Or giving a treat to someone who's been working hard—because everyone deserves a pick-me-up, even if it's just a candy bar.

And my absolute favorite? Just being kind. You don't need to wait for a special occasion to do something nice. Put your cart away at the store. Smile at strangers, even when you're having a bad day. Let someone in when you're stuck in traffic—because hey, it's just a few seconds of your life, and it might make someone else's day a little easier. Hold the door for people. Say "hello" to the staff at the coffee shop, and *actually* mean it. These little things? They matter more than you think.

In the end, being a good human is all about looking up from your own world, recognizing when someone else needs a hand, and just doing the right thing—whether it's big or small. So, let's all take a page out of Bobby's book and keep our eyes up. You might just be surprised at what you find.

Adam's Story: The Power of the Reset

So, here's a gem of a story that I'll never forget. Adam **(THE TEACHER)**, while coaching me through a tough moment, shared something profound that honestly made me rethink a lot of things. He said, "It's been years since I've thought about this, but when I was younger, in our division one soccer league, my coach used to tally points every time we brought the ball back instead of pressing forward."

Pause. You're probably thinking, "Wait, isn't the whole point of soccer to *keep moving forward*? What's this 'taking a step back' business?" I had the same thought. But as he continued, it all started to click.

He explained that sometimes, moving forward led to mistakes or errors, while bringing the ball back or passing to a defensive teammate acted as a reset. Sure, it felt like a step backward in the moment, but 9 out of 10 times, after that reset, they'd score. Sounds a little counterintuitive, right? But it made so much sense.

Now, this story stuck with me, because it's such a perfect metaphor for life. We're all so caught up in constantly moving forward—pushing, striving, and sometimes stumbling along the way—because we think we're supposed to keep going no matter what. But here's the thing: Sometimes, it's okay to *reset*. It's okay to take a step back, reflect, and give yourself the space to learn, grow, and adjust.

We all have those moments when we're stuck, comparing ourselves to others, caught up in our egos, or just unsure of where we're headed. It feels like there's no room to breathe or to retreat, but sometimes that's exactly what we need. That "reset" isn't a failure—it's the moment that allows you to get back on track and move forward, but this time with more clarity, purpose, and direction.

And let's be honest—who hasn't been in a situation where taking a step back was the best move? You know those times when everything's a mess, and the best solution is to pause, breathe, and recalibrate. Think about it: How many times has a little breather or a tiny shift in perspective helped you see things in a new light?

So, the next time you feel like you're about to stumble, or that your ego's holding you back from making a change, just remember—sometimes, the best move is a reset. Take a step back. Reflect. Learn. Then move forward with a clearer, more powerful direction. Because, in the end, that small adjustment might just be the thing that leads you to your next big win.

Unconditional love isn't about never messing up; it's about giving yourself the grace to reset, regroup, and move forward—no matter how many times it takes.

Ego and Humility:

His story also speaks to the role of *ego* in decision-making. We often push forward because of our ego, striving for success, validation, and approval from others. When we "reset" and step back, it requires a degree of humility—recognizing that we don't always have all the answers and that it's okay to reassess and change course. This act of resetting can be an expression of personal growth, acknowledging the imperfections within ourselves, and being open to improvement without fear of judgment.

Gus: The Unexpected Messenger:

35.5628° N, 106.1309° W

So, picture this: I'm sitting in my car, parked outside a mini-mall, soaking up the sunshine and nibbling on my lunch. It's one of those moments where you think, "Nothing's gonna happen here—just a little me-time." But then, I glance over, and there he is. This blonde Italian guy, casually hanging up suits in the back like he's some kind of expert. For a second, I think, "Huh, this is weird... but also strangely familiar." I introduce myself, he replies Hi, I'm Gus.

He was like a reminder from the universe—a little nudge, a gift from God. See, I had just had an accident and was thinking about life, as one does when you've got a little extra time on your hands. And the thought hit me: "*You know, there are really only five people in life who would drop everything to help you in a time of struggle.*" And I had been giving, and giving, and giving without making sure there was balance. And you know what? It hit me like a ton of bricks: Maybe I haven't been good at asking for help. Maybe I needed to be a little more direct about what I needed—because it turns out people can't read your mind, no matter how much you *think* they should.

My default mode is to give, give, give. But here's the thing—I'm not talking about just money. I'm talking about giving all of myself, my time, my energy. It's like I want to love people so hard that I end up acting like their unpaid therapist, giving unsolicited advice, and coaching them through life. And the thing is, they didn't even ask for it. It's like I've taken on this "big sister" role I never applied for. It's sweet, but also... Why am I doing this to myself?

Okay, fast forward. I'm on my way to get acupuncture (because, of course, that's what you do when you've got a bum leg and this is a last stitch effort for life). I take a long drive to clear my head, and, as I'm sitting at a stop sign, I glance up and see *GUS* in big letters on a building. I start laughing. It felt like a wink from the universe. And then, to make it even better, I look in my rearview mirror and see a car with a red temporary handicapped tag hanging from the rearview. Just like I have hanging from my mirror. The literal reflection looking back at me. Now that's a funny metaphor, isn't it? *"Just temporarily stuck."* It made me laugh because it was like life was telling me: "Hey, it's okay to be temporarily stuck. You'll get out of it."

And that's when the real magic started to happen. Gus and I had talked about long drives and how they can be a form of therapy, and here I was, about to embark on another one into the unknown. Little did I know, that drive was going to lead to a seriously healing experience.

As I drove, the thought from the man who had stopped me in the hallway at work and asked to pray for me the day before came rushing back. He'd told me that in the Bible, God says we need to stop retreating into darkness and spend time with Him, away from the chaos and noise. Sometimes, to move forward, you need to take five steps back. That lesson came up again, right when I needed it.

Then, as if on cue, a song came on my phone—*Revival*, a country gospel track that set the tone for my ride. It made me think of Maren Morris, and I remembered once when Damon had asked me if I liked country music. I replied "Of course, I do—I'm from the country, after all." But what I didn't realize was that this music was about to unlock something even bigger for me. And then it unlocked the memory of Mr. Killa, who once said, **"You should be a country singer."** Shocked, I replied, "WHAT?"

He said *"The way you belt out country songs, that's really coming from your heart, it's in your soul."* At the time, I was stunned, but now it made sense. Country music was part of my heart, and in that moment, I realized that God was sending me all these little messages— through people, music, and moments—that I wasn't alone. The community, my church, my family—they were all there to hold me up.

I was reminded that sometimes you don't have to be the founder or the one in charge to make a difference. Sometimes, it's about being a leader in your own way—supporting the team, growing for the greater good, and being in sync with God's plan.

Oh, and by the way—*highly recommend* long drives. Seriously. They're therapeutic. And who knows? You might just get a wink from the universe, too.

CHAPTER FORTY TWO

ECHOES OF LOSS.

The Angel of Death: A Comedic Take on Grief and Unconditional Love

I had this weird realization one day—after a string of losses in my life, I started calling myself the "Angel of Death." It wasn't a name I gave myself for dramatic flair or because I thought it made me sound like a gothic character from a teen novel. No, it was more like a coping mechanism. Let's rewind a bit...

First, it was my great grandpa. That one hit hard, but I was still in my early years, still trying to understand life and death. Then came my mom's mom—my grandma. She was *the* best. She'd been a staple in my family.

Then my other grandma passed away, my dad's mother. She'd always been the rock in his family, the one you could turn to for advice, love, or a hilarious story from the past. Watching her struggle in the end, though, was a whole different experience. She had Alzheimer's, and eventually, she didn't even know who I was. It broke my heart. But then, just as I thought I couldn't take any more, it was my grandpa. And that's when I witnessed something that, to this day, I can't shake: he died of a *broken heart*.

I didn't even know that was a *real* thing until Johns Hopkins Medicine confirmed it: **"Broken Heart Syndrome"**—or, as I like to call it, "the saddest diagnosis ever." Apparently, when you experience a *major* emotional shock—like losing the love of your life—your heart can literally weaken and expand, making it hard to pump blood. And just like that, Grandpa was gone. Watching him die from something so heartbreaking made me realize just how deep love runs—how deeply it can wound when you lose it. It's a wild thing to experience.

"They say death comes in threes." And just when I thought life couldn't throw anything more at me, it kept coming. First, one to hit home was Ben, and our house pet bird Jordyn, then it was a couple of friends who passed away by suicide. Then came my uncle, and right after, my cousin—leaving behind his wife and kids. I was starting to feel like grief was my unofficial career path. It was almost like I had a front-row seat to the worst reality show ever.

But here's the kicker: through all of this, I became *too familiar* with death. It became so much a part of my life that, honestly, it didn't faze me as much anymore. You get used to it, you know? Then, during my nursing years, I had my own share of helping people cross over—or even bring some back. You'd think that would have made me more jaded, but oddly enough, it gave me a sense of peace. I was doing something to help others in their final moments, to bring comfort or closure.

And then, of course, *cue the pandemic*—when death felt like it was everywhere, it was almost as if I was living in a "death bubble." It seemed like people were dropping like flies, and it was impossible to keep up. I remember thinking, "Am I *the* angel of death now?"

But here's the thing: For every death, there's a birth. *Yes, there is.* And I'm not just saying that as some fluffy, feel-good line. It's true! For every person who dies every second, roughly four people are born on average. That's about 4.3 births per second globally. Do the math, and that means for every death, there are about *two births*. Isn't that wild? It's like the universe's way of balancing the scales. For all the pain and heartache we experience, there's always something new to begin with.

So yeah, I've seen a lot of loss, and it's shaped me in ways I didn't expect. But that's where unconditional love comes in. Love doesn't stop when someone leaves. It's the things we carry from those who are no longer here—the lessons they taught us, the love they shared, and the memories that stay with us. So, maybe "I *am* the Angel of Death?"—Just in the sense that I've learned to navigate through it all. But I know, in the bigger picture, there's always something new on the horizon. For every goodbye, there's a hello waiting somewhere in the world.

It's all part of the circle of life, and whether we're ready for it or not, we're all in this beautiful, messy, unpredictable ride together.

CHAPTER FORTY THREE

INVESTING IN HUMANS.

Why I Find Myself in Leadership Roles: A Humbling Journey

I don't know about you, but I've always been the type of person who can't resist learning every position in the room. Whether it's a company, a project, or a new endeavor, I dive into every role just to understand the whole picture. It's like I have this superpower to see all sides and connect the dots between worlds. Sounds cool, right? But here's the catch—it can sometimes get a little out of hand.

I used to get caught up in the idea of being a founder. The *founder*—that's the dream, right? The title. The vision. The power. I thought that was the only way I could have an impact. So, I'd rack my brain thinking, "What should I start? What should I build? What can I create from scratch?" But then, after a lot of overthinking and my not-so-successful 6 last attempts, I started asking myself the real question: *"Why do I need to be the founder?"*

Why can't I lead in something that's already successful? Why does it have to be about creating something new? Maybe I'm better off helping something that's already thriving, where my efforts can be an asset. I realized that leadership doesn't have to be about owning the whole ship—it can be about steering it in the right direction, helping it grow, and making sure everyone on board is moving toward the same goal.

And let's talk about ego for a second—because *wow*, it sure knows how to show up. I spent a lot of time thinking my role had to be bigger, louder, and more noticeable. But here's the kicker: I've started to learn that humility is a pretty powerful tool. Sometimes, I've had to swallow my pride, let go of my "founder fantasies," and just listen. *Listen*, not speak. Be a student, not a teacher.

It's funny how hard that is sometimes—especially when you feel like you *know* what's best or think you can do it better. But guess what? There's always more to learn. Even in leadership roles, it's about balancing confidence with the humility to accept that you don't know everything—and that's okay.

The real growth comes when you can step back, let go of the ego, and simply be part of something bigger than yourself. And while I still struggle with it (a *lot*), I'm learning that true leadership isn't about being at the front of the pack. It's about lifting others up and knowing when to step aside and let someone else take the lead.

So, maybe I'm not meant to be the founder of something new. Maybe I'm here to help steer what's already in motion. And that, my friends, is a superpower too.

FAR AWAY: LIFE LONG

One of the most heartwarming experiences I treasure is realizing that long-time friends have seen you through so many versions of yourself, and yet, they still love you unconditionally through it all. Every few months, I get this queenly instinct to check in with my lifelong besties from all over the country. We catch up on everything—life updates, new relationships, how the kids are growing, career leaps, who's in their inner circle, and all that fun stuff. It's a two-way street, of course, but what I truly value is how, no matter where life has taken us, we still manage to lift each other up through every season.

Find those friends you can cherish through all the years and changes. Keep inspiring each other, live vicariously through each other's lessons, share wisdom, and just shower them with love. Cheer them on from afar, send them prayers, and when they randomly cross your mind, check in! A simple "how are you?" can brighten their day. Life is so much richer when you feel valued, and there's something truly special about that connection. So, whenever you can, just spread some joy and let them know you care.

Emotional Regulation:

Lifelong friendships act as an anchor during challenging times, helping to regulate emotions by providing reassurance, encouragement, and perspective. Positive relationships are linked to higher life satisfaction, and life feels "richer" when we feel valued—suggesting that emotional nourishment through connection is a key factor in our happiness.

Unspoken Bond:

Lifelong friends can stay connected across distance and time, without needing constant physical proximity, a depth of love that transcends conditions or circumstances. Our relationships don't require frequent interaction to remain strong, the bond is steady, and it remains intact because it's rooted in something deeper than surface-level exchanges.

Investing in Friends: The Best ROI You Never Expected:

You know that feeling when you're hanging out with your friends, laughing so hard your stomach hurts and you're just grateful for the moment? That's what I call the "best investment"—because every time you invest in your friends, you're really investing in yourself.

Think about it: the bachelorette parties, the birthdays, the camping trips, the road trips. It's like these little nuggets of joy tucked away in your memory bank. And let's be real, those are the moments that get you through the tough days. You know, the ones where you're stuck in traffic or staring at your inbox, wondering if you'll ever find time to breathe again. But then, *ding!*—you remember that one time you all piled into a car, drove for hours just to get lost, and somehow ended up at a taco truck. Magic. Those memories are priceless.

But here's the thing—life gets busy, right? Before you know it, it's been months since you've checked in. Why? Because... well, life. You've got work, errands, appointments, and just *adulting* in general. It's easy to get swept up in the chaos and forget to call your bestie. But guess what? There's no time like the present to hit that "call" button.

Trust me, that phone call, even if it's just to hear the voice of someone who's been through the same crazy ride as you, will remind you of what really matters. You need that laughter. You need that support. You need to make plans to do it all over again—whether it's for a spontaneous weekend getaway or just a night of pizza and gossip.

So, next time life gets busy (which it will), take a moment to reach out. Invest in those friendships because, in the end, those are the relationships that keep you grounded. Plus, they're the ones who'll remind you to *stop working for five minutes* and actually enjoy life.

You'll thank yourself later—and your belly will thank you too. Laughter truly is the best investment you can make.

This book is a reflection of the light that guides us through communication, connection, and community. At the core, we're all just searching for others who resonate with us—a place we can truly call "home," a home we've chosen, and continue to choose.

As I walk down these unexpected roads, I'm discovering beauty in the smallest moments. Sometimes it's as simple as stopping to smell the roses. It's about keeping your "eyes up"—because you never know what beauty is right in front of you, or who you might meet along the way.

It's like when you're driving, focused on staying in your lane, missing the view that the passenger has, or the walker who gets to see the city's buildings and landscapes from the streets.

We're all searching for something bigger than ourselves—constantly teetering on the edge of missing the present moment. But it's in those moments we find the beauty of creation, the beauty of connection.

Full Circle

Back in the **wild Wilmington days**, Mr. Killa and the squad were up to our usual mischief—bouncing between shows, hyping up DJs, and stirring up just enough **good trouble** to keep things interesting. The air was thick with bass, neon lights flickered like electric dreams, and there I was, twirling my hula hoop like some kind of rave fairy, sprinkling chaos and encouragement in equal measure.

And then—**bam!** Destiny, in the form of a world-touring, Wilmington-born DJ, strolled into the scene.

MK, wide-eyed and buzzing, nudged me like a kid spotting his superhero in real life. *"You know who that is, right?!"* he whispered, practically vibrating.

Naturally, I did what I do best. I smirked, turned to MK, and with the kind of reckless confidence that only comes from believing in the magic of the moment, I said, *"Well then... let's bring him back to the studio!"*

Because really, what's better than **"afters"** at the studio? Nothing. That's what.

Somehow, through sheer enthusiasm (and maybe a little hula-hoop-induced hypnosis), we **made it happen**. We lured that DJ back to our creative cave, where he and MK conjured music deep into the early morning. Beats spilled like secrets, ideas tangled in the air like smoke, and when the sun finally peeked through the blinds, the DJ looked at me—**grinning, glowing, utterly mind-blown**.

MK said to me, "I can't believe you pulled that off... again."

I replied, "Oh, my friend. You underestimate my powers."

MK and I kept in touch over the years—just those occasional, unplanned **"hey, how's life?"** kind of calls. By then, I had packed up my memories and moved to Cali, but Wilmington still pulsed in my bones.

And then, one day, out of nowhere, MK hits me with:

"Ohhh, I have the best news!"

I braced myself—because MK and *good news* usually meant something wild.

"Remember that night we brought 'said DJ' back to the studio?"

"Of course," I laughed. "How could I forget?"

*"Well... he left his label. Came back to Wilmington for a while. And guess what? We've been making **non-stop music together** ever since. I just thought you should know. And... thank you—for always believing, for making those connections. You're the best."*

And just like that, I **beamed through the phone**, warmth spreading in my chest like the golden hour.

"Wow... thank you, I really appreciate you taking the time to tell me that. That really makes me happy to hear."

Funny how these **small, spontaneous decisions**—the late nights, the right words at the right time, the tiny ripples we don't even think twice about—can turn into **waves**. Lifelong investments really can pay off.

Somewhere in Wilmington, music was still being made because of **one night, one chance, one fearless "why not?"**

What an incredible revelation. I'm so grateful to also keep such a loving friendship with MK, after years. No matter wherever in the world he is, I'll always be so proud of him.

CHAPTER FORTY FOUR

MOMENTS YOU NEED.

DINNER YOU DIDN'T KNOW YOU NEEDED:
34.0195° N, 118.4912° W

As I reflect on this past Thanksgiving, it was a time to appreciate the people we're grateful for—the ones we've shared deep moments with, the ones who will always have a piece of your heart. To those we've lost, whether physically or spiritually, they're never far from us. I was honestly surprised by how grounded I felt that day. God kept me centered. He's my anchor, always guiding me through life's unpredictable waters.

That day, I didn't have a game plan—just one of those spontaneous tracks that always leads me to something beautiful when I stop trying to control everything. I realized how much I tend to stress over the little details. The table settings, the napkin folds, making sure everyone is happy and everything looks "just right." I'm always trying to make sure that things go according to plan, even when life has other ideas. You stress over things you can't control, like whether people will actually show up when they say they will.

But this year, I let it go. I decided to let God take over, which was a peaceful shift. A few days before Thanksgiving, I shared this reflection with my mom. "I've got no plans," I said. "And sometimes, I think that's the best way. Whatever's meant to happen will find me."

Then, I got a text from my church group about a flag-football game on Thanksgiving morning. I knew it'd be fun, even though deep down, I wasn't exactly thrilled about getting up early. I wanted to sleep in, find an excuse to back out. But something told me I should go. So I pulled myself out of bed, hopped in the car, and drove down the 101 towards

Burbank, with the sun shining and my car filled with the upbeat vibes of some bumping house music.

As I cruised through the mountain peaks, I realized I rarely get to see this view—usually, I'm driving at night. When I arrived, I saw a few friends, and we all gathered our blankets and snacks. Everyone was happy to see each other, and the guys got ready to dominate the flag-football field while the rest of us ladies enjoyed from the sidelines. Becoming the best cheerleaders, while we enjoyed small talk, snacks, and coffee.

That's when I met Cassi **(THE REMINDER).** We started talking about community—how important it is to surround yourself with diverse, healthy people, and how changing your perspective can teach you so much. It's all about the people you choose to be around.

A couple of hours later, Nikki (**THE EMPOWERER)** asked about my plans for the day. I shrugged and said, "Nothing much, just working on my book and maybe catching up with a friend later." She said, "Come over. Bring anything or nothing—we've got it covered."

At first, I almost bailed. But deep down, I knew I needed to show up. God often speaks through the voices of others, and I trusted I'd hear something I needed, something I couldn't get on my own. I'm a woman of my word—I don't make excuses. If I say I'm coming, I show up. I'd been craving good company, and I knew this was an opportunity I couldn't miss.

When I got there, I was overwhelmed with joy. The details were all taken care of—the cute glasses, the charcuterie boards, stuffed Bree cooking in the kitchen—and the energy was just right. The company was incredible. We all sat down to eat together and shared what we were carrying forward into the New Year.

I talked about my book, but when it came to the last person's turn to share, I was floored. Stephanie **(THE REMINDER)**, told a story that hit home for me—a lesson I'd learned before, but with a fresh perspective that felt so relevant to what I was going through right now. It was like the universe had delivered exactly what I needed at that moment.

She shared the story of her family being back in Miami, where they had lived for a while. Before they moved, her pup had been sick, but once they were settled in, he thrived surrounded by the other dogs and the family. However, one day, she knew it was time to leave. So, they packed up and moved across the country to California. But by then, the dog was clearly in decline. He wanted to be with the pack back home.

That's when she made the decision to return to Florida for a month, to be with him during his final days, letting him pass in a peaceful, familiar environment. She talked about how animals are like humans—they need different types of love from different relationships, much like how a child finds a unique connection with their grandma, or how a father needs different forms of love from his family. "*I'm going to let him be with whoever he needs in the end,*" she said.

"**Love is a sacrifice**," she added. And when she said that, it hit me deeply.

As she continued, she explained how she had always tried to control things. But with healing, she's learning to let others help and use their gifts, trusting that their way may be the best way. Letting go of control, she said, has been difficult. But she's starting to accept it. She knows that soon, she will be on her own. No one prepares you for the end of someone's life. "I don't even know who I am without them," she said. "I don't know what I'm going to do. There's a new chapter ahead... and I'm not sure what that looks like."

We all go through hardships, but most of us don't allow ourselves to be vulnerable enough to release the weight and let others support us. In that moment, I realized that what she was sharing, her story, was meant for me. Nikki turned to look directly at me, and we shared a quiet smile. I said, "Thank you for sharing your story. I needed to hear that. I empathize—I've been right where you are, and I know the storm you're about to face. I'm here for you, if you need anything."

Sometimes, we think we need community, but in return, community needs us, too. Each person brings something special. It's truly remarkable. You can't choose your family, but you can choose your friends. You can choose your chosen family.

LOVE LANGUAGE:

Remember at the beginning of the book when I talked about the importance of understanding love languages—not just how you receive love, or how you *think* your partner will receive it, but the beautiful (and sometimes hilariously unexpected) ways love actually shows up?

Well, I figured it's only right to take a moment and share some of my favorite memories—those little snapshots of life where love spoke fluently, effortlessly, and sometimes in ways I never saw coming. Because love isn't always candlelit dinners and poetic declarations... sometimes, it's someone saving you the last slice of pizza or tolerating your terrible taste in reality TV.

So, let's dive in—into the messy, magical, and ridiculously heartfelt ways love languages have shown up in my life. ♡

My love language: When "he" cooks for me, Not just a meal, but a feast, you see.

When his apron's on and the kitchen's his stage, I know I'm in for something that'll engage.

A sprinkle of spices, a dash of delight, each bite is a hug, each taste feels just right.

Ray, with his Caribbean background, loved cooking. He was so proud of his heritage, and I was more than happy to enjoy the plantains. Every bit of love and intention he put in—it made my heart melt. Oof, my heart was eating right out of the palm of his hands.)

Even Marseillesl and Vasenna know this is the way to my heart. Nothing beats a good meal, filled with joy and flavor that makes my taste buds dance.

Music: When "he" has a good ear for music, too. Like he's tuned into the playlist of my soul—who knew? He'll send me a song, and I'll smile real wide, because it's exactly what I needed inside. A melody that fits, a beat that feels right, It's like he's reading my heart in the dead of night. Not just a generic mix, oh no, my friend, it's a curated selection, from start to end.

Songs that get me, that speak to my soul, like you've tapped into my Spotify goal. When you share music that hits just right, you're speaking my language, all day and night.

Mr. Kila, hands down, took the cake with this one. As a musician, he knew my heart and soul. Fawk, over time and with consistency, has been the longest-raging champion in this era of music development. I cherish it so much.

GIFTS: And then there's the **thoughtful gift**, oh so sweet, a little surprise that sweeps me off my feet. It could be a trinket, a book, or a note, but it's the thought behind it that really gets my vote. When "he" knows me so well, like he's a mind reader, I didn't even know I needed it, but now it's a keeper. **"I Was Thinking of You" Gift Cards.** Not just any present, but a digital gift, like, "I saw this, and thought of you, here's a Lyft." An Amazon voucher, or a cute Etsy find, shows you're tuned into my quirky mind. Gift cards aren't tacky when they come with care,

They say, "I see you," and "I'm always there."

MY FAVS: Coffee, Sushi, Bookstores, Chocolate, Movie Dates:

Grab a bouquet at the coffee shop: roses and sunflowers to be exact. Thank you very much!

Or yes, feed me chocolates underneath the moonlight, or just in bed. Take me to brunch, and let's sip on chai, or champagne. Whatever fits the mood best. A bacon, egg, and cheese with a side of your grin, slap some sriracha on me, and let's enjoy an egg roll together.

Surprise me with a new bookstore, or the way to my heart: storytelling— let's watch a movie together, boo. Now that's the kind of love language I'm all in.

Mr. J took my breath away once when I shared with him that (at the time) flowers reminded me of death, and I'd rather have sushi. One Valentine's Day, the store was out of sushi, but he knew how much it would mean to me. So, he went to the chocolate section, bought a heart-shaped box, took the candy out piece by piece, and added sushi inside, giving me the chocolates on the side. It was such a thoughtful, cherished moment.

Damon was super sweet with this one. I hinted that I loved flowers, and one day, he came over and said, "I didn't forget. I know you love flowers, but I was in such a rush to see you, I didn't have time to stop. But I promise I will next time." And sure enough, the next time, he brought me the most beautiful bouquet of yellow sunflowers and other flowers, along with wine, and pizza—his commitment and care made me feel so loved.

Inside Jokes (and Spontaneous Memes):

A quirky text, a meme, or a "HELLO GORGEOUS" text. You've found the perfect one to share—I bet it. It's our little thing, an ongoing joke, that no one else gets—except us, I hope!

We laugh 'til we snort, roll on the floor, because humor, my love, is what makes me adore.

Take the Lead: The "No Need to Ask" Texts:

When I'm hungry, and you just know,

You send me a text with, "Pizza on the way, yo!" (veggie or pepperoni—with pineapples—and white wine: pinot grigio, chardonnay—you can *never* go wrong with champagne!)

No need for me to drop hints or plead, you feel me, and that's all I need.

Yes, it's nice to be asked, but just make an executive decision and pick it up!

Don't go back and forth with me; I've got enough tough business decisions during the day. We don't need to waste good brainpower on that! Feel free to put my favorite food items, what I can eat and what I can't in your phone. Places I like the most, whatever makes it easier for you. Plus your phone can just be your personal assistant. You just get it—and that's how love flows, through pizza, Thai, and sushi that glows.

THE FINAL PIECES

I say all of this to reflect on the deepest relationships I've had—those that lasted longer than a few months. How does one make it last with another person in this fast-paced dating world? And why am I moving so quickly with people, only to realize it's not the right pace?

It makes me question: "how does one love another person for a whole lifetime?" I do believe love like that exists. A part of me still holds love for those I've lost, and I love everyone deeply. But still, the question lingers: "Is there really one person for me? Does my match truly exist? And if so, can we find that hope together?"

The real question is not when I'll find him, but how we'll continue to choose each other through life's ups and downs. Anyone can love when it's easy, but who will hold us through the hardest of times?

I guess that's what the journey is all about—staying present, loving fully, and keeping my eyes open. I'll keep following my heart, dancing to the beat of my own drum, until our hearts can reunite as one. Until then, I'll continue to love everyone unconditionally and serve others with all my heart. The one thing I can control is my reaction, my perspective, and my commitment to making tomorrow better than today.

That's how I've stayed grounded, and that's how I'll keep walking the path toward unconditional love, with everyone. It's a journey that seems to last forever.

You Belong in Cali

"You belong in Cali." I hear these words all the time—from friends, family, and sometimes even strangers. They always say it's something about my attitude, my essence, or my fashion sense that screams "**California.**" I can't deny it. There's something about LA that just suits me at this point in my life.

It all started when I visited my childhood friend during a summer get-together. As we sat chatting, she looked at me and said, "You're glowing in California. It just suits your personality. You're pursuing so much more here. I never felt that when you lived in North Carolina. Honestly, I wondered why you stayed there so long."

I smiled and responded, "Thank you. I do feel like I belong in Cali. But I think I needed to be in North Carolina first. It was the perfect place for me at that time. It allowed me to grow, to see things more clearly, and to get the experiences I needed."

Months later, I had a similar conversation with my mom. I was describing how much of an illusion California can be. The world sees Hollywood and thinks it's this magical place. But in reality, it's a ghostly representation of forgotten dreams—a place where homelessness is rampant, where trash litters the streets, and where pollution fills the air. Chemtrails, car exhaust, and the smog from traffic make the skies look more like a dystopian movie than the bright, glamorous city everyone imagines.

Mom listened quietly and then asked, "So why are you there? Why do you stay in California if it's all like that?"

I paused and thought about it for a moment before responding, "Because I love the culture. The diversity here is unlike anywhere else. Every day, I meet someone with a completely different background, and it humbles me. It's an opportunity to grow as a person, to stay open to new experiences. That kind of growth pushes me to be better. The views here are incredible—one moment, I'm at the ocean, and an hour later, I'm in the mountains. The weather is perfect, and I get to live the life I always dreamed of—dancing, singing, performing."

I smiled as I spoke, feeling the energy of it all. "Coming to California wasn't just about me. It's like God called me here for a bigger purpose. There's a light I'm meant to bring to this place, to a world that sometimes feels dark. I'm here to help others, maybe even people I haven't met yet. This is the place where doors open for me to fulfill my purpose."

My mom nodded. "You know, you can find positives and negatives everywhere. I've had my own thoughts about North Carolina, and even Wisconsin, but you're right—if you were to move back to Wisconsin, your soul would shrivel. You'd stop listening to God, and you wouldn't be living up to your potential. You'd be playing small."

She paused, reflecting for a moment. "This isn't the place for you. You're meant for more."

I looked out the window, thinking about how everything had led me here. The signs—big and small—that had shown me California was where I was meant to be. The universe had been nudging me, but I hadn't fully listened until now. I'd ignored the whispers, thinking I had all the time in the world to figure it out.

But God moved things out of my way.

I remember a lesson my pastor shared with me once, a lesson that still echoes in my mind like a song I can't quite shake off. It was about the voice of God, and how, if you're a little hard-headed (guilty as charged), you might hear that call but choose to ignore it. He said, "If you're stubborn, the universe might whisper, 'Go to Thailand,' but you'll brush it off because your partner is here, your life's comfortable, and hey, things seem *perfect*."

But then—*boom*—out of nowhere, the relationship ends. And suddenly, you're standing there, scratching your head, thinking, *What just happened?* Why did everything fall apart? You can't quite figure it out.

Here's the thing: The universe doesn't make mistakes. If you're not listening, it starts removing all the distractions, piece by piece. Your partner, your job, maybe even that comfy couch you've grown so fond of. It feels like everything's falling apart, but it's not. It's the universe clearing your path so you can finally hear the call.

And when you finally hear it—when that clarity hits, like a thunderclap in a quiet room—and you say, "Alright, God. I'm listening now. I'll move," that's when the blessings start pouring in. It's like the universe says, *"About time!"*

I smiled to myself, like someone who'd just figured out the punchline to a joke they've been telling wrong all their life. "Okay, God. I hear you. No need to take anything else away. I'm ready. Let the blessings rain down."

And just like that, I felt lighter. Not in the "I-lost-five-pounds-on-a-diet" kind of way, but in a deeper, spiritual sense. Like I was where I was supposed to be, at exactly the right time.

And that's how I ended up in California—not just for the palm trees and the celebrity sightings, but for something bigger, something I couldn't quite put into words until now. There were bumps, detours, and moments when I didn't quite understand why everything felt like it was falling apart. But now, looking back, I see that it was all part of a bigger plan.

Sometimes, life has to give us a little push—a big shove, even—to make us listen. To make us grow. And to remind us that where we're meant to be is exactly where we are.

God's got a plan. And when you finally listen? Everything falls into place.

Self-Actualization:

The process of realizing and fulfilling one's potential. According to Maslow's hierarchy of needs, self-actualization represents the pinnacle of psychological growth, where a person becomes the best version of themselves. Moving to California is symbolic of the moment I stepped into a space where I could achieve my fullest potential. California aligns with my personality, growth, and aspirations, reinforcing that finding an environment which supports our values and goals can facilitate a deeper sense of self-fulfillment.

CHAPTER FORTY FIVE

RE-ROOTED.

Re-routed: A Snowed-In Airport Story (childhood lesson)

Being re-routed always seems to remind me of another time I was stuck in an airport, but this time it was around a holiday. A massive snowstorm had hit Denver, and I remember wishing our flight would get canceled, because—let's be real—I didn't want to go back to school. The vacation had been amazing, and I wasn't ready for the reality check of returning to the grind.

But of course, I didn't realize the other side of that wish. The reality of being stranded at an airport overnight in a snowstorm wasn't quite as glamorous as I had imagined. The whole airport was buzzing with frustrated travelers, and as soon as we were stuck there, the family drama started. You know the kind. My brother and I were fighting like cats and dogs, really needing space from each other, yet stuck in close quarters. It was the kind of tension that only being trapped together for hours could bring.

Meanwhile, my parents were doing their best to navigate the storm—my mom suggested we go grab some food to calm the storm brewing within us, while my dad was off on a hunt for the bathroom (because, of course, he was trying to avoid the drama too). The whole situation was comically bad.

As we sat there, eating overpriced airport food and trying to keep it together, I realized something: Sometimes, being re-routed isn't about just getting somewhere faster. It's about being forced to pause, reflect, and re-evaluate your situation. At that moment, I realized that maybe the frustration wasn't just about the delay—it was about what we all needed to learn from it.

What if we could step back from the chaos of our lives, take a breather, and think about what we could do to make things better? What would happen if we used moments like these—the delays, the re-routes—to look inward, to reflect, and to work on improving how we react to life's little bumps?

Looking back, it was funny how something as frustrating as being stuck in an airport could offer me the clarity I needed. The "vehicle" I was in—literally and figuratively—was meant to slow me down, to hold me in that moment and give me a chance to reflect. It's not always about the destination; sometimes it's about what happens when you're forced to stay put, even when you don't want to.

So, that snowy night in Denver became a funny, albeit slightly chaotic, reminder that life's re-routes are often the perfect opportunity for growth. And maybe, just maybe, those delays were a blessing in disguise.

Life has a funny way of making us pause when we don't expect it. When things go off track or get delayed, take a moment to reflect—what can you learn from the situation? It's not always about where you're going, but what you can gain along the way.

Sometimes You Get Rerouted- AGAIN:

32.897480 -97.040443

Sometimes, you take a different vehicle to get to your destination. It might be unexpected, but it's often the new experience you need. And sometimes, that means hopping on a plane for a faster route.

It's the eve of Christmas Eve, and I'm in a whirlwind of packing. I double-check my flight details and, of course, an email pops up with a

"Record Locator" for my ticket, plus a strange warning about storms in Dallas. "Hmm," I think, "That's odd. I've never gotten a pre-flight warning like this before." But I shrug it off. Tomorrow's problem, right?

Later, my dear ANA, stops by with Thai food, she's notorious for fueling me emotionally and physically. We often spent sunset picnics together, gym dates, walks, and heart to hearts. She's a god given angel, has a passion for love and support of people even if they've wronged her. With her beautiful dark brown curly hair, and Spanish background, we spend the evening catching up, praying over our meal, sharing stories, and laughing until my stomach hurts. After she leaves, the pain in my hips starts to creep in as the meds wear off. Cue Damon, the guy with the magnetic pull. I know, I know, I've promised myself to let go of him, but it's hard when he's right there, offering comfort. He sees the pain in my face and starts rubbing my body, easing the tension away.

The night unfolds in a blur of emotions, and hot, messy intimacy. But as I hold him and breathe him in, something clicks. *This is it, again, THIS IS FOR REAL THE LAST TIME!* I'm done with the on-again, off-again dance for far too long, and it's time to close that door for good. No more back and forth. *Cut the cords, spit on them, burn this sexual energy away.* I'm done.

At 4:00 AM, the alarm blares. It's time to get moving for my flight. Damon, of course, is ready to bolt. He didn't sleep a wink—he's not a fan of cats, especially Cleo, who adores him. He's also not fond of my pillows, and my late-night rambling keeps him awake. He helps me with the last bits of packing, kisses me lightly on the forehead, and wishes me safe travels. "No time for another sad goodbye," I tell myself. *Turn the page. Move on.*

I know no matter where we are we'll have love and care for eachother. He is something remarkable. I know we'll always be a part of each other's story somehow. We just needed to close the book and start a new story.

I uber off to the airport on Christmas Eve morning. I wheel myself through security, which actually isn't as bad as I thought. With a little help from Dan, my "assistant driver" from the Philippines, I breeze through the process. He even stops for Starbucks so we can enjoy a gingerbread coffee—a special treat this time of year. As I take that first sip, a wave of joy washes over me. Dan notices. "Warms your soul, doesn't it?" he says with a smile.

"It's the little things," I responded, my heart a little lighter. I pull out my cane from my backpack, just in case I need extra support as I walk. Dan helps me get to the gate, and I'm first in line. But then a cute little lady in a mask approaches me, telling me she has the window seat. Without hesitation, she offers to swap seats so I can have it. I'm floored. *People can be so kind.*

The plane boards, and as I settle into my middle seat (which I never, ever choose, but here we are), I'm a little cramped. As the plane fills up, a woman with curly brown hair approaches and tells me she's in the window seat, but noticing my situation, she suggests I take it. *Yes! A window seat on a full plane!*

As we take off, I'm quickly lulled to sleep by the exhaustion of the night before. But then, in the middle of my slumber, I'm jolted awake by an announcement: "We're rerouting to Denver due to thunderstorms in Dallas." My eyes fly open. "Wait, what?" I look to my left, and then— oh! There's my gingerbread coffee, still sitting there, warming my soul all over again.

The captain comes on the intercom and starts fumbling over his words. It's awkward, and people start to murmur. After a half-hour of confusion, they announce that if we get off the plane in Denver, we won't be able to reboard, and there are no flights out of Denver until Friday morning. It's Wednesday. *I'll miss Christmas,* I think, and then, with a deep sigh, I brace myself for what's next.

Suddenly, people begin to complain loudly on their cell phones, venting to friends and family about missed connections and lost luggage. One woman even mentions she needs $400 for a new flight. Everyone is stressed, but I can't help but notice: *we're all in this together.* No one's situation is more important than anyone else's.

As I make my way to the bathroom, I overhear a flight attendant apologizing to another passenger, and I can't help myself. I turn to her with a smile and say, "Merry Christmas! And hey, don't worry about it. Sometimes in life, you just have to be rerouted."

Her eyes widened a little, surprised by my positivity. "I appreciate that," she says. "Thank you."

"You're welcome," I replied. "We might not know why we're stuck or frustrated in the moment, but there's always a bigger picture. Maybe this detour saved us from something else, who knows? It's all about perspective."

I feel the tension in the cabin ease just a little. Sure, everyone's still annoyed, but my words seem to make a difference. "*Find the good. The silver lining. It's all going to be okay.*"

I text Daniel, who's still with me in spirit, and nod. "It's all going to work out," I say, "One way or another. Life gets uprooted sometimes, but it's all about how you respond. People will have different experiences based on their circumstances, but we can't control that. The key is to be kind to each other and be intentional with how we react."

Daniel replies back at me. "That's right. It's Christmas after all."

And just like that, I'm reminded: Life is unpredictable. You can't always control what happens, but you can control how you respond. So why not choose kindness, perspective, and a little bit of joy, even in the middle of rerouting?

Life is full of detours, but how you respond to them is what matters. You can always find a silver lining—sometimes, it's as simple as a warm cup of coffee or a kind word. **Stay kind, stay open, and remember: things will work out.**

And I stayed optimistic..

Until dreadful hours of uncontrolled narratives continued the saga.

"Bad Luck Chuck." —Christmas Disaster

Lucky for me, one disaster has a way of leading to another, and then another, like dominoes in a poorly constructed game of life. After waking up in Denver when I was supposed to land in Dallas for my layover, was an immediate shock to the system—like a caffeine jolt without the caffeine. Calm as a cucumber (or so I told myself), we endured the five-hour shuffle back to Dallas, only to arrive and have my connecting flight times pushed back not once, not twice, but *seven* times. It felt like being stuck in a poorly written sitcom, except no one was laughing.

The ADA attendant, bless his heart, dropped me off at the wrong location and left me to fend for myself in a sea of equally frazzled travelers. It was chaos, but in the spirit of communal suffering, I found solace. I ended up seated next to a lovely couple who kindly bought me dinner (again, silver linings). As flights continued to get delayed and shuffled like a never-ending game of airline roulette, the crowd started to form a makeshift community. We were all in this together, bound by a shared sense of exasperation. I even gave a fellow traveler two protein bars—my humble contribution to the cause.

But then, at 10:30 p.m. on Christmas Eve, the inevitable happened: my flight was canceled. There I was, slumped in a wheelchair the airline provided, abandoned in a corner of the terminal that now echoed with silence. It was a ghost town of forgotten souls and lost luggage. Humans who had once packed the terminal were now scattered across the airport like pieces of a puzzle no one cared to finish.

Shuffled once more, this time into the ADA line, I waited until 1:30 a.m., only to be told there was no transportation available. They offered me a hotel—how generous—except it was too late to actually get there, and again I was in a wheelchair (great thanks). That's when I met Cinthini **(THE REMINDER)**, a warm soul from Chile who quickly became my line buddy and, dare I say, Christmas miracle.

As we waited together, she confided in me that she was a recent widow. "I don't like Christmas anymore," she admitted softly. "I used to spend all my time with him, and now that he's gone, I don't have anywhere to go. I don't want to intrude on anyone." She explained she was only in the States to sell some land, a bittersweet errand during what used to be a season of joy.

Then she looked at me and said something that cracked my heart wide open. "If I were at home, I'd probably be alone, sad, and crying. But instead, I'm here, stuck with you." She smiled—a real, warm smile—and in that moment, the chaos and exhaustion seemed to fade just a little.

"I hope Santa brings you whatever gift you want," she said with a twinkle in her eye.

I smiled back and replied, **"He already did. It's you."**

We hugged, two weary travelers finding a sliver of magic in the midst of the mayhem.

Of course, the airline staff continued their reign of incompetence, leaving us to scavenge for food vouchers and a place to sleep in the airport. After a restless night on cold benches, Cinthini eventually made her way to her gate. My saga, however, was far from over. The ADA service continued to be a disaster, leaving me stranded, frustrated, and exhausted. At one point, I had no choice but to wheel myself backwards in my rollator (yes, my *cane with wheels*) like some kind of desperate, backwards superhero.

Eventually, I made it to my gate and, by some Christmas miracle, onto a flight to Wisconsin. Moral of the story? Airlines treat the disabled like an afterthought. But amidst the frustration and exhaustion, I found a glimmer of humanity—a stranger who turned a night of chaos into a memory of warmth and connection.

Sometimes, the best gifts aren't wrapped in shiny paper; they're found in unexpected places, like an airport terminal on Christmas Eve.

UNEXPECTED FIRES:

After surviving the drama of the airport, Christmas with my family was pleasant—I spent it mostly in bed or rocking in a chair like a certified grandma. By the time I made it back to LA, I was off the pain meds (hallelujah!) and ready for some normalcy. But life had other plans.

One morning, I woke to a barrage of messages: wildfires had broken out, swallowing most of the Palisades in Los Angeles. Updates poured in every ten minutes, each more chaotic than the last. The air was thick with ash; it coated my porch, my car, and, metaphorically, my patience.

Marseilles,(**THE ETERNAL**) who was supposed to come by the day before to help me around the house, ended up arriving on Wednesday instead—by some divine act of God. Standing outside for only a few minutes, her eyes burned from the ash-filled air. "You need a mask just to breathe out here," she said, squinting at the smoky sky.

Inside, she helped me with meal prep while we watched the updates from the "Watch Duty" app, hoping for a miracle. Then came the update we'd been dreading: the fire had spread to the Hollywood Hills. "Okay," I said, half-joking but mostly panicked, "My mom was right. I've gotta get out of here."

I had told myself I'd leave if the fire reached a certain part of the map, and there it was—crossing that invisible boundary. Being handicapped and living alone, there was no way I could evacuate on my own. Marseilles sprang into action, helping me pack up the essentials, loading the car with everything I could carry. Smoke filled the air even through my N95 mask as we worked quickly. My car was packed, my nerves were fried, and I took off just an hour before our neighborhood's mandatory evacuation was announced.

The roads were packed with other cars fleeing the fire, traffic crawling as smoke loomed in the rearview mirror. Driving through LA parts of town were in a blackout and others were whipped off the map. After a few hours of driving, around 12:30 p.m., I pulled up Google Maps and picked the first hotel I could find. When I arrived, I froze.

It was *the same hotel* I had evacuated to the year before during another LA disaster—a hurricane. **LOVEKIN BLVD. 33.6088° N, 114.6059° W**

I couldn't believe it. A strange sense of comfort washed over me, a gentle nudge from the universe saying, *"You're in the right place"*. My first "God wink."

Of course, Cleo, my cat, was not as impressed. Pets weren't allowed, so she had to stay in her carrier. Every few hours, I'd let her out to pee—no rest for either of us as I popped pain meds, constant fire updates, and waded through messages from concerned friends and family.

The next day, I finally made it to my grandparents' home in Arizona. Relieved, I let Cleo out of her carrier, but she bolted for a hiding spot like a cartoon character fleeing the scene. She disappeared into Nana's **(THE ETERNALS)** closet, leaving me to fish her out.

That's when I saw it. Hanging on the door of the closet was a sign, one of those heartfelt gifts from another grandchild. It read:

"Nana- A constant source of unconditional love. One who teaches, motivates, and encourages. One who gives warm, big hugs, tells great stories, and is the best cook ever. Loved beyond words."

I stared at it, my second "God wink." A message as clear as day about unconditional love: I was where I was meant to be. Smiling, I pulled Cleo from the closet, feeling an odd sense of peace settle over me. Those words were only a small beacon of her essence, but they were all 100% accurate.

Life has a funny way of shaking you up and then placing you exactly where you need to land. From the ashes of wildfires to the safe embrace of my grandparents' home, I realized that sometimes the chaos is just a detour to unconditional love.

Analyzing:

This demonstrates the connection between life's unpredictability and the unconditional love that can ground and guide us through difficult times. The psychological concepts of emotional resilience, attachment, faith, and the healing power of unconditional love intertwine to show that, even in the chaos of life, we are constantly being led to spaces where love—pure, unchanging, and unconditional—can heal and restore us. Just as the narrator eventually finds comfort and peace with their grandparents, unconditional love has the power to transform pain and uncertainty into a sense of belonging and peace.

Beyond Illusions: A Reflection on Love, Loss, and Humanity

Everything I've written is an invitation to look beyond the illusions that cloud your judgments, life, and uncover the truths that guide you back to the path of unconditional love. It's a call to step outside your own experiences, to free yourself from forms of oppression that may bind you, and to look deeper—beyond the surface and between the lines.

Every place you live and every moment you experience comes with its share of positives and negatives. It's all about perspective—how you choose to see the downfalls. Through these stories, I hope to offer you a lens to see past the rose-colored glasses, even when I wore them myself. Learn to notice the **RED FLAGS** that warn you and follow the **GREEN FLAGS** that lead you toward success and fulfillment.

Humanity falters when we rely on misconceptions, like thinking, "*Oh hey the rich, finally got what they deserved*," when tragedy strikes. Some people dismiss Los Angeles as a playground for the wealthy, but in truth, it's a city of contradictions. Behind the glamour of Hollywood lies a much harsher reality.

According to a google search: "As of 2023, Los Angeles had a population of over 3.8 million, making it the second-largest city in the U.S. But behind its size and allure is a sobering statistic: 13.9% of its residents—around 1.3 million people—live below the poverty line." California, despite its wealth, continues to lead the nation in poverty, with rates that disproportionately affect Black and Latinx communities. Beneath the palm trees and bright lights, countless individuals are simply fighting to survive.

I remember a conversation with a friend who questioned "*Why do people care about the rich people of Los Angeles and not Asheville.*" Their comment stung, rooted in misunderstanding, because I've seen the struggles of both places. I lived in North Carolina and year after year we were hit with devastation. In 2024, I watched Asheville endure devastation, its beauty scarred by nature's wrath. My LA church even sent a relief team to help. My pastor's wife was also from NC. We almost took the pain of loss personally. Not long after, Los Angeles faced its own disaster—the 2025 wild fires that consumed everything in their path (That was not an "act of god"- as Insurance companies would say). It wasn't natural at all. Nature didn't cause that trauma, foul play- arson did. Nevertheless, a disaster is still a disaster.

On social media, I saw comments dripping with scorn: "*Good, the rich got what they deserved.*" But the reality is far more complex. Yes, affluent neighborhoods were hit, but so were immigrant communities, small businesses, and countless people living paycheck to paycheck. Fires don't discriminate. They destroy and steal memories, homes, animals, and lives.

When evacuation orders came, I packed what I could—only the irreplaceable things. I thought about those who didn't have that chance, who had to flee with nothing but the clothes on their backs. It's in these moments of crisis that we're reminded of what truly matters. Material things can be replaced, but the lives and stories behind them cannot.

The devastation was overwhelming, but amidst the destruction, I witnessed something incredible: **humanity coming together. Strangers helping strangers, communities uniting, and the resilience of people determined to rebuild. It's a reminder that even in a disaster, there's beauty—a "beautiful disaster," as I've come to call it.**

Los Angeles is a city of dreams, but it's also a place of profound struggle. Many residents live in overcrowded conditions, juggling multiple jobs just to stay afloat. For some, the idea of leaving California—or even imagining a different life—feels impossibly out of reach. Trapped in a relentless cycle of survival, they remain confined to the boundaries of their reality. The job market itself can be a dead end, tangled in inefficient application systems and impersonal recruiting platforms, leaving many unable to secure work that covers even basic living expenses in one of the most expensive regions in the country. While the city boasts immense wealth and success for a fortunate few, it stands in stark contrast to the sacrifices and hardships endured by millions barely scraping by on minimum wage.

The fires took so much—land, homes, and lives. But they also revealed something profound: the capacity for creation and connection in the face of destruction. It's in these moments of rebuilding, of coming together, that we find the essence of humanity.

So, as you navigate your own life, I encourage you to slow down and reflect. Look beyond the illusions, see the truths that lie between the lines, and cherish the connections that bring us together. Life's challenges may be daunting, but they also offer opportunities for growth, understanding, and, ultimately, love.

"There is perfection in everything. Strive to see the perfection. In other words, in the midst of the greatest tragedy, see the glory of the process."
—**Conversations With God: Neal Donald Welsh**

Empathy and Compassion Amidst Tragedy:

Some people dismissing the fires as "what the rich deserved," reveals a disconnect between empathy and societal perceptions of fairness. This highlights a fundamental psychological issue: **group-based biases and scapegoating**. In this case, some people see disaster as a form of karmic justice. However, I challenge that perspective by pointing out that **disasters do not discriminate**, and the pain is felt universally, whether by the wealthy or the marginalized. By empathizing with those who have lost everything we can show **unconditional love**. Love, in this case, is not bound by who "deserves" it but rather flows freely to everyone, especially in their moments of greatest need.

"In a moment of great tragedy, the challenge always is to quiet the mind and move deep within the soul."
—Conversations With God: Neal Donald Welsh

Resilience and Collective Healing:

This describes witnessing the **resilience of humanity** during the fires—strangers helping strangers, communities uniting, and people coming together to rebuild. This speaks to the psychological concept of **collective trauma** and healing. Despite the devastation, people's ability to connect and support one another highlights the human capacity for **compassionate action** and solidarity. Unconditional love is often reflected in these collective moments of mutual aid, where people extend care and compassion to others without expectation of return. This is reminiscent of the psychological benefits of **prosocial behavior**—engaging in acts of kindness not only helps others but also promotes the well-being of the giver, as it creates a sense of purpose and connection.

"Fear not, for I am with you." "That is what poetry has to say to the person facing tragedy. "In your darkest hour, I will be your light. In your blackest moment, I will be your consolation. In your most difficult and trying time, I will be your strength. Therefore, have faith! For I am your shepherd; you shall not want. I will cause you to lie down in green pastures; I will lead you beside still waters. I will restore your soul, and lead you in the paths of righteousness for My Name's sake. And yea, though you walk through the valley of the Shadow of Death, you will

fear no evil; for I am with you. My rod and My staff will comfort you. I am preparing a table before you in the presence of your enemies. I shall anoint your head with oil. Your cup will run over. Surely, goodness and mercy will follow you all the days of your life, and you will dwell in My house—and in My heart— forever.
—**Conversations With God: Neal Donald Welsh**

REVELATION:

As I've walked, run, driven, and flown through the ever-evolving journey of life, I've come to understand that the true meaning of unconditional love holds many faces, many truths, and many stories for those who seek it. It has meant different things to different people, and for me, it has been a path of both joy and sorrow. I've been in love, I've battled, I've been bruised and broken, only to rise again, open-hearted, ready to love once more.

Throughout my life, I'll continue to search for new ways to give and receive love in its purest form, ever striving to shine with compassion and understanding. And yet, deep in my heart, I know that one day, when I am reunited with my Creator, I will be embraced by a love beyond words—a love that transcends all understanding, felt only in the soul, shown only through action. A love so vast, it cannot be matched by anything earthly.

I am grateful to be a beacon of light, showing that love can be a gift to all who cross my path. In the quiet reflection of my journey, I've realized that even some of my pain wasn't mine to bear alone; it was there to show others beauty, grace, and hope. Pain, too, has its purpose—to remind us that even in the darkest days, *we can stand tall, and the light will always lead us through.*

Sometimes, **suffering isn't about us at all.** It's a way of offering pieces of God's love to those around us, reminding them that there is a **bigger story unfolding**, a plan far grander than we can comprehend. We may not have all the answers. In truth, sometimes we don't like the answers we get. But when we slow down, when we reflect, the clarity begins to unfold, revealing deeper truths that were hidden before.

And then, there are moments when we meet someone—someone with whom we think we are meant to share a significant part of our lives, whether romantically or emotionally. But sometimes, we realize that our purpose in their life was not to stay, but to connect them with someone else. We were the bridge, the link, the thread in a much grander tapestry. We are all connected, like the six degrees of separation, each of us touching the lives of others in ways we may never fully understand.

Through all these trials of love, sorrow, grief, and the repeating cycles of life, I've learned to romanticize every moment, to embrace each lesson, and to never forget to "stop and smell the roses." For, in the end, it is always better to have loved—deeply, passionately, unconditionally—than to have never loved at all.

SUNSET REFLECTION:

As I gazed out the window of my grandparents' house, my breath caught in wonder. The sunset unfolded like a masterpiece, each moment unveiling hues so vivid they seemed otherworldly. The fiery reds melted into warm oranges, embraced by the soft glow of yellow, all draped beneath a sky of delicate cotton candy clouds. It was a slow transformation; each shift a gentle reminder of nature's patience—majestic and serene.

Here, in this quiet sanctuary, time seemed to stretch. The sparse houses in the neighborhood only deepened the sense of stillness. Mornings began with the melodic chirping of birds, and afternoons carried that same tranquility. As I watched a small group of students pass by, I was swept back to memories of my childhood in the country. Life there felt like an eternal stretch, each year lingering endlessly—and yet, in a blink, those days were gone.

Love, in contrast, feels so fast-paced in Los Angeles. It moves in tandem with the whirlwind of the environment, urging you to keep up, to never pause. But what happens when you slow down? Truly slow down. In those moments of stillness, reflection blooms. You begin to grow—not hurriedly, but deeply—gathering wisdom in a way that feels rooted and intentional. Slowing down allows you to disentangle yourself from the chaos of the world we've created, a culture so often driven by distraction and frenzy.

That's why my parents chose for us to grow up in a peaceful place, a refuge where life could unfold gently. And now, looking back, I see the gift in experiencing both worlds. There's beauty in finding balance, in harmonizing the stillness of the country with the momentum of the city. Each season of life serves its purpose—some meant to ground us, others to propel us forward. It's all interconnected, a symphony of growth and transformation.

To truly embrace this, you have to slow down. Not just in action, but within yourself. Only then can you hear the quiet whispers of God, the universe, or the Creator—guiding you toward joy and fulfillment. These moments of pause offer clarity, stripping away confusion and distraction, leaving only the profound beauty of existence. Life, after all, is not a race but a journey, and the most meaningful steps are often the ones taken in stillness.

A Day of Blessings and Bouquets

It was one of those days where the universe seemed to be sprinkling its magic everywhere, despite a bumpy start to this new chapter of life. GOD, in His infinite wisdom, always knows how to close one door and open another, placing you exactly where you're meant to be.

The day began with plans to meet Yaya **(THE EMPOWER)** for lunch, but the stars had their own agenda. Schedules collided, and dinner plans became the compromise—a divine delay that allowed me to tackle errands galore. First stop: Phoenix. A quick visit to the bank where I had a heart to heart with the bank teller about my life struggles of the "disabled disaster relief vitamin." She opened up to tell me about her son who had just passed on due to an overdose of a "bad batch of fentanyl." We shared our grievances with love and support. I believe that I was supposed to meet her, the amount of trouble it took for me just to deal with the online banking, I knew that she was the secret sauce. Her first day back to work in 3 weeks, and it fit just perfectly for to stop at that location. **(THE REMINDER)**

Then I went on to have a small victory in the form of an eyebrow wax (life-changing, truly). It's the little things, people. Brows snatched, errands checked off, and a triumphant visit to the grocery store for a restock of fresh fruit.

As I wandered through the aisles, my gaze landed on the flower section, where vibrant blooms seemed to wink at me. I'd been craving flowers all month, and today was the day. Three bouquets went into my cart—one for Nana, my sweet rock who'd taken such good care of me and Cleo during this whirlwind. Words couldn't express my gratitude, but flowers? They could speak volumes. The other two bouquets would serve a purpose later, their destiny yet to be revealed.

Driving to Scottsdale to meet Yaya was pure bliss, thanks to a solid 30 minutes of Griz—electronic beats layered with a soulful saxophone. As I pondered the thoughts of his recovery —from a recent "retirement." Is there a better soundtrack to life? (Spoiler: there isn't.) Mid-drive, the DMV called to inform me I was exempt from a smog regulation needed for my California plates. Talk about divine timing! I'd tried to handle that chore right before the evacuation, thinking I'd be back the next day (ha, jokes on me).

Arriving at the restaurant Yaya and I agreed upon, I was greeted by a vision in black—an absolute goddess glowing with her signature radiance. Yaya's energy is like sunshine bottled, and seeing her always feels like a hug from the universe itself.

The evening turned into something extraordinary as I attended a keynote meeting with some of the greatest leaders in our industry. Hugging and reconnecting with my Arizona business partners, mentors, and friends was the highlight of my entire evacuation saga. It was a reminder of why I do what I do—proof that even in chaos, there's room for celebration and connection.

And then came my signature move: the flower distribution. The "Jenny Squared" duo, as I affectionately call them, were my chosen recipients. One Jenny, a blonde bombshell with piercing blue eyes and a baby on the way, practically glowed in her baby-blue blazer. The purple flowers I handed her felt like an accessory to her radiance. The other Jenny, a strong, athletic brunette with a heart of gold, lit up the room with her mere presence. Naturally, she received sunshine-yellow blooms to match her aura.

Their husbands? Absolute gems—kind, generous, and men of impeccable character. First-class humans all around. As I handed out flowers, I realized I wasn't just spreading joy; I was soaking in it, too.

Heading home that night, my heart was full. Laughter, gratitude, and bliss swirled together like the perfect cocktail, closing this chapter with poetic finality. It felt like a fitting ceremony to mark the end of one saga and the start of something new. I followed my heart back to back to LA to help rebuild, restore, and claim my dreams (with the best soundtrack guiding me home).

Until the next book, my friends. *"The future is bright."*

Unconditional love is this magical thing, isn't it? It's the kind of love that's profound and selfless, with no strings attached. It's the love you give without expecting anything in return. It's not based on conditions or even on whether the other person meets all your expectations. Instead, it's about seeing someone for who they truly are, flaws and all, and still choosing them every single day.

It's that beautiful acceptance—the kind that embraces every little imperfection and still says, "I love you just as you are." And then, there's the selflessness. You put their happiness and well-being before your own, not because you have to, but because you genuinely want to. It's like, "I've got you, no matter what."

Forgiveness plays a huge role too. It's that willingness to let go of past mistakes, not carrying grudges with you like unnecessary baggage, and just moving forward. And don't forget support. Unconditional love doesn't only show up when everything's perfect; it's there during the tough times too. Whether you're celebrating the high moments or working through the low ones, it's all about being there, unwaveringly.

Commitment is another key part. It's about sticking with someone even when life gets tough and the road ahead feels uncertain. And empathy— oh, empathy! It's being able to feel what the other person feels, to truly understand them without judging, no matter what they're going through.

Then there's patience. Unconditional love isn't about rushing someone to change or grow. It's giving them the space and time they need to evolve on their own terms. Compassion follows closely, always showing care and concern for what the other person is going through, even when it doesn't affect you directly.

And let's not forget non-judgment. It's about accepting others fully, no matter their quirks, and letting go of the need to criticize. Respect is the final ingredient—valuing them as an individual, letting them be themselves, and honoring their boundaries and autonomy.

Unconditional love is often easy to spot in the bond between parents and children, but it can also be found in friendships, romantic relationships, and all kinds of human connections. It's the kind of love that stands the test of time and transcends circumstances. It's deep, lasting, and always there, no matter what life throws at you. It's the love that says, "I'm with you, always."

Remember, the journey of love is never linear—it's full of twists, turns, and heart-opening moments. But every step, every page, and every little act of love counts.

Now, go forth and love like you've never loved before. 🌼 💖

Interloop

My hope is that this book challenges, inspires, and educates you through these stories, ideas, and facts. I want you to discover the beauty in your own journey, just like I found mine through music. Music became my means of connecting to something deeper, a way to experience unconditional love. It's like the sound waves, perfectly orchestrated by a maestro, creating a rhythm that resonates with the heart. Guiding me through all of the stories and paving my own way through the driver's seat to reflections. May your journey be full of bliss, wonder, and boldness.

In this book, we've explored the fact that understanding your health and wellness is a deeply personal and ongoing journey. It requires patience, self-reflection, and a commitment to caring for both your mind and body. Remember, true transformation begins by acknowledging where you are now and taking intentional steps toward the future you desire.

For more guidance on analyzing your health and wellness, visit my website at Contact - Aire Stillman Lifestyle. There, you'll find valuable resources to assist you on your path to better health and a more balanced life.

About the Author

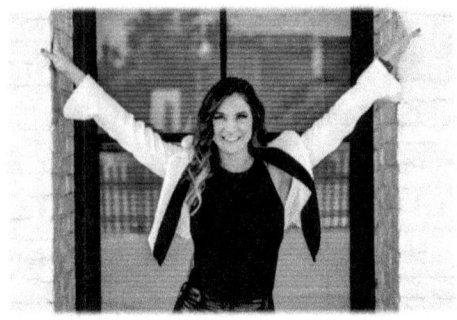

Aire Stillman is dedicated to fostering human connection and communication, with a deep passion for creating vibrant, loving communities. Her book, The Reflections of Unconditional Love, explores life stories from both strangers and her own experiences, offering insightful reflections on the essence of love.

With a background in crafting engaging content, Aire has written blog posts, press releases, and marketing materials for various businesses, including ES Lifestyle Consulting, Healing Leaves and WTRK. She is also an accomplished host and speaker, having appeared on "Up To Date," a dating game show at EDC Vegas, Conga Kids, CBT Studios, News & radio stations, and numerous podcasts.

An avid storyteller, Aire channels her passion for music through songwriting, singing, and dancing. Her mission is to bridge worlds and create healing spaces through the power of words, sound, and movement, enriching any community she joins.

LinkedIn: www.linkedin.com/in/aire-stillman-29549a223
Facebook: https://www.facebook.com/EricaStillmanConsulting/
Instagram: https://www.instagram.com/aire_stillman/
Website: https://ericastillman.com/

Congratulations on completing this journey toward understanding the transformative power of unconditional love. You've taken the first step toward living a life rooted in connection, compassion, and growth. But this is just the beginning. There is so much more for you to discover, and I want to be part of your next chapter.

What's next for you?

If you're ready to take this transformation to the next level and apply the principles of love, communication, connection, and community in your own life, I invite you to **connect with me**. Here's how:

1. **Join the Movement:** Sign up for my newsletter and get exclusive access to insightful resources, personal growth tips, and inspiration to keep you aligned with the path of unconditional love. You'll also receive updates on upcoming workshops, webinars, and coaching sessions that can take your journey to the next level.

2. **Transform with Coaching:** If you're feeling ready for deeper, more personalized guidance, let's work together. Whether it's one-on-one coaching, group sessions, or a transformative workshop, I am here to help you unlock the next phase of your personal growth. **Let's schedule a consultation today** and start creating the life and relationships you've always dreamed of.

3. **Connect with a Like-Minded Community:** I believe that when we surround ourselves with a supportive and loving community, magic happens. By joining my community, you'll be surrounded by others who are on the same path of growth, healing, and unconditional love. Together, we can share experiences, support each other, and create lasting connections that uplift us all.

Why take action now?

By embracing these next steps, you're committing to a life filled with more joy, fulfillment, and love. The tools and resources you gain will guide you on your journey of growth, not just for today, but for the rest of your life. Don't wait for the "perfect" moment to begin your transformation—there's no better time than NOW.

Ready to make love the foundation of your life?

It's time to create the life you deserve. I can't wait to continue this journey with you. Together, we'll unlock your highest potential.

Schedule your consultation or
sign up for the newsletter to get started today!
Aire Stillman Lifestyle Consulting - www.ericastillman.com